How-to Manual for Pacemaker and ICD Devices: Procedures and Programming

How-to Manual for Pacemaker and ICD Devices

Procedures and Programming

Edited by

Amin Al-Ahmad
Texas Cardiac Arrhythmia Institute
Austin, TX, USA

Andrea Natale
Texas Cardiac Arrhythmia Institute
Austin, TX, USA

Paul J. Wang
Stanford University School of Medicine
Stanford, CA, USA

James P. Daubert
Duke University Medical Center
Durham, NC, USA

Luigi Padeletti
IRCCS MultiMedica
Milan, Italy

WILEY Blackwell

This edition first published 2018
© 2018 John Wiley & Sons, Inc.

The right of Amin Al-Ahmad, Andrea Natale, Paul J. Wang , James P. Daubert and Luigi Padeletti to be identified as the authors of the editorial material in this work has been asserted in accordance with law.

Registered Offices
John Wiley & Sons, Inc., 111 River Street, Hoboken, NJ 07030, USA

Editorial Office
9600 Garsington Road, Oxford, OX4 2DQ, UK

For details of our global editorial offices, customer services, and more information about Wiley products visit us at www.wiley.com.

Wiley also publishes its books in a variety of electronic formats and by print-on-demand. Some content that appears in standard print versions of this book may not be available in other formats.

Library of Congress Cataloging-in-Publication Data

Names: Al-Ahmad, Amin, editor. | Natale, Andrea, editor. | Wang , Paul J., editor. | Daubert, James P., editor. |
   Padeletti, Luigi, editor.
Title: How-to manual for pacemaker and ICD devices : procedures and programming / edited by Amin Al-Ahmad,
   Andrea Natale, Paul J. Wang , James P. Daubert, Luigi Padeletti.
Description: Hoboken, NJ : John Wiley & Sons, Inc., 2018. | Includes bibliographical references and index. |
Identifiers: LCCN 2017049884 (print) | LCCN 2017050275 (ebook) | ISBN 9781118820865 (pdf) |
   ISBN 9781118820742 (epub) | ISBN 9781118820599 (pbk.)
Subjects: | MESH: Pacemaker, Artificial | Defibrillators, Implantable | Equipment Safety–methods |
   Cardiovascular Surgical Procedures–methods
Classification: LCC RC684.P3 (ebook) | LCC RC684.P3 (print) | NLM WG 26 | DDC 617.4/120645–dc23
LC record available at https://lccn.loc.gov/2017049884

Cover Design: Wiley
Cover Images: (X-ray) © Science Photo Library - ZEPHYR./Gettyimages;
(Circles: From top to bottom) © RandyJayBraun/Gettyimages;
Courtesy of Brett Atwater; © Jan-Otto/Gettyimages

Set in 10/12pt Warnock by SPi Global, Pondicherry, India
Printed and bound by CPI Group (UK) Ltd, Croydon, CR0 4YY
C9781118820599_040124

v

Contents

List of Contributors

Amin Al-Ahmad, MD, FACC, FHRS, CCDS
Texas Cardiac Arrhythmia Institute
St. David's Medical Center
Austin, TX, USA

Brett D. Atwater, MD
Duke University Health System
Durham, NC, USA

Yousef Bader, MD
Tufts University School of Medicine
Tufts Medical Center
Boston, MA, USA

Giuseppe Bagliani, MD
Department of Cardiology and Arrhythmology
Foligno General Hospital
Perugia, Italy

April Bain, RN
Medtronic Inc.
Nashville, TN, USA

Advay G. Bhatt, MD
Boston Medical Center
Boston University School of Medicine
Boston, MA, USA

Maria Grazia Bongiorni, MD
Second Division of Cardiovascular Diseases
Cardiac-Thoracic and Vascular Department
Azienda Ospedaliero Universitaria Pisana
Pisa, Italy

Noel G. Boyle, MD, PhD
UCLA Cardiac Arrhythmia Center
Ronald Reagan UCLA Medical Center
Los Angeles, CA, USA

Jason S. Bradfield, MD
UCLA Cardiac Arrhythmia Center
Ronald Reagan UCLA Medical Center
Los Angeles, CA, USA

Chad Brodt, MD
Cardiac Electrophysiology & Arrhythmia
Service
Stanford University Medical Center
Stanford, CA, USA

Daniel H. Cooper, MD
Cardiovascular Division
Department of Medicine
Barnes-Jewish Hospital
Washington University School
of Medicine
St. Louis, MO, USA

George H. Crossley, MD, FHRS, FACC
Vanderbilt Heart and Vascular Institute
Nashville, TN, USA

James P. Daubert, MD
Division of Clinical Cardiac
Electrophysiology
Duke University Medical Center
Durham, NC, USA

Andrea Di Cori, MD
Second Division of Cardiovascular Diseases
Cardiac-Thoracic and Vascular
Department
Azienda Ospedaliero Universitaria Pisana
Pisa, Italy

Lucy Ekosso-Ejangue, MD
J.W. Goethe University
Frankfurt, Germany;
Department of Medicine – Cardiology
Evangelical Hospital Bielefeld
Bielefeld, Germany

N.A. Mark Estes III, MD
Tufts University School of Medicine
Tufts Medical Center
Boston, MA, USA

Roger A. Freedman, MD
Division of Cardiovascular Medicine
University of Utah Health Sciences Center
Salt Lake City, UT, USA

Alessio Gargaro, MS
Biotronik, Clinical Research Department
Vimodrone (MI), Italy

Carola Gianni, MD
Texas Cardiac Arrhythmia Institute
St. David's Medical Center
Austin, TX, USA

Michael R. Gold, MD, PhD
Division of Cardiology
Medical University of South Carolina
Charleston, SC, USA

Nora Goldschlager, MD
Professor of Medicine
San Francisco General Hospital
San Francisco, CA, USA;
University of California, San Francisco, CA, USA

Edoardo Gronda, MD
Cardiovascular Department
IRCCS MultiMedica
Sesto San Giovanni
Milan, Italy

Michael C. Giudici, MD, FACC, FACP, FHRS
Professor of Medicine
Director of Arrhythmia Services
University of Iowa Hospitals
Iowa City, IA, USA

Shrinivas Hebsur, MD
Michigan Heart and Vascular Institute
Ann Arbor, MI, USA

Donald D. Hegland, MD
Duke University Medical Center
Durham, NC, USA

E. Kevin Heist, MD, PhD
Cardiac Arrhythmia Service
Massachusetts General Hospital
Boston, MA, USA

Patrick M. Hranitzky, MD
Texas Cardiac Arrhythmia
Austin, TX, USA;
WakeMed Heart and Vascular Center
Raleigh, NC, USA

David T. Huang, MD
Division of Cardiology, Department of
Clinical Cardiac Electrophysiology
University of Rochester
Rochester, NY, USA

Carsten W. Israel, MD
J.W. Goethe University
Frankfurt, Germany;
Department of Medicine – Cardiology
Evangelical Hospital Bielefeld
Bielefeld, Germany

Kevin P. Jackson, MD
Division of Clinical Cardiac
Electrophysiology
Duke University Medical Center
Durham, NC, USA

Winston B. Joe, BA, MD
Stanford University School of Medicine
Stanford, CA, USA

Michael G. Katz, MD
Division of Cardiology, Department of
Clinical Cardiac Electrophysiology
University of Rochester
Rochester, NY, USA

Rachel Lampert, MD
Yale University School of Medicine
New Haven, CT, USA

Giosuè Mascioli, MD, FESC
Unit of Arrhythmology and
Cardiac Pacing
Cliniche Humanitas Gavazzeni
Bergamo, Italy

Kevin M. Monahan, MD
Boston Medical Center
Boston University School
of Medicine
Boston, MA, USA

Javid Nasir, MD
Division of Cardiovascular Medicine
Stanford University School of Medicine
Stanford, CA, USA

Andrea Natale, MD, FACC, FHRS, CCDS
Texas Cardiac Arrhythmia Institute
St. David's Medical Center
Austin, TX, USA

Leenhapong Navaravong, MD
Division of Cardiovascular Medicine
University of Utah Health Sciences Center
Salt Lake City, UT, USA

Brian Olshansky, MD
Professor Emeritus
University of Iowa
Iowa, USA;
Cardiac Electrophysiologist
Mercy Hospital-North Iowa
Mason City, Iowa, USA

Luigi Padeletti, MD
IRCCS, MultiMedica
Sesto San Giovanni
Milan, Italy

Margherita Padeletti, MD
Cardiology Unit
Borgo San Lorenzo Hospital
Florence, Italy

Luca Paperini, MD
Second Division of Cardiovascular Diseases
Cardiac-Thoracic and Vascular Department
Azienda Ospedaliero Universitaria Pisana
Pisa, Italy

Marco V. Perez, MD
Cardiac Electrophysiology & Arrhythmia
Service
Stanford University Medical Center
Stanford, CA, USA

P. Pieragnoli, MD
Heart and Vessels Department
University of Florence
Florence, Italy

Edward Platia, MD
Medstar Washington Hospital
Center/Georgetown University
Washington, DC, USA

Sean D. Pokorney, MD, MBA
Duke University Medical Center
Durham, NC, USA

Anil Rajendra, MD
Division of Cardiology
Medical University of South Carolina
Charleston, SC, USA

G. Ricciardi, MD
Heart and Vessels Department
University of Florence
Florence, Italy

Attila Roka, MD, PhD
Cardiovascular Institute of the South
Meridian, MS, USA

Stefania Sacchi, MD
Institute of Internal Medicine and Cardiology
University of Florence
Florence, Italy;
International Centre for Circulatory Health
National Heart and Lung Institute
Imperial College
London, UK

Pasquale Santangeli, MD, PhD
University of Pennsylvania
Philadelphia, PA, USA

Claudio Schuger, MD, FACC, FHRS
Cardiac Electrophysiology
Henry Ford Hospital
Detroit, MI, USA

Luca Segreti, MD
Second Division of Cardiovascular Diseases
Cardiac-Thoracic and Vascular Department
Azienda Ospedaliero Universitaria Pisana
Pisa, Italy

Win-Kuang Shen, MD
Division of Cardiovascular Diseases
Mayo Clinic Arizona
Phoenix, AZ, USA

Kalyanam Shivkumar, MD, PhD
UCLA Cardiac Arrhythmia Center
Ronald Reagan UCLA Medical Center
Los Angeles, CA, USA

Gurjit Singh, MD
Cardiac Electrophysiology
Henry Ford Hospital, Detroit, MI, USA

Jagmeet Singh, MD, PhD
Cardiac Arrhythmia Service
Massachusetts General Hospital
Boston, MA, USA

Ezio Soldati, MD
Second Division of Cardiovascular Diseases
Cardiac-Thoracic and Vascular Department
Azienda Ospedaliero Universitaria Pisana
Pisa, Italy

Dan Sorajja, MD
Division of Cardiovascular Diseases
Mayo Clinic Arizona
Phoenix, AZ, USA

Rachel Tidwell, RN, MSN, CCDS
Medtronic Inc.
Nashville, TN, USA

Gaurav Upadhyay, MD
Heart Rhythm Center
University of Chicago Hospital
Chicago, IL, USA

Emilio Vanoli, MD, PhD
Cardiovascular Department
IRCCS MultiMedica
Sesto San Giovanni
Milan, Italy;
Department of Molecular Medicine
University of Pavia Margherita
Pavia, Italy

Santosh C. Varkey, MD
Boston Medical Center
Boston University School of Medicine
Boston, MA, USA

Stefano Viani, MD
Second Division of Cardiovascular Diseases
Cardiac-Thoracic and Vascular Department
Azienda Ospedaliero Universitaria Pisana
Pisa, Italy

Paul J. Wang, MD
Stanford University School of Medicine
Stanford, CA, USA

Seth J. Worley, MD, FHRS, FACC
Medstar Heart & Vascular Institute
Washington Hospital Center
Washington, DC, USA

Paul C. Zei, MD, PhD
Brigham and Women's Hospital
Harvard Medical School
Boston, MA, USA

Giulio Zucchelli, MD, PhD
Second Division of Cardiovascular Diseases
Cardiac-Thoracic and Vascular Department
Azienda Ospedaliero Universitaria Pisana
Pisa, Italy

About the Companion Website

This book is accompanied by a Companion Website:

The URL to the Website is **www.wiley.com/go/al-ahmad/pacemakers_and_icds**

The Website includes:
- Videos

Part One

1

How to Access the Cephalic Vein Using a Cut-down Approach

Carola Gianni[1], Pasquale Santangeli[2], Andrea Natale[1], and Amin Al-Ahmad[1]

[1] Texas Cardiac Arrhythmia Institute, St. David's Medical Center, Austin, TX, USA
[2] University of Pennsylvania, Philadelphia, PA, USA

The cephalic vein has been used for access and lead placement ever since transvenous leads were developed. The cephalic vein offers relatively easy access into the central venous system with a very low risk of complications [1]. There is essentially no risk of pneumothorax with the cephalic vein cut-down compared with axillary or subclavian puncture. In addition, lead longevity with cephalic access is superior to that of other common techniques such as access via axillary or subclavian veins [2]. This is because of a more gentle angle of entry with cephalic access and a lower risk of subclavian crush to the lead when compared with subclavian access [3,4].

Some physicians use cephalic access for all device implants, while others use it only for selected patients. All physicians should become proficient with implants via cephalic access as it can be useful in patients with access challenges, such as those who have a high risk of complications such as pneumothorax, as well as patients where the longevity of the lead is of prime importance such as young patients.

In this chapter we describe the techniques to gain access into the cephalic vein as well as some of the potential challenges and pitfalls.

Procedure Description

An important aspect of the cephalic vein cut-down procedure is an understanding of the anatomy of the pectoralis and deltoid muscle areas as they relate to the location of the vein. The cephalic vein runs in the deltopectoral groove. On the skin, this is the groove where the shoulder meets the chest and is visible and palpable in most people (Figure 1.1). The incision can be made either parallel to the deltopectoral groove, or perpendicular. Care should be taken to ensure that the incision is close enough to the groove that access to the vein is unencumbered. An incision too medial will lead to a difficult dissection of the cephalic vein. An incision directly on the groove can also be uncomfortable for the patient. A typical incision is approximately 1 cm (or 1 finger's breadth) medial to the groove, approximately 1–2 cm (or 1–2 finger's breadths) below the clavicle. An incision that is too low can make for a challenging dissection and can be too close to the axilla in some individuals.

Once the incision has been made, dissection is carried through to the pectoral fascia using blunt dissection and electrocautery. A fat-pad located in the deltopectoral groove can now be easily identified in most people. The vein is located within the fat-pad (Figure 1.2). Using only blunt dissection with a small clamp (such as a "mosquito" clamp) or a pair of Metzenbaum dissecting scissors allows for removal of the fat and identification of the vein. In the fat-pad area, the use of electrocautery should generally be avoided as it can destroy the vein and render it useless for access. The vein will be thin, white, or have a blue hue in some cases. The vein may also be flat or should become flat when lifted gently. Care should be made to avoid the artery that in some cases runs adjacent to the vein. The artery can be identified as it is thicker, more rounded, and white in color. When the artery is manipulated it may constrict and pulsations can be seen during systole. Occasionally, the artery is positioned such that access into the vein is challenging; in these cases, using the clamp or pick-ups (Debakey forceps), the artery can be moved away from the vein and a small application of electrocautery in the "cautery" mode applied to the metal of the clamp will destroy the artery.

How-to Manual for Pacemaker and ICD Devices: Procedures and Programming, First Edition. Edited by Amin Al-Ahmad, Andrea Natale, Paul J. Wang, James P. Daubert, and Luigi Padeletti.
© 2018 John Wiley & Sons, Inc. Published 2018 by John Wiley & Sons, Inc.
Companion website: www.wiley.com/go/al-ahmad/pacemakers_and_icds

(a)

(b)

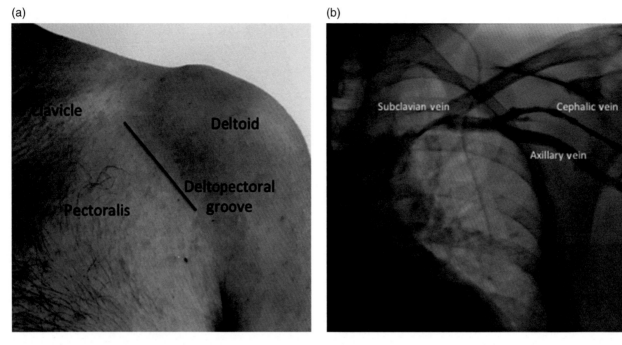

Figure 1.1 (a) Deltopectoral groove. (b) Venogram demonstrating the relationship between the bony landmarks and the cephalic vein. Also, the relationship to the axillary and subclavian veins can be appreciated.

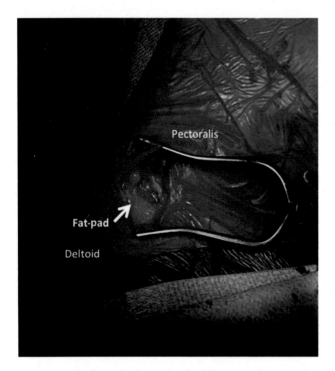

Figure 1.2 The fat-pad is located in the deltopectoral groove. The cephalic vein is within the fat-pad.

Figure 1.3 Cephalic vein isolation using a small clamp.

A right-angle clamp can be used to dissect around the vein to ensure that the vein can be lifted free from any tissue in the groove. At this point the vein is inspected to ensure that any adherent tissue is removed so that only the vein is manipulated (Figure 1.3). Using the right-angle clamp, two pieces (approximately 10 cm) of non-absorbable suture (0 silk or 0 Ethibond) are brought around the vein to maintain control of the distal and proximal aspects of the vein (Figure 1.4). The vein can then be manipulated and accessed.

Figure 1.4 Sutures loops are placed around the vein to maintain control of the proximal and distal aspects of the vein.

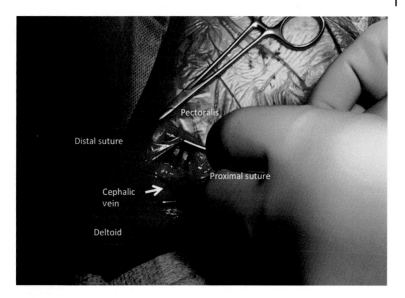

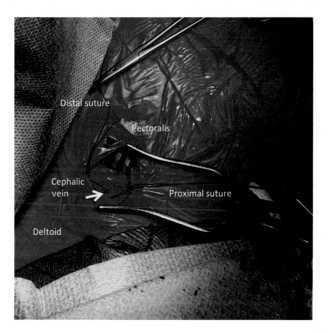

Figure 1.5 Lifting the distal suture to show the cephalic vein. This allows access either by direct venotomy or with a small Angiocath needle.

More than one technique can be used to access the vein. A commonly used technique utilizes a scalpel to make a small venotomy. This is best done while lifting the more distal suture gently as this reduces the amount of bleeding from the vein (Figure 1.5). The scalpel should have a straight blade (typically, number 11 blade) and should cut the vein initially placed in a horizontal position and lifted vertically once the vein has been pierced (Figure 1.6). Care should be taken not to make the venotomy too large so that the integrity of the vein is compromised. In addition, it is important to ensure that the venotomy cuts into the vein rather than only the adventitia surrounding it. Typically, a small amount of blood escapes and the lumen of the vein should be visible. Once the vein has been cut, a vein pick is placed at the lip of the incision and used to lift the lip of the incision to expose the lumen of the vein. Now, under direct visualization, a small (4 French, Fr) sheath can be advanced a small amount into the vein and a hydrophilic glide wire advanced via the sheath into the venous system under fluoroscopic guidance (Figure 1.7).

An alternative approach to using a scalpel and vein pick is direct puncture into the vein with an Angiocath or a micropuncture needle. The Angiocath needle is commonly used to obtain peripheral percutaneous vascular access, while the micropuncture needle is used for central percutaneous vascular access. Once vascular access is obtained with the Angiocath needle, the catheter is advanced gently into the vascular space. With the micropuncture technique, after obtaining vascular access with the needle, a micropuncture wire is advanced into the vein and the micropuncture dilator (5 Fr) is advanced over the wire. Then, through the Angiocath catheter or the micropuncture dilator, a hydrophilic glide wire may be advanced into the central venous system.

Once the wire has been advanced, the small 4 French sheath or the Angiocath catheter is removed and the wire can be used to place a larger peel-away sheath for the lead delivery. This wire needs to support placement of a larger sheath, so a stiff angled tipped glide wire is often the best choice for this job (e.g., Glidewire). The same wire can be used for both sheath placements in the case of a dual chamber system. In this situation, the first sheath is oversized to retain the wire while placing the lead (Figure 1.8). After removal of the sheath, a second sheath can be placed over the wire and advanced.

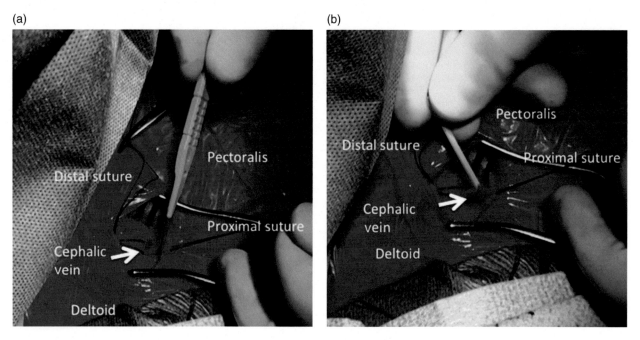

Figure 1.6 (a) Venotomy using an 11 blade with the sharp aspect of the blade pointing upwards. (b) A vein pick (yellow) is placed in the vein to maintain the opening so that a wire can be inserted.

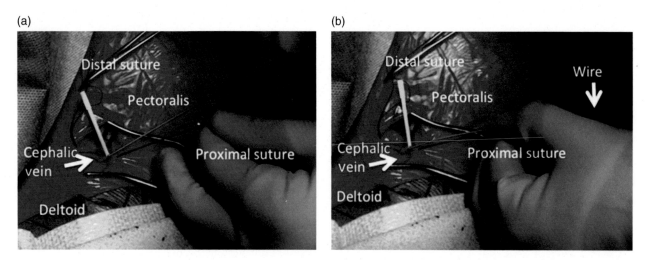

Figure 1.7 (a) Introduction of the 4 Fr sheath. (b) The hydrophilic guide wire is placed via the 4 Fr sheath and advanced into the vein. It can be advanced into the heart under fluoroscopy.

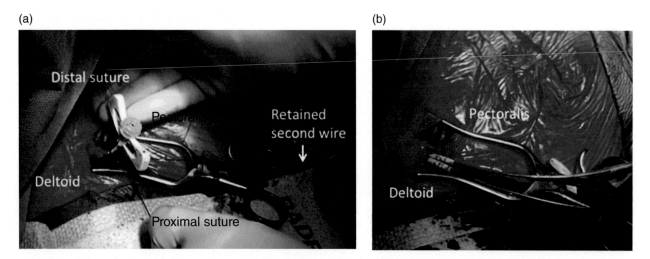

Figure 1.8 (a) The proximal suture is tied to limit "forward" bleeding. Also, a second wire can be inserted by the side of the sheath. This wire can be inserted within the first sheath and then the sheath can be removed retaining two wires in the vasculature. This wire can be retained for placement of the second sheath. (b) Two leads can be easily placed and sutured to the fascia in this location.

The choice to retain the wire with the second sheath is often based on physician preference, with the advantage of keeping the wire being that access is maintained until both leads are placed. Alternatively, once the first sheath is placed, another wire can be advanced in the case of a dual chamber system and the sheath then removed, leaving two wires in place that can each be individually accessed with a sheath. In this case, there is no need to use an oversized sheath.

Potential Pitfalls and Complications

A common challenge is seen in patients who are overweight. In these patients, the deltopectoral groove is not always easy to see, so this may result in an incision that is too lateral or medial. This makes the dissection much more difficult, especially given the large amount of fat and the depth of the dissection needed. In these patients, taking the time to perform deep palpation and finding the area where the deltopectoral groove lies is of utmost importance. Typically, the operator begins palpation at the shoulder and "walks" his or her fingers over the deltoid muscle towards the chest until finding the "deepest" area. This is the deltopectoral groove.

In very thin individuals the surface landmarks are typically easy to find; however, the fat-pad area may be devoid of any fat. In these patients, examining the muscle fiber orientation of the pectoralis and the deltoid muscles leads to identification of where the cephalic vein should run.

Occasionally, the cephalic vein is very small which makes it a challenge to access. Presence of a small vein should not necessarily result in abandoning the approach, as often one can still place two leads via a small cephalic. The use of a small amount of local anesthetic (lidocaine) may help increase the girth of the vein, as sometimes manipulation of the vein can result in some spasm. Typically, a few drops of local anesthetic directly on the vein helps. Once a wire is placed through the cephalic and advanced into the right atrium, or preferably the inferior vena cava, a sheath can be advanced through the vein. In these cases, the vein will be destroyed with advancement of the sheath, but this rarely causes any long-term problems. In some cases, the vein cuff is tight around the sheath causing difficulty with sheath advancement and lead–lead interactions. The use of electrocautery to cut the vein cuff will allow the sheath to be advanced. In some cases, the vein needs to be dilated with progressively larger dilators until the sheath can be placed. The use of a stiff wire such as a "super-stiff" Glidewire can be useful to help advance the sheath. Occasionally, even after the vein is dilated and the sheath advanced, there can be significant interaction between the leads placed together in the cephalic. In these patients, care not to dislodge a lead when removing a sheath and manipulating the other lead is critical. Sometimes, the interaction is too severe and can impact implant success. In these cases, a separate subclavian or axillary puncture for the second lead can simplify the procedure significantly. In devices with three leads, while they can all be placed via the cephalic vein, it is generally preferred to place the smaller of the leads in the axillary or subclavian vein. This is commonly the left ventricular pacing lead.

When the vein is very large, the main problem is bleeding around the leads. This back bleeding can become an issue in patients with a large cephalic vein and high venous pressures, such as those with congestive heart failure. Often, simple manual pressure at the entry site of the cephalic vein is adequate to quell the bleeding after the leads have been placed. In some cases, a purse string suture may be needed. This should be placed carefully with an absorbable suture to ensure that the lead is not compressed within the suture or otherwise damaged by the suture needle. A reasonable approach is to place the purse string suture prior to placement of the leads when significant back bleeding is anticipated.

Conclusions

The cephalic vein cut-down procedure is a simple technique to gain access for lead placement, with very low risks and a high success rate. Once the operator becomes proficient, it can be performed as quickly as an axillary or subclavian puncture. Understanding the potential difficulties, the operator can usually succeed in obtaining access using this technique.

References

1 Chang HM, Hsieh CB, Hsieh HF, Chen TW, Chen CJ, Chan DC, *et al.* An alternative technique for totally implantable central venous access devices: a retrospective study of 1311 cases. Eur J Surg Oncol 2006;32:90–93. doi: 10.1016/j.ejso.2005.09.004

2 Gallik DM, Ben-Zur UM, Gross JN, Furman S. Lead fracture in cephalic versus subclavian approach with transvenous implantable cardioverter defibrillator systems. Pacing Clin Electrophysiol 1996;19:1089–1094.

3 Roelke M, O'Nunain SS, Osswald S, Garan H, Harthorne JW, Ruskin JN. Subclavian crush syndrome complicating transvenous cardioverter defibrillator systems. Pacing Clin Electrophysiol 1995;18:973–979.

4 Parsonnet V, Roelke M. The cephalic vein cutdown versus subclavian puncture for pacemaker/ICD lead implantation. Pacing Clin Electrophysiol 1999;22:695–697.

2

Extrathoracic Subclavian Vein Access

Paul C. Zei[1] and Javid Nasir[2]

[1] Brigham and Women's Hospital, Harvard Medical School, Boston, MA, USA
[2] Division of Cardiovascular Medicine, Stanford University School of Medicine, Stanford, CA, USA

Placement of traditional transvenous cardiac rhythm management (CRM) devices requires access to the venous system for endocardial lead positioning in the right-sided cardiac chambers. Given the typical placement of modern CRM devices in the pectoral region, vascular access to the upper extremity venous system is required. Several techniques can be used to access the venous system for CRM devices. Prior to the development of peel-away sheaths almost all devices were implanted using a cephalic cut-down; subsequently, subclavian access became much more prevalent. Most recently, with the development of percutaneous, extrathoracic techniques to access the venous system (e.g., extrathoracic subclavian and extrathoracic axillary access), these presumably safer techniques have become the standard approach. Cephalic cut-down and the traditional intrathoracic subclavian access are discussed elsewhere; here we focus on access of the extrathoracic subclavian vein and briefly discuss accessing the extrathoracic axillary vein.

There are several advantages particular to extrathoracic subclavian vein access. Given the typical placement of the pulse generator, these veins can often provide the most direct and, as a result, least stressing course for lead travel into the venous system. Unlike the cephalic vein, the subclavian vein is generally large enough to accommodate multiple leads and, when performed correctly, does not carry the risk of pneumothorax or subclavian crush inherent with traditional subclavian access techniques. Therefore, in most operators' assessment, the extrathoracic subclavian vein is considered the preferred approach to obtaining venous access.

Venous Anatomy

The axillary vein is the segment of the venous drainage system from the upper extremity beginning as a continuation of the basilic vein in the axilla (when it crosses the teres major). It continues to course just inferiorly to the clavicle until it reaches the lateral margin of the first rib and becomes the subclavian vein. While, technically speaking, the portion of the vein that overlies the first rib is the extrathoracic portion of the subclavian vein, in clinical practice, many refer to this as the medial axillary vein to differentiate this type of access from traditional subclavian access [1]. The rationale for this distinction is that if performed correctly, access of the extrathoracic subclavian vein does not carry the same risk of pneumothorax or subclavian crush as true subclavian vein access.

A typical venogram demonstrating left upper extremity venous anatomy is illustrated in Figure 2.1. The axillary vein typically is projected over the lateral edge of the ribcage between the second and third ribs and then crosses over the first rib just inferior to the clavicle. The vein tends to be more cranial in location in men and patients with higher body mass index (BMI), and tends to lie more caudally in Caucasians. A more caudal axillary vein course (lateral to medial) has also been reported in those with a history of congestive heart failure [2]. As a "bookkeeping" note, all subsequent anatomic and technical descriptions will by default refer to the left upper extremity venous system. For right-sided implants, specific considerations will be addressed additionally.

How-to Manual for Pacemaker and ICD Devices: Procedures and Programming, First Edition. Edited by Amin Al-Ahmad, Andrea Natale, Paul J. Wang, James P. Daubert, and Luigi Padeletti.
© 2018 John Wiley & Sons, Inc. Published 2018 by John Wiley & Sons, Inc.
Companion website: www.wiley.com/go/al-ahmad/pacemakers_and_icds

(a)   (b)

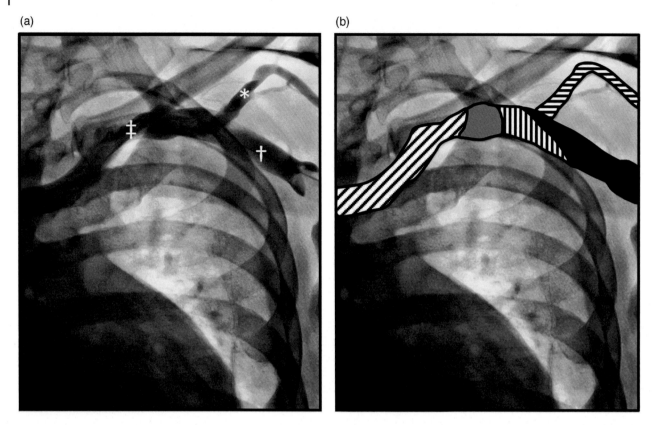

Figure 2.1 (a) Venogram demonstrating the typical course the cephalic, axillary, and subclavian veins. (b) The venous anatomy has been marked with the extrathoracic axillary vein colored black, the cephalic vein with horizontal stripes, the thoracic axillary vein with vertical stripes, the extrathoracic subclavian with gray and the subclavian with diagonal stripes.

Accessing the Extrathoracic Subclavian Vein

Access to the central venous system via the extrathoracic subclavian vein was first described by Byrd as an alternative approach to failed intrathoracic subclavian access [3]. He subsequently described his experience accessing the extrathoracic subclavian vein preferentially in 213 consecutive patients with a 98% success rate with no complications [4]. This approach was later prospectively evaluated in 2001 in 200 patients randomized to either a cephalic cut-down or a contrast-guided extrathoracic subclavian approach [5]. In this study, when compared with a cephalic cut-down, extrathoracic subclavian access resulted in a higher success rate (99% vs. 64%; p <0.001), shorter procedure time (86 ± 22 vs. 98 ± 35 min; p <0.01), less blood loss (55 ± 13 vs. 115 ± 107 mL; p <0.01), and no difference in the rates of complications (6% vs. 11%; p = 0.2).

With this approach, the vein is accessed superficially to the first rib and lateral to the clavicle. This allows access to the vein with a shallow angle, providing a less strained lead course and should eliminate the risk of subclavian crush associated with more medial access and risk of second rib fatigue fractures with more lateral access.

Additionally, if performed correctly, the risk of pneumothorax is no greater than with cephalic cut-down [5], as the first rib will be encountered if the vein is missed, providing the underpinning for one descriptor of this technique as a protected first rib approach.

Consent

Informed consent should include a comprehensive assessment of the patient's risks and benefits, which should be tailored to the planned access method. Access-related complications discussed with the patient should include pneumothorax, bleeding, venous thrombosis, arterial puncture (including risk of AV fistula formation, and lead fracture. Other complications, not related to access, are discussed elsewhere.

The assessed risk of pneumothorax should be tailored to the planned access technique. With cephalic, extrathoracic subclavian, or extrathoracic axillary access, the published rates of pneumothorax are approximately 1% compared to 2% for traditional subclavian access [6]. Risk of significant pneumothorax requiring a chest tube in cephalic and traditional subclavian access has been reported as 0.2% and 1.2%, respectively [7].

The risk of pocket hematoma is likely similar with the various available access techniques and is related primarily to both surgical technique and patient medication use (e.g., antiplatelet or anticoagulants); however, this risk may be slightly increased with use of the retained wire approach. Hemothorax is a rare complication usually related to injury to great vessels. By avoiding medial, non-compressible needle sticks the risk of this complication can be mitigated.

The risk of lead failure is related to access technique. Accessing the intrathoracic subclavian vein can cause subclavian crush or fracture of the lead in an anatomically restricted space between the first rib and clavicle. This is likely related to soft tissue entrapment by the subclavius muscle and can be avoided by accessing the venous system more laterally [8]. The stress on leads is also likely increased with extrathoracic axillary techniques because of the extreme angulation required for extrathoracic access of the axillary vein and can lead to second-rib related fatigue fractures. While data are wanting, this was most evident when the Canadian Heart Rhythm Society retrospectively examined the data for 3169 Sprint Fidelis leads and found that axillary access was one of the strongest risk factors for lead fracture [9].

Pre-procedure

Prior to implantation of the CRM device, a careful history and physical examination should be performed. The presence of hemodialysis shunts or catheters may preclude venous access to the ipsilateral axillary vein. Similarly, prior lymph node dissection and excision, typically seen in mastectomy, will increase the risk of impaired venous return if leads are placed in the ipsilateral vein. Additional contraindications (relative and/or absolute) to performing access for lead implantation include known venous thrombosis in the upper extremities, ongoing infection, coagulopathy, and known contralateral pneumothorax.

If the patient is undergoing an upgrade, with addition of one or more leads to an existing pacing system, generally the first choice approach is to utilize the venous system ipsilateral to the existing system. However, there is always the possibility that the existing lead system has already resulted in chronic venous occlusion, so a careful examination of the ipsilateral chest surface for the presence of superficial venous collateral vessels should be performed. Additionally, consideration should be made to perform ipsilateral venography prior to incision, in order to plan for this scenario and still allow for a successful outcome. This may involve abandonment of the existing system and placement of an entire new system on the contralateral pectoral region, accessing the venous system on the contralateral side and tunneling the proximal portion of the lead across the chest superficial to the sternum and ribs to the existing system, ipsilateral venoplasty, or lead extraction to allow venous access on the ipsilateral system.

Prior echocardiography should also be reviewed to ensure no congenital abnormalities are present and there is no evidence to suggest persistent left-sided superior vena cava (SVC; e.g. dilated coronary sinus). An assessment of renal function, coagulation status, and electrolytes should be performed. In patients with renal insufficiency, pre-hydration and/or premedication with *N*-acetylcysteine can be considered [10]. With significant renal dysfunction, contrast can usually be avoided for pacemaker or implantable cardioverter-defibrillator (ICD) implantation with extrathoracic subclavian or cephalic access, but usually a small amount of contrast is needed for implantation of leads in the coronary sinus. If difficulty accessing the extrathoracic subclavian is encountered and one wishes to avoid the use of contrast, a coronary wire can be placed through a peripheral IV in the upper extremity to illustrate the path of the venous anatomy.

Regarding medications, oral diabetic medications and short-acting insulin should be held. We also tend to hold diuretics while the patient is NPO. We generally will continue aspirin in the perioperative period but will hold clopidogrel for 5 days if the patient has not undergone percutaneous coronary intervention (PCI) in the last 12 months. Management of warfarin in the perioperative period is more complex. If there is no compelling indication for continuous anticoagulation (e.g., mechanical heart valve, pulmonary embolism, atrial fibrillation with high risk of thromboembolism, left ventricular thrombus) we usually stop warfarin 3 days prior to the procedure and resume upon discharge or within 48 hours. If there is a compelling reason for anticoagulation, most operators are comfortable performing device implantation in patients on warfarin with an international normalized ratio (INR) ≤3.0 at the time of implantation; however, patients on heparin or enoxaparin are transitioned to warfarin, if possible, to minimize the risk of pocket hematoma. Birnie *et al.* [11] demonstrated patients on therapeutic warfarin instead of heparin or enoxaparin bridge had significantly lower rates of clinically significant pocket hematoma (3.5% vs. 16.0%; p <0.001). Some operators will perform implantation while patients are continuing with novel oral anticoagulants (NOACs); however, the data on this practice are currently sparse and there may be increased rates of serious complications [12], so most operators will hold NOACs in the perioperative period [13]. We generally discontinue NOACs 2–3 days prior to implant and restart typically within 1–2 days post implant if excessive bleeding is not seen.

Preparation

Access is typically performed with a pectoral region pulse generator placement in mind. Therefore, the pectoral region should be prepped in a typical surgical sterile fashion. Consideration should be made whether to prep the unilateral or bilateral pectoral region, in case one side must be abandoned and implant will proceed on the contralateral side. In our practice, bilateral pectoral regions are prepped. In that regard, at least medium bore (20 G or less) IVs are placed in the bilateral distal upper extremities to allow for venograms on either side if needed.

Relative hypovolemia can result in venous under filling and a resultant smaller target vein. This may increase the risk of missing the vein entirely or going through-and-through the vein. We typically administer a small IV saline bolus (the volume depends on the patient's condition and how long they have been NPO) just before access is attempted.

Incision and Creation of the Pocket

Most operators create an incision that both runs medial to and parallel to the deltopectoral groove, or inferior and parallel to the clavicle. The advantage of the former incision is that is allows better exposure of the deltopectoral groove if a cephalic vein cut-down is being considered and tends to produce a more cosmetically appealing scar. Disadvantages of creating the incision parallel to the deltopectoral groove result from having to dissect medially to make the pocket to prevent the generator from lying too close to the axilla, while still allowing access to the extrathoracic subclavian vein. That being said, to allow for the option to access the cephalic vein and for improved cosmetics, we typically create an angled incision approximately 1 cm inferior and medial to the deltopectoral groove.

In patients presenting for a lead revision or upgrade with an existing system, the location of the new incision may be placed directly overlying the pre-existing scar from prior incision(s), or a new incision can be made entirely. While efforts are made to use an existing incision, if there are concerns regarding the location of the existing scar, we will make a new incision. Potential concerns include the prior incision not being in a location suitable for access to the venous system, device migration (typically, inferiorly and laterally) which may lead to difficulty accessing the prior device and/or leads, or inadequate soft tissue at the incision site to allow for a well-healed scar. Otherwise, we tend to create an incision at the prior incision if feasible. Excision of the prior scar and other cosmetic techniques are available, but these are not discussed here.

After we have decided on the location of the incision, the patient prepared, and the venogram performed, we administer light conscious sedation with fentanyl and midazolam (if general anesthesia is not being used) and inject copious local anesthetic along the intended incisional line both superficial and deep. An incision is then created with a No.10 blade taking care to cut through the entire skin thickness with one smooth incision. Using Weitlaner retractors and electrocautery, the incision is continued through the adipose and connective tissues until the muscular fascia is seen, with care being take to avoid disrupting the fascia. We will then inject another 10–20 mL of local anesthetic just superficial to the fascia and along the floor of the pocket where access and suturing is anticipated, and we will create a pocket for placement of the pulse generator at this time. While some will defer creation of the pocket until after access has been obtained or the leads have been secured, we advocate for creation of the pulse generator pocket at this time, as this will allow adequate time to assess for persistent bleeding that should be addressed.

Venography

Although in general the vein takes a relatively well-defined and predictable course, there is enough patient-to-patient variation such that we almost universally perform venography to visualize the venous anatomy prior to access. However, access to the extrathoracic subclavian can be obtained using only fluoroscopy. Only 4 of 213 of the patients in Byrd's series required venography and access without venography was successful in 245 of 250 of the patients in Gardini and Benedini's series [4,14]. Hence, many operators will "walk" the access needle along the first rib blindly until the extrathoracic subclavian vein is accessed and only use venography if the vein is not easily found. However, venography should always be performed if old leads are present, if there is suspicion for vascular abnormality (e.g., persistent left SVC or large coronary sinus on echocardiography), or if access is not easily obtained.

Prior to performing venography, the fluoroscopy camera should be positioned so that that image encompasses the vertebral bodies medially, clavicle superiorly, and deltopectoral groove laterally (Figure 2.2a,b). In addition to visualizing the extrathoracic subclavian vein, this positioning will allow examination for the presence of a persistent left SVC and show the position of the extrathoracic axillary vein and cephalic vein in case alternate approaches are chosen (e.g., extreme anterior displacement of clavicle). Oftentimes, operators will place the access needle at or near the anticipated access path at the surface of the pectoral muscle prior to venography so access can be performed after cineography but prior to the contrast leaving the vein.

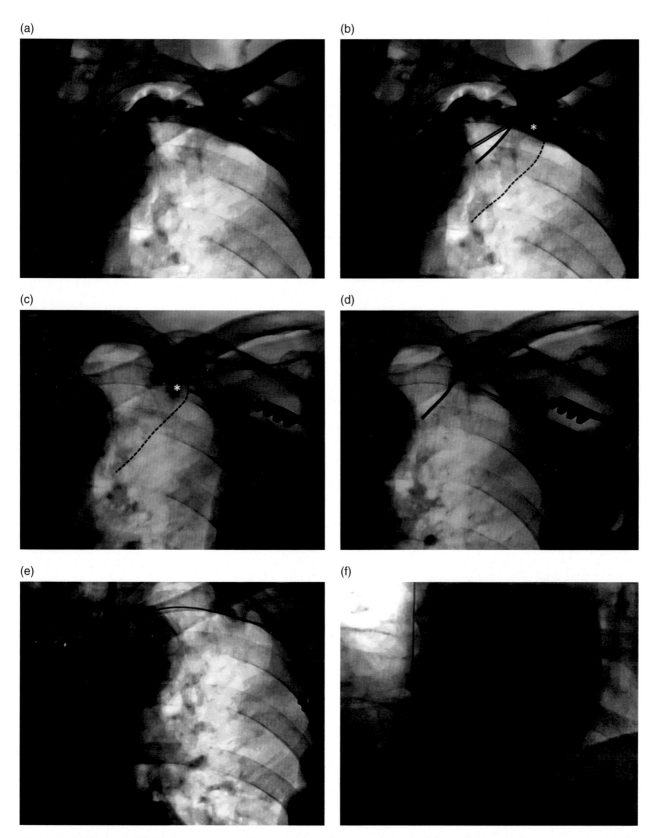

Figure 2.2 (a) Venogram of left upper extremity. (b) The anatomy relevant for accessing the extrathoracic subclavian has been marked with the inferior margin of the clavicle identified with a solid double line, the lateral margin of the first rib with a dotted line, and the medial margin of the first rib with a thick solid single line. The target for accessing the extrathoracic subclavian has been marked with an asterisk. (c) The lateral margin of the first rib has been marked with a dashed line and the extrathoracic subclavian with an asterisk. (d) The access needle is above the first rib and approaching the medial margin of the first rib which has been identified with a thick black line. The medial margin of the first rib should not be violated with the access needle unless you are intentionally accessing the intrathoracic subclavian vein. (e) Access has been obtained and a J wire advanced into the intrathoracic subclavian vein. (f) The J wire has been advanced into inferior vena cava (beneath the diaphragm and on the left side of the vertebral body in AP view) ensuring you have not inadvertently accessed the arterial system.

After correct positioning of the camera, 20 mL of a 1:1 contrast:saline mixture should be injected through in the ipsilateral upper extremity followed immediately by at least 10–20 mL saline. A larger bore (≥20 G) IV in the distal ipsilateral upper extremity is used for injection. If the proximal upper extremity is used, care should be taken to avoid the cephalic vein as the axillary vein may not be opacified well. Short pulses of fluoroscopy are then used until contrast is seen entering the extrathoracic axillary artery and then cineography is performed. During cineography, if existing leads are present we will pan the table towards the SVC–right atrium (RA) junction to ensure no occlusion or stenosis is present. The resultant venogram can then be displayed as a "roadmap" for "offline" access to the vein.

Vascular Access

After the creation of the pocket and venography, we proceed to access the extrathoracic subclavian and/or axillary vein(s). The access needle (typically either 18 gauge or a micropuncture needle) should be attached to a 10 mL Luer Lock syringe and filled with 1–2 mL saline. We choose an access point on the floor of the pocket at least 2 cm from the lateral edge and advance the needle bevel up superficially while applying gentle negative pressure until the lateral margin of the first rib is reached (Figure 2,2c). The rationale for a relatively medial entry point is to ensure an adequate area to secure the leads to the pectoral muscle. Typically, our angle of entry is approximately 30 degrees, adjusted according to body habitus and anatomy. We will decrease the angle in thin patients or if we anticipate there will significant distance to travel. A more acute angle may be used if significant soft tissue in this region suggests a deeper vein location. Once the lateral margin of the first rib is reached (as seen on fluoroscopy), we change our angle to approximately 60 degrees and advance until we make contact with the first rib, reach the medial border of the first rib, or the vein is entered (Figure 2.2c,d). If the vein was not accessed, the needle should be slowly drawn back with continued gentle negative pressure. If the vein was punctured through-and-through, most often a flash will be seen during needle withdrawal as the needle once again enters the lumen of the vein. If the vein is not accessed with withdrawal of the needle, the needle should be repositioned to either follow a steeper angle (if the first rib was not encountered prior to reaching the medial margin of the first rib) or either more cephalad or caudal (if the first rib was encountered) until access is obtained, using a saved frozen image of the venogram as an anatomic guide. We recommend attempting to access the vein directly through the "front wall" of the vein,

rather than a "through and through" Seldinger technique. The latter increases the likelihood of continuing to advance the needle well past the vein, risking pneumothorax or other complications if it is not suspected that the vein has already been entered and passed.

At this point, the syringe is removed, and a wire is advanced through the needle into the vein. If no significant resistance to advancement is perceived, the wire can be safely advanced several centimeters without fluoroscopy (Figure 2.2d). Once the wire is reasonably secure within the vein, fluoroscopy is used to guide advancement of the wire past the subclavian vein, the SVC, and into the RA. At this point, we recommend further advancement of the wire into the inferior vena cava (IVC; rightward of the spine and beneath the diaphragm in AP: Figure 2.2e). Advancing the wire past the diaphragm will ensure that the arterial system has not been inadvertently entered, potentially leading to erroneous lead placement within the left ventricle. Additionally, by placing the wire within the IVC it will not interfere with lead implantation in a more secure position. The access needle is removed, and the wire is then secured externally using a clamp to avoid dislodgement and/or migration of the entire wire into the venous system, a potentially significant complication. Typically, we use a 60 cm 0.035" J wire given its soft atraumatic tip but will occasionally use a St. Jude Medical 0.035" Tigerwire or Covidien 0.025" Whorley wire if a steerable wire is needed to cross an area of stenosis or tortuosity. In general, hydrophilic wires should not be used for initial access, as pulling the wire back to any degree within the needle may result in shearing of the hydrophilic coating at the needle edge.

Subsequent Venous Access

If two or more leads are planned, either separate access points are obtained for each lead, a retained wire approach is used to maintain access as each lead is sequentially placed, or a hybrid approach is used. We generally favor a hybrid approach for CS lead placement, in which a retained wire technique is used for the RA and RV leads, while a separate access is used for the CS lead, if needed. This will minimize lead–lead interaction for the CS lead, while somewhat reducing the number of separate punctures required.

If more than one access point to the vein is desired, we recommend keeping additional access sites remote from the initial access site to minimize interaction between leads and crowding during suturing of the leads. In general, additional contrast is not needed, as the wire just placed can be used as a fluoroscopic landmark. The advantages of separate access points for each lead are the minimization of lead–lead interactions during lead manipulation, and possibly reduction of bleeding from axillary vein back bleeding. The downside of an approach utilizing separate access points for each lead is that with each pass of the access needle comes an additional risk of pneumothorax if the medial margin of the first rib is inadvertently violated.

Alternatively, a retained wire technique can be used. Once the access wire is placed, that same site can be used for subsequent lead placement by placing a sheath that is large enough bore to accommodate both the lead and a wire. The lead is then advanced through the sheath with the wire still within the sheath. Once the lead enters into the RA, the sheath is peeled before positioning the lead to minimize interactions between the lead and wire, and wire retained for subsequent access. This retained wire approach can be then repeated as needed for subsequent leads. While the retained wire technique may decrease the risk of pneumothorax by limiting the number of needle passes, this approach may also increase the risk of axillary venous back bleeding and result in significant lead–lead interaction during manipulation of the leads.

Another option to minimize needle passes and avoid oversized sheaths is to advance a small (e.g., 5 Fr) sheath over the initial access wire. Once the dilator is removed, additional wire(s) are advanced through the sheath back into the venous system (all the way to the IVC again). The sheath can then be withdrawn, and the sheath intended for the first lead to be placed is advanced over one of the two-plus in situ wires. The advantages of this approach are that it allows for the smallest necessary sheath sizes to be used for each lead and minimizes needle passes. The disadvantages are that multiple additional steps are needed, there may be a higher rate of bleeding because of multiple leads passing through a single vein puncture, and an increased risk of lead–lead interactions.

Whether using separate sticks or a retained wire technique, we recommend advancement of at least the first sheath, if not all sheaths, under fluoroscopic visualization. This will confirm the sheath tracks along the access wire; otherwise, the sheath may easily tear the vein. This is particularly important in right-sided implants, as the course of the right subclavian vein into the SVC is more acute, rending it more difficult for the sheath to track along the acutely angled wire.

Hemostasis

One of the more significant causes of pocket hematoma is access vein back bleeding, especially in patients with elevated venous filling pressures, as often is the case in patients undergoing cardiac resynchronization therapy (CRT) placement. Once all the desired wires are placed into the venous system, we favor placement of a suture that encompasses the puncture site(s) at the pectoral muscle, at least 1 cm proximal to the wire exit point from the muscle. This suture is clamped and not tied off until the leads have been secured and tested. At that point, this "back bleed control" suture is tightened around the pectoral exit site such that any back bleeding from the axillary vein will be minimized, if not eliminated. We always use an absorbable suture, typically 2-0 Vicryl, which allows for good hemostasis initially but avoids permanent tension on either the pectoral muscle or the leads.

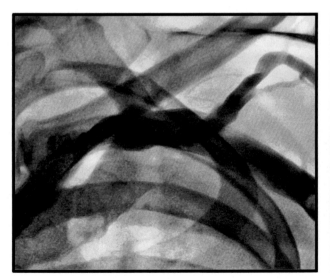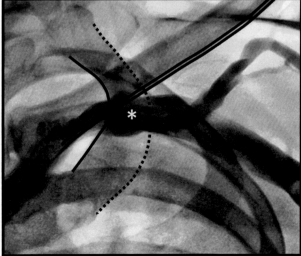

Figure 2.3 Venogram demonstrating dimpling of the extrathoracic axillary vein with access.

Extrathoracic Axillary Access

Many operators utilize a lateral axillary vein access site. With this technique the vein is accessed at the lateral margin of the rib cage just cephalad to the intersection of the inferior border of the second rib and superior border of the third rib (Figure 2.3). A needle approach angle of 45 to nearly 90 degrees is typically used. Using fluoroscopic landmarks alone, Burri *et al.* [15]reported a 61% success rate without venography and 95–99% success rate with venography.

The primary advantage of this technique is minimization of pneumothorax risk, as the needle should never pass over the projection of the ribs and hence the lung fields; however, there are significant drawbacks to this approach. The placement of leads near the axilla may result in patient discomfort, as the leads and potentially pulse generator may sit within the axilla, subject to movement and irritation from arm movement. Additionally, the acute angulation of the access needle may result in increased risk of lead fracture [11].

References

1 Belott P. How to access the axillary vein. Heart Rhythm 2006;3(3):366–369.
2 Hsu JC, Friday J, Lee BK, Azadani PN, Lee RJ, Badhwar N, *et al.* Predictors of axillary vein location for vascular access during pacemaker and defibrillator lead implantation. Pacing Clin Electrophysiol. 2011; 34(12):1585–92.
3 Byrd CL. Safe introducer technique for pacemaker lead implantation. Pacing Clin Electrophysiol 1992;15(3):262–267.
4 Byrd CL. Clinical experience with the extrathoracic introducer insertion technique. Pacing Clin Electrophysiol 1993;16(9):1781–1784.
5 Calkins H, Ramza BM, Brinker J, Atiga W, Donahue K, Nsah E, *et al.* Prospective randomized comparison of the safety and effectiveness of placement of endocardial pacemaker and defibrillator leads using the extrathoracic subclavian vein guided by contrast venography versus the cephalic approach. Pacing Clin Electrophysiol 2001;24(4 Pt 1):456–464.
6 Aggarwal RK, Connelly DT, Ray SG, Ball J, Charles RG. Early complications of permanent pacemaker implantation: no difference between dual and single chamber systems. Br Heart J 1995;73(6):571–575.
7 Kirkfeldt RE, Johansen JB, Nohr EA, Moller M, Arnsbo P, Nielsen JC. Pneumothorax in cardiac pacing: a population-based cohort study of 28,860 Danish patients. Europace 2012;14(8):1132–1138.
8 Magney JE, Flynn DM, Parsons JA, Staplin DH, Chin-Purcell MV, Milstein S, *et al.* Anatomical mechanisms explaining damage to pacemaker leads, defibrillator leads, and failure of central venous catheters adjacent to the sternoclavicular joint. Pacing Clin Electrophysiol 1993;16(3 Pt 1):445–457.
9 Birnie DH, Parkash R, Exner DV, Essebag V, Healey JS, Verma A, *et al.* Clinical predictors of Fidelis lead failure: report from the Canadian Heart Rhythm Society Device Committee. Circulation 2012;125(10):1217–1225.
10 Zagler A, Azadpour M, Mercado C, Hennekens CH. N-acetylcysteine and contrast-induced nephropathy: a meta-analysis of 13 randomized trials. Am Heart J 2006;151(1):140–145.
11 Birnie DH, Healey JS, Wells, GA, Verma A, Tang AS, Krahn AD, *et al.* Pacemaker or defibrillator surgery without interruption of anticoagulation. N Engl J Med 2013;368:2084–2093.
12 Kosiuk J, Koutalas E, Doering M, Sommer P, Rolf S, Breithardt OA, *et al.* Treatment with novel oral anticoagulants in a real-world cohort of patients undergoing cardiac rhythm device implantations. Europace 2014;16(7):1028–1032.
13 Nascimento T, Birnie DH, Healey JS, Verma A, Joza J, Bernier ML, *et al.* Managing novel oral anticoagulants in patients with atrial fibrillation undergoing device surgery: Canadian survey. Can J Cardiol 2014;30(2):231–236.
14 Gardini A, Benedini G. Blind extrathoracic subclavian venipuncture for pacemaker implant: a 3-year experience in 250 patients. Pacing Clin Electrophysiol 1998;21(11 Pt 2):2304–2308.
15 Burri H, Sunthorn H, Dorsaz PA, Shah D. Prospective study of axillary vein puncture with or without contrast venography for pacemaker and defibrillator lead implantation. Pacing Clin Electrophysiol 2005; 28(Suppl 1):S280–283.

3

Subcutaneous Implantable Cardioverter-Defibrillator

Anil Rajendra and Michael R. Gold

Division of Cardiology, Medical University of South Carolina, Charleston, SC, USA

Since its advent in 1980 and widespread commercial use in 1985, implantable cardioverter-defibrillators (ICDs) have been a very effective therapy in aborting sudden cardiac arrest (SCA) as well as improving survival in high-risk patients. Conventional ICDs utilize a transvenous approach to lead implantation in the endocardium for arrhythmia detection and defibrillation. Although this approach was a major advance compared with the early systems which required patches placed on the heart via a thoracotomy, there are numerous potential complications associated with transvenous lead implantation. Procedural complications include pneumothorax, hemothorax, cardiac perforation, and tamponade, whereas, more chronically, lead failure and malfunction can lead to inappropriate therapies and require lead revisions. Device infections are associated with serious morbidity and mortality and require extraction of the leads, a procedure that is associated with substantial morbidity and mortality.

Recently, an entirely subcutaneous ICD (S-ICD) was developed with the goal of avoiding the complications associated with transvenous ICDs. In early human trials, the optimal electrode and generator placement was determined, with the generator placed in the left lateral axilla and the coil in the left parasternal position [1]. In this configuration, the proximal sensing electrode is adjacent to the xiphoid process, and the distal sensing electrode is at the manubriosternal junction. Three sensing vectors can be derived with this lead placement: primary (proximal electrode to can), secondary (distal electrode to can), and alternative (distal electrode to proximal electrode). In studies of induced arrhythmias, S-ICD has been shown to be highly sensitive (100%) and specific (98%) for arrhythmia discrimination, with better discrimination of supraventricular arrhythmias than with transvenous devices [2]. In addition, the S-ICD achieved high success in defibrillation during ventricular fibrillation (VF) testing at implant [3]. In this chapter, we seek to describe optimal patient selection and implant techniques.

Patient Selection

The S-ICD has been approved broadly for patients meeting previously established guidelines for primary or secondary prevention of SCA who do not have a pacing indication. This device should be avoided in patients who require pacing for bradycardia, ventricular tachycardia, or cardiac resynchronization therapy. This device is most commonly used for patients who are poor candidates for a transvenous system for a variety of reasons. Such groups include patients with congenital heart disease with no or limited venous access, hemodialysis patients, and those with previous bacteremia including endocarditis. Patients with previous transvenous device infections, whether systemic or localized, are frequently treated with an S-ICD.

Transvenous ICD leads have a high long-term failure rate [4]. This often results in the need for further transvenous leads, increasing the risk for venous occlusion, or to lead extraction, which carries substantial risks. Therefore, young patients with a long life expectancy may benefit from a subcutaneous approach to avoid these potential complications. Similarly, patients with inherited disorders associated with sudden death, including channelopathies, are often young with no pacing indications. They are another excellent group to consider for an S-ICD. Such conditions include hypertrophic cardiomyopathy, Brugada syndrome, and long QT syndrome.

How-to Manual for Pacemaker and ICD Devices: Procedures and Programming, First Edition. Edited by Amin Al-Ahmad, Andrea Natale, Paul J. Wang, James P. Daubert, and Luigi Padeletti.
© 2018 John Wiley & Sons, Inc. Published 2018 by John Wiley & Sons, Inc.
Companion website: www.wiley.com/go/al-ahmad/pacemakers_and_icds

Despite ideal as well as poor candidates for S-ICD, the majority of ICD candidates do not fit into one of these categories. Thus, patient selection for this device continues to evolve and other factors influence the choice of device, such as the need for remote monitoring, battery longevity, costs, and, importantly, patient preference.

Patients need to be screened to ensure appropriate identification and discrimination of arrhythmias. The lead is placed subcutaneously; the sensing vector resembles the signal of a standard surface ECG, thus leaving it susceptible to oversensing of cardiac signals (i.e., T waves) and noise. To prevent this issue, the sensing algorithm has a threshold that adapts to the amplitude of the QRS complex and decays over time. To ensure that the sensing algorithm can be effective, cutaneous ECG screening is performed prior to implant to ensure an adequate R to T wave ratio. The three electrodes are placed where the subcutaneous pulse generator and lead electrodes would be positioned rather than at traditional ECG locations. If the R to T wave ratio is inadequate, then implantation is discouraged, as the patient is at increased risk of inappropriate shocks.

Anatomic Landmarks for Implantation and Prepping

The implantation of an entirely subcutaneous ICD can be performed completely by anatomic landmarks without the use of fluoroscopy. The major landmarks are the left lateral mid axillary line, the xiphoid process, and the manubriosternal junction. The pulse generator (i.e., can) sits in the left mid axillary line, with small incisions at the xiphoid process and manubriosternal junction. Prior to prepping the skin, fluoroscopy can be used to identify the apex of the heart or this can be identified by palpation, because the ICD can should be placed at that level. The site for the can may be indicated with a marking pen prior to the skin being prepped to ensure the appropriate location for the incision (Figure 3.1).

Care should be made to prep an adequate area for the implant, as it is a larger area than conventional transvenous implants. The skin should be clipped from just right of the sternum to the posterior axilla, and from the chin to the epigastrium. The same area should be prepped with a typical skin cleansing solution. It is important to prep far enough posterior to decrease the risk of infection. To improve visualization and access to the axilla, a roll or wedge can be placed under the patient's left side so that it is slightly elevated or a rotating surgical table can

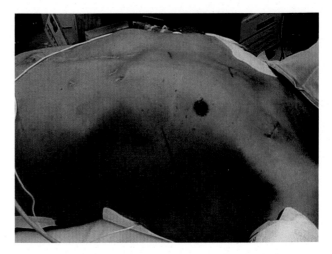

Figure 3.1 Photograph of a patient from the left side. The sites for the incision (left axilla, xiphoid process, and manubriosternal junction) are marked with a blue pen prior to the skin prep and draping.

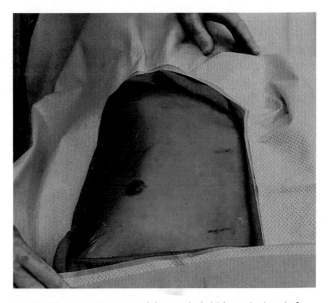

Figure 3.2 A superior view of the sterile field from the head of the bed. Note that a wide surgical field is draped to allow access to the incision sites.

be used. The left arm will need to be extended out to the side on an arm board so that it does not obscure the axilla and is not in the operative field.

As with skin preparation, placement of the sterile drapes should be wide enough to provide an adequate operative field (Figure 3.2). The entire axilla to the sternum and the xiphoid process to the sternal notch should be included in the sterile operative field. With the left arm extended out to the side, an additional drape will need to be placed over the arm to maintain good sterility.

Implantation Procedure

After the patient has been adequately prepped and draped using a sterile technique, the pocket should be made in the left lateral axilla. The can should reside at the apex of the heart, above the level of the diaphragm in the left axilla. A good landmark for the diaphragm is the xiphoid process (i.e., the can should not sit lower than the xiphoid process). Placement of the can in an anterior location can lead to inadequate defibrillation so erring toward the posterior axilla is preferable. Typically, the incision for the pocket is made in the lateral axilla and dissected posteriorly until an adequate pocket size is achieved. Numerous cutaneous vessels reside in the area, and care must be taken to ensure adequate hemostasis. As with transvenous systems, dissection should be performed to the fascia, in this situation of the latissimus dorsi muscle, and care should be taken to avoid interruption of that fascia to prevent excessive bleeding.

Once the pocket for the can has been made, attention should be turned to the smaller incisions along the sternum. An incision about 2 cm in length should be made just left of the xiphoid process. There is no clear consensus whether a vertical or horizontal incision is preferred. The lead should lie along the left parasternal border, so the incision should be made about 1 cm left of the xiphoid process. The fascia should be sufficiently uncovered with dissection. Using 2-0 silk, a suture is tied to the fascia; another 2-0 silk suture is tied to the fascia 1 cm lateral from the initial suture. The strands of these two sutures should be left in place, as they will be used to tie the suture sleeve in place later. Another incision is made 1 cm left of the manubriosternal junction. This landmark can be found by palpating the sternal notch. Similar to the previous incision at the xiphoid process, the subcutaneous tissue should be dissected and the fascia revealed. Using a 2-0 silk, a suture is tied to the fascia.

Next, the tunneling trochar is placed in the incision at the xiphoid process at the level of the fascia. The trochar is then tunneled along the fascia laterally toward the inferior border of the lateral pocket until it breaks through the tissue and penetrates the pocket (Figure 3.3). The trochar has a small hole at the end, through which a 2-0 silk suture is tied. A long strand should be preserved and is then tied to the end of the lead so that the lead is attached to the trochar. This set-up allows the lead to be pulled with the tunneling device. The trochar is then pulled from the handle through the incision at the xiphoid process until the lead is pulled through that incision as well (Figure 3.4). There is a sensing electrode 1 cm proximal to the coil on the lead. A suture sleeve with two grooves is attached to the lead 1 cm proximal to the sensing electrode. The sutures that were tied to the fascia

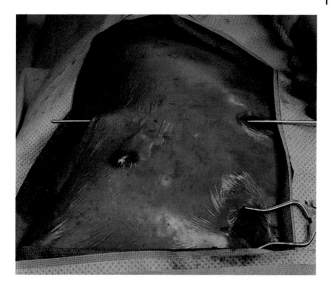

Figure 3.3 The trochar has been tunneled from the xiphoid incision to the lateral pocket.

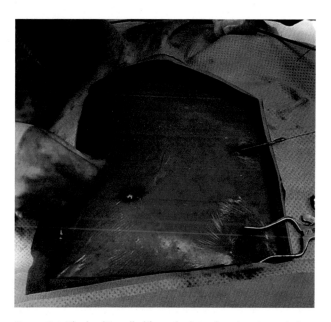

Figure 3.4 The lead is pulled from the lateral pocket through the xiphoid incision via the silk tied to the trochar.

previously are used to secure the lead to the fascia with the suture sleeve. The trochar, with the lead still attached via the silk suture, is then inserted into the incision at the xiphoid process again, but this time directed cranially toward the superior parasternal incision. When the trochar breaks through the tissue at the manubrium, the lead is then pulled into the incision with the silk tie that was attached to the tip. The silk tie is then cut so that the lead is freed from the trochar. The 2-0 silk that was sutured to the fascia previously is then placed through the hole in the end of the lead, and the lead is secured to the fascia.

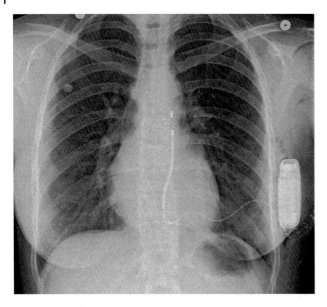

Figure 3.5 A chest X-ray of the subcutaneous implantable cardioverter-defibrillator (S-ICD) after implantation, showing the proper lead and can position.

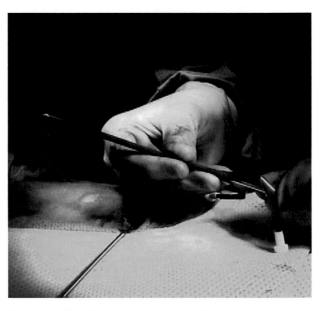

Figure 3.6 The 11 Fr sheath on the tunneling trochar.

The lead is now in place, running along the left parasternal border and across to the lateral pocket (Figure 3.5). A suture is then placed in the floor of the pocket at the cranial end and tied to the fascia. The lead is placed in the header of the can, and the set screw is tightened. The suture that was tied to the fascia of the pocket is attached to the can through a hole in the header. The pocket is then closed in the usual fashion. The smaller incisions along the sternum are also closed in the usual fashion.

Two-Incision Technique for Implantation

The above technique was developed for good lead stability as the lead is secured in three locations, leaving little room for lead dislodgement. However, the superior parasternal incision is conspicuous, thus having cosmetic disadvantages. In addition, more incisions increase the risk of infection and prolong the implantation procedure. Consequently, a technique that eliminates the incision at the manubriosternal junction was developed [5]. This technique was evaluated in 39 patients, with a mean follow-up of 18 months. There were no lead dislodgements and no patients required lead revisions, demonstrating the technique to be safe and viable.

The two-incision technique eliminates the superior parasternal incision. The pocket and incision at the xiphoid process are fashioned in the same manner as described above. Once the lead has been tunneled to the inferior

parasternal incision and tied to the fascia, the silk tie connecting the lead to the trochar is cut. The tunneling device is then placed through an 11 French peel-away sheath (Figure 3.6). The trochar is then tunneled cranially toward the manubriosternal junction along the left sternal border. Once the trochar has reached the superior landmark, the sheath is advanced over the trochar to that landmark. The sheath is held in place as the tunneling device is then removed. The sheath is now in place along the left sternal border up to the manubriosternal junction. The lead is placed through the sheath until it has been advanced completely into the sheath. The end of the lead typically can be felt in its superior location. The sheath is then peeled away while the lead is held in place by applying external pressure to the tip of the lead to keep it steady. The lead is now in its final position again along the left parasternal border. The lead is attached to the can and the incisions closed as described above.

Defibrillation Testing and Device Programming

Once the S-ICD has been implanted, the device automatically selects the optimal sensing vector to prevent double counting and T-wave over-sensing. This can be changed manually if necessary. At the end of the initial implant procedure, arrhythmia detection and termination can be tested using a 65 joule shock to ensure an adequate (15 J) safety margin. For spontaneous arrhythmias, the device delivers 80 J shocks only, with the polarity automatically switching for failed shocks. A shock zone is programmed in all devices that is analogous to the VF zone in transvenous systems. An optional "conditional" zone can also be programmed from 170 to 240 bpm that will apply rhythm discrimination algorithms to differentiate VT from SVT. This arrhythmia discrimination algorithm applies morphology template matching that is similar to transvenous systems but evaluates up to 41 points on the QRS complex to increase resolution. Several studies have shown that that two-zone programming markedly reduces the incidence of inappropriate shocks [6].

Final device programming options are minimal. Shock therapy, a conditional zone, rate cutoffs for the zones, and post-shock pacing are the only programming capabilities with shock output and polarity being automated.

Conclusions

The S-ICD is a new defibrillator for the prevention of sudden death. It has been shown to be a safe and effective alternative approach to the traditional transvenous implant. Although the implant technique is quite different from the transvenous approach, it can be easily learned and carried out relatively quickly and safely. For certain patient populations, the S-ICD is a viable and often preferable option.

Acknowledgments

We thank Dr. Peter Belott for sharing some of the photographs in this article.

References

1 Bardy GH, Smith WN, Hood MA, Crozier AG, Melton IC, Jordaens L, *et al.* An entirely subcutaneous implantable cardioverter-defibrillator. N Engl J Med 2010;363:36–44.

2 Gold MR, Theuns DA, Knight BP, Sturdivant JL, Sanghera R, Ellenbogen KA, *et al.* Head-to-head comparison of arrhythmia discrimination performance of subcutaneous and transvenous ICD arrhythmia detection algorithms: the START study. J Cardiovasc Electrophysiol 2012;23:359–366.

3 Weiss R, Knight BL, Gold MR, Leon AR, Herre JM, Hood M, *et al.* Safety and efficacy of a totally subcutaneous implantable cardioverter-defibrillator. Circulation 2013;128:944–953.

4 Borleffs CJ, van Erven L, van Bommel RJ, van der Velde ET, van derWall EE, Bax JJ, *et al.* Risk of failure of transvenous implantable cardioverter-defibrillator leads. Circ Arrhythm Electrophysiol 2009;2:411–416.

5 Knops RE, Olde Nordkamp LRA, de Groot JR, Wilde AAM. Two-incision technique for implantation of the subcutaneous implantable cardioverter-defibrillator. Heart Rhythm 2013;10:1240–1243.

6 Gold MR, Weiss R, Theuns DAMJ, Smith W, Leon A, Knight BP, *et al.* The use of discrimination algorithm to reduce inappropriate shocks with a subcutaneous ICD. Heart Rhythm 2014;11:1352–1358.

4

Internal Jugular Venous Access and Lead Implantation for Cardiac Implantable Electronic Devices

Michael G. Katz and David T. Huang

Division of Cardiology, Department of Clinical Cardiac Electrophysiology, University of Rochester, Rochester, NY, USA

Patients with cardiac implantable electronic devices (CIEDs) frequently require upgrading procedures. Greater awareness of pacemaker syndrome and the benefits of cardiac resynchronization therapy have resulted in more frequent and earlier implantation of additional functional leads. At the same time, implanting physicians encounter subclavian vein obstruction more frequently because of prolonged patient survival and the presence of multiple pre-existing leads [1]. Implantation of a separate pacemaker or defibrillator system is a strategy that can be reasonably employed. However, this results in significantly more endovascular leads and abandoned leads that crowd the venous return, including the critical superior vena cava (SVC). Accessing an occluded or severely stenosed subclavian venous system can be associated with increased risks of vascular injury, dissection, inadvertent arterial access, and collateral injury including pneumothorax.

The stenosis or occlusion involved with transvenous implantable cardiac devices typically occurs at the level of subclavian–axillary juncture or at the venous access sites. When occlusions are present, obtaining access at sites distinctly separated from the same venous system will allow implantation with vascular entry on the ipsilateral side as the remaining functional leads and device. The internal jugular (IJ) vein drains a separate venous return plexus and often remains patent even in patients with multiple leads in the subclavian system. Access via the IJ permits a direct path to the right cardiac chambers for implant of cardiac device leads.

Patient Selection and Preparation

Implanting a lead via the IJ approach requires percutaneous access to the vasculature at the neck, opening the pectoral device pocket, tunneling from the pocket across the clavicle, and ultimately pulling the lead across the clavicle into the pocket via the tunnel. An adequate amount of subcutaneous tissue is vital to prevent erosion as the lead crosses the clavicle under the subcutaneous tissue. It is also important to recognize the anteriorly displaced clavicle, which is frequently associated with kyphosis in elderly women. The risk of serious vascular or brachial plexus injury is high if the lead is accidentally tunneled under rather than over the clavicle.

Contrast venography should be considered in any patient with pre-existing leads, when venous patency is in doubt, or if abnormal anatomy is suspected. When a peripheral, left-sided, occlusion is noted in patients with devices already implanted via the left subclavian, it may be helpful to perform right-sided venography to evaluate for the presence of central occlusion at the SVC or innominate veins, potentially precluding the IJ approach. Bilateral venography may also reveal other potential targets for contralateral central venous access. We generally perform the venography immediately prior to the planned procedure, after the patient is positioned on the table, but prior to the antiseptic preparation, so that the anatomy is representative of the patient's anticipated positioning during the procedure and draped so as to offer a wider operative window as necessary.

How-to Manual for Pacemaker and ICD Devices: Procedures and Programming, First Edition. Edited by Amin Al-Ahmad, Andrea Natale, Paul J. Wang, James P. Daubert, and Luigi Padeletti.
© 2018 John Wiley & Sons, Inc. Published 2018 by John Wiley & Sons, Inc.
Companion website: www.wiley.com/go/al-ahmad/pacemakers_and_icds

The use of contrast dye for venography requires careful attention to pre-procedural renal function to avoid contrast-induced nephropathy (CIN). Although it is beyond the scope of this chapter to discuss the pathophysiology of CIN and the evidence base for prophylactic procedures, it is important to consider that even modest amounts of dye (<20 mL) can result in renal dysfunction in an unprepared patient. Patients are risk stratified for potential CIN, taking into account factors such as advanced age, chronic kidney disease, diabetes, and severe reduction in left ventricular ejection fraction (LVEF) (<0.40) [2]. If patients have multiple risk factors for CIN, they are instructed to hold diuretics and angiotensin converting enzyme inhibitors on the day of the procedure. While randomized control trials have not provided clear evidence on the best type of periprocedural hydration, normal saline or sodium bicarbonate is administered as a bolus 1 hour prior to the procedure and several hours afterwards.

When the decision to proceed with IJ implantation of the lead has been made, the surgical site should be widely prepared and draped. In addition to scrubbing the pectoral area of the chest with chlorhexidine and alcohol solution, we also prepare up to the hairline, behind the ear, and to the mandible on the side ipsilateral to the device. Once the area has been scrubbed, the area of interest is surrounded by surgical towels and covered with a sterile see-through plastic adhesive drape, which is impregnated with iodoform solution. We modify a standard device drape by extending the window with suture scissors. We secure the superior edges of the newly extended window with several occlusive transparent dressings (Tegaderm) (Figure 4.1). It is important to insulate the superior edges securely to both maintain sterility and prevent fire in the surgical suite. Electrocautery may ignite the supplemental oxygen in use and the 70% alcohol-based scrubs may serve as fuel if the skin surface is not completely dry.

The technique described can be accomplished with the components of a standard pacemaker instrument tray and two lead introducer kits. It is useful to have a long-stemmed instrument, such as a Bozeman uterine dressing forceps, for tunneling purposes. Additionally, we utilize vascular ultrasound to establish venous access as described next.

Procedure

Once the device area and ipsilateral neck are prepared and draped, a site for IJ venous access is selected approximately two finger breadths above the cranial edge of the clavicle along the lateral edge of the sternal head of the sternocleidomastoid muscle. This approach

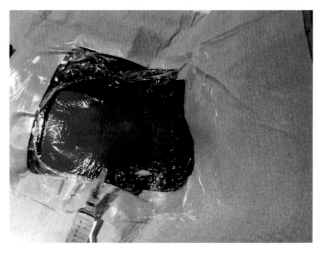

Figure 4.1 The pectoral and neck region is prepared widely, with adequate room (at least two finger breadths) above the clavicle. A standard drape can be modified by cutting out a portion of the drape to allow access to the neck. Care must be taken to secure the modified drape to ensure sterility and to avoid ignition of supplemental oxygen by electrocautery.

helps to avoid pneumothorax and allows for adequate distal separation of the IJ from the internal carotid artery and at the same time minimizes the tunneling distance. Numerous studies of central venous access demonstrate that ultrasound guidance has been shown to increase the success of first-time wire placement and to decrease the risk of complications. We utilize vascular ultrasound with a sterile sleeve to directly visualize the compressible IJ, immediately lateral to the pulsatile carotid artery. This area is then infiltrated with 1% lidocaine solution. Using the components from a standard peel-away sheath kit, a 5 cm 18-gauge needle is inserted at an angle of about 20 degrees to the skin, in the direction of the ipsilateral nipple. After venous access is obtained, the J-shaped end of the wire is introduced into the needle and advanced into the IJ vein. The free end of the wire is temporarily secured with a mosquito or mini Kelly clamp. Delaying sheath placement, as the conclusion of the Seldinger technique prior to the tunneling, avoids distortion of the anatomy of the neck.

Attention is turned to opening the device pocket. Typically, our pectoral incision is positioned around two finger breadths below the caudal border of the clavicle. Efforts are made to coordinate the incision over the cranial aspect of the device, with care not to make the incision too caudal. This site of incision will allow for minimized tunneling of the lead to be inserted (Figure 4.2; Video 4.1, 0:04).

The tunneling process starts at the inner, medial, and cranial edges of the pocket lip. To avoid skin erosion and bleeding complications, it is essential to tunnel just on top of the fascial layer and clavicle, with as much

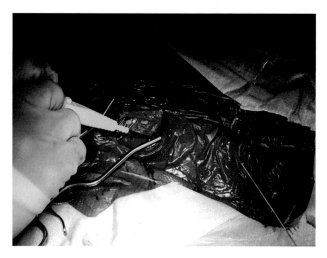

Figure 4.2 The incision to open the pocket is made cranial to the device to reduce the tunneling distance from the internal jugular (IJ) entrance site.

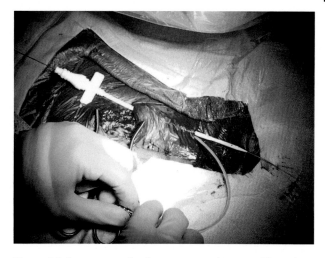

Figure 4.4 Bozeman uterine forceps are used to tunnel from the pocket, over the clavicle, and towards the guidewire exiting the IJ.

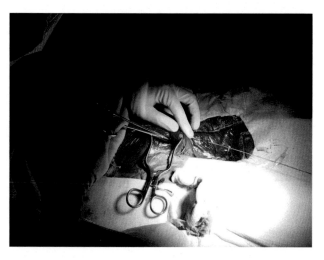

Figure 4.3 Electrocautery can be used to nick the upper lip of the pocket so that tunneling can be initiated directly anterior to the prepectoral fascia.

overlaying subcutaneous tissue as possible. For control and visualization of the tunnel entrance, electrocautery can be used to make a small nick at the desired entrance site (Figure 4.3; Video 4.1, 0:22). With the curved angle facing anteriorly (i.e., towards the ceiling), the Bozeman forceps are introduced to the entrance of the tunnel and bluntly dissect along the subcutaneous tissue to create a tunnel over the clavicle, towards the skin entrance of the secured guidewire. The upward curve of the forceps prevents inadvertent tunneling into the muscle or under the clavicle (Figure 4.4). Once the instrument reaches the clavicle, the angle of the forceps is turned downward (i.e., towards the floor) to conform to the anatomic curve of the clavicle. As the tunneling passes over the clavicle,

the forceps are once again turned upward or anteriorly directing towards at the site of the J wire retained in the IJ.

The Seldinger technique is then completed and the peel-away sheath along with the dilatator are inserted into the IJ over the J wire. Once in place, the wire and dilator are removed en bloc, leaving the sheath within the IJ. The lead is then inserted into the sheath and implanted in a fashion similar to traditional percutaneous implantation via a subclavian–axillary venous access in the pectoral pocket. The silicone elastomer collar of the lead is temporally removed. Iris scissors can be used to make longitudinal cut along the collar to remove it. Care must be applied so as not to injure the lead insulation (Video 4.1, 0:29).

At this point, the sheath remains "unbroken," and acts to protect the newly implanted lead from trauma as the Bozeman forceps is inserted from the pocket into the newly formed tunnel, again with the curve facing upwards. The tips of the forceps should exit the skin surface where the sheath enters the skin (Video 4.1, 0:51). A skin nick with a scalpel can be helpful if the tips do not easily exit the subcutaneous tissue and the skin surface. One end of sheath guidewire is then grasped by the forceps and pulled back to the pocket through the tunnel (Video 4.1, 1:20). The end result is wire that enters at the IJ sheath site and exists into the pocket. The sheath is then broken and peeled away (Video 4.1, 1:58).

A Seldinger maneuver is utilized again as a sheath and dilator, enough to accommodate the terminal pin end of the lead (e.g. a 9 Fr sheath for 7 Fr pacemaker leads or an 11 Fr sheath for 9 Fr IS-4 ICD leads), are passed into the tunnel, over the wire, entering through the cranial edge of the pocket and exiting at the newly fashioned IJ lead insertion site (Figure 4.5). The wire and dilator are, again, removed en bloc. The free terminal end of the implanted

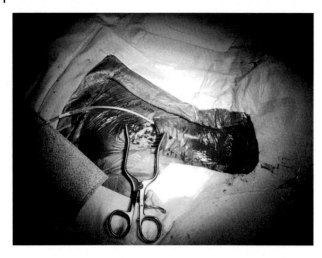

Figure 4.5 Once a standard J-guidewire has been pulled back through the tunnel by the Bozeman forceps, a sheath can be advanced over the wire, through the tunnel. Once the dilator and wire are removed, the lead terminal can be secured in the free end of the sheath.

lead should fit snugly into the nearby tip of the sheath. Once the terminal is fitted securely within the sheath, the lead can be pulled back to the pocket by the sheath, via the tunnel. Gentle traction on the lead will result in reduction of the proximal loop formed at the skin surface and this will smoothly tuck underneath the skin surface (Video 4.1, 2:17). The end result is a lead that enters the IJ vein, tunnels subcutaneously across the clavicle, and enters the pocket. The silicon collar that was initially removed from the lead may be carefully re-applied to the free end of the lead, as it exits the pocket. The lead may then be secured to the pectoral fascia, via the silicon collar, allowing enough slack for the lead to be secured to the header. The pocket can then be closed in the usual

fashion. A small amount of surgical skin adhesive can be applied to the IJ puncture site following hemostasis.

Long-Term Outcome

In the presence of peripheral occlusion of the axillary or subclavian veins, our institution has found lead implantation via the IJ vein to be safe, straightforward, and durable with regard to lead performance. Of 14 leads implanted via the IJ at the University of Rochester from 2000 to 2011, 7 remain in use and are followed at our institution, with excellent thresholds, sensing, and surgical results. There has been no report of erosion at the IJ site or over the clavicle. No patient discomfort has been noted. Five patients were subsequently followed at other institutions, but no problems were reported. Two leads were removed. One lead was removed as a result of device infection 2 weeks after implant. An implanted left ventricular lead was extracted without complications in the context of high capture thresholds and the presence of a separate shock lead fracture. Both of these leads were removed relatively early after implant, using simple traction. The course and curvature of the lead as it travels over the clavicle and enters the IJ would generally prohibit the co-axial use of telescoping or laser-utilizing extraction sheaths.

Given the morbidity burden of most patients undergoing device upgrade, the ability to add another lead via a patent IJ affords an alternate opportunity to implant a revised system on the side ipsilateral to the existing system. Importantly, this technique avoids extensive vascular dilation and/or ballooning and has been demonstrated to be safe and associated with longer term survival of the system.

References

1 Lickfett L, Bitzen A, Arepally A, Nasir K, Wolpert C, Jeong KM, *et al.* Incidence of venous obstruction following insertion of an implantable cardioverter-defibrillator: a study of systematic contrast venography on patients presenting for their first elective ICD generator replacement. Europace 2004;6(1):25–31.

2 Mehran R, Aymong ED, Nikolsky E, Lasic Z, Iakovou I, Fahy M, *et al.* A simple risk score for prediction of contrast-induced nephropathy after percutaneous coronary intervention: development and initial validation. J Am Coll Cardiol 2004;44(7):1393–399.

 To watch the videos, please log in to the Companion Website: www.wiley.com/go/al-ahmad/pacemakers_and_icds

5

Implantation of the Left Ventricular Lead

Shrinivas Hebsur[1] and Edward Platia[2]

[1] *Michigan Heart and Vascular Institute, Ann Arbor, MI, USA*
[2] *Medstar Washington Hospital Center/Georgetown University, Washington, DC, USA*

Venous Access

Whether implanting a fresh biventricular pacing system or upgrading a pre-existing dual chamber system, obtaining venous access must be carried out with forethought. It is highly advisable to have separate access points for each lead. This will help increase maneuvering and positioning of leads. At the very least, the access point for the left ventricular (LV) lead should be separate. In cases where coronary sinus (CS) access is straightforward and lead placement goes smoothly, the need for a separate access point may seem conservative. There are considerably more potential challenges of successful CS lead implantation, and to ensure the maximum freedom of catheters, it is best to have a separate venous access point to allow easier manipulation of the sheath, guiding catheters, and lead. If venous access is obtained via the subclavian approach, LV lead guiding catheters must negotiate between the subclavius muscle, the costocoracoid ligament, and the costoclavicular ligament. The access of axillary or cephalic vein will allow easier manipulation of the LV lead system, and therefore it is our recommended access site for LV lead implantation.

If venous access to the target vessel is difficult to obtain, simple solutions include giving intravenous fluids, raising the patient's legs, or applying traction on the patient's arm. Another option is using the internal jugular vein. This technique is best suited if the device is on the right-hand side as the left internal jugular vein poses difficulty for the LV lead to traverse the various bends. It is recommended to use ultrasound guidance for proper visualization of the vessel. Once the lead is placed into the CS at the desired location, it may be tunneled in a subcutaneous fashion using standard blunt instrumentation to the pulse generator located in the infraclavicular fossa (Table 5.1).

Especially for patients in whom there has been pre-existing access or intervention of the venous system, it is imperative to perform a venogram to determine vessel patency. For patients for whom there is moderate to severe stenosis of the venous system, venoplasty may be considered.

Each implanting physician has his or her preference, but it is often helpful to have at least the right ventricular (RV) lead in place first. This offers several advantages, including pacing back-up and to provide a landmark to aid in locating the CS os.

Coronary Sinus Catheter

The basic platform assembly for LV lead implantation involves an outer guide catheter and an inner telescoping catheter for target vein access. If a short 9 Fr vascular access sheath is used, the guide catheter is usually a 9 Fr sheath with a 7–8 Fr inner catheter, which can deliver a 5–6 Fr lead. Table 5.2 shows a variety of guide catheters based on operator preference and patient anatomy. Most guide catheters are preformed to allow the greater curvature to rest against the free wall of the right atrium and act as a fulcrum to allow easy manipulation of the catheter toward the CS. Larger or extended curve guide catheters are available from each company to help with access in patients with severely dilated atria (Figure 5.1). Some guides now come with two curves. The primary curve is large, which allows the guide to rest on the right atrium. The secondary curve bends in a posterior plane, which allows for easier access to posterior structures, such as the CS. Many operators choose not to use an inner telescoping catheter, relying on the outer guide or using a 0.035 inch soft wire to probe for the CS.

How-to Manual for Pacemaker and ICD Devices: Procedures and Programming, First Edition. Edited by Amin Al-Ahmad, Andrea Natale, Paul J. Wang, James P. Daubert, and Luigi Padeletti.
© 2018 John Wiley & Sons, Inc. Published 2018 by John Wiley & Sons, Inc.
Companion website: www.wiley.com/go/al-ahmad/pacemakers_and_icds

Table 5.1 Order of lead placement.

Right ventricular (RV) lead first	Left ventricular (LV) lead first
Advantages: • Allows back-up pacing • Fluoroscopic landmark of tricuspid annulus and interventricular septum	Advantages: • Easier sheath, guide catheter manipulation • Coronary sinus will not be obstructed by the RV lead

Table 5.2 Outer guide catheters.

Brand: Product line	Types of catheters offered
Biotronik: Selectra	Straight, Standard, Extended, Right, Amplatz, MP
Boston Scientific: Acuity Break-Away	Straight, Standard, Extended hook, Right, Amplatz, MP
Pressure Products: SafeSheath CSG	Standard, Jumbo, 90°. Note this is a peel-away sheath. Dilators come preformed in 45°, 90°, 180° angles
Medtronic: Attain Command	Straight, Standard, XL, Multipurpose, Amplaz, Right Sided, Deflectable. Attain Prevail® is steerable
St. Jude: CPS Direct	Straight, Wide, X Wide, 135°, 115°, Right. CPS Luminary™ is deflectable

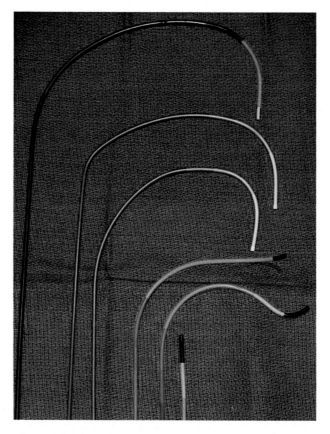

Figure 5.1 From left to right: St. Jude CPS Direct SL II X-Wide; Boston Scientific Acuity™ Break-Away Extended; Boston Scientific Acuity™ Break-Away Right; Medtronic™ Attain 3D catheter; Medtronic™ Attain Amplatz; Medtronic™ Attain 50 Strait.

Some operators use a deflectable tip electrophysiology catheter as the telescoping catheter. This technique can be particularly useful in difficult cases. Inner catheters are also manufacturer specific, and there are many different varieties. Some are steerable or deflectable. The inner catheter can also be a standard coronary angiographic catheter, such as an Amplatz or multipurpose catheter.

Coronary Venous Anatomy

Implantation of the LV lead requires good knowledge of cardiac anatomy, in particular the opening of the CS, structures surrounding or obstructing the CS, and the general course of the CS and its various tributaries. The CS arises in the posteroinferior aspect of the right interatrial septum. The orifice tends to be roughly 5–10 mm in size. The valve of the CS is the Thebesian valve, which varies in extent of coverage of the CS os. The Eustachian ridge is the thick muscular structure contiguous with the crista terminalis, which starts at the os of the inferior vena cava (IVC) and terminates on the interatrial septum just posterior to the CS os. A prominent Eustachian ridge can obstruct or misdirect the guide catheter from the CS. Often times in patients with dilated cardiomyopathy, the ostium and the proximal portion of the CS will point in a more cephalad fashion, creating a more acute angle for cannulation and also tortuosity of the mid and distal coronary venous segments.

Fluoroscopy can help in the location of the CS os. The CS lies in the atrioventricular fat-pad. Using right anterior oblique (RAO) cine, the fat-pad can be located, which may help locate the level of the CS. In standard AP fluoroscopy, the os is located along the left border of the spine, 1 cm above the contour of the diaphragm. One of the advantages of placing the high-voltage RV lead in first is that the proximal edge of the shocking coil is usually immediately inferior to the CS os in standard AP view.

Although there is a great deal of variation in the anatomy of coronary venous drainage, a knowledge of normal anatomy in several views will help the implanting physician find the best site for LV pacing (Figure 5.2).The optimal site for pacing should be a posterolateral and basal location on the LV. The left anterior interventricular vein (AIV) runs alongside the left anterior descending artery. It drains the anterolateral left ventricle, and where there are small secondary and tertiary tributaries going more lateral, this may

(a)

(b)

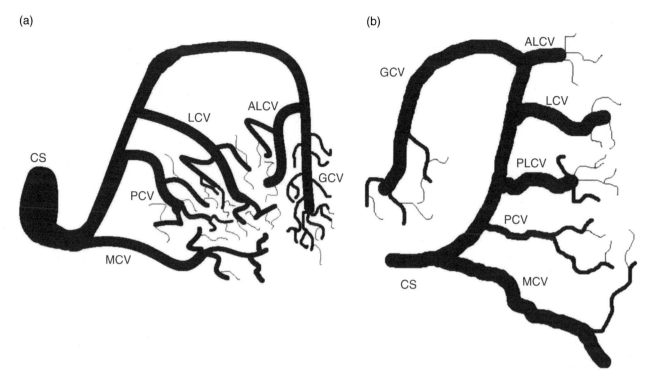

Figure 5.2 (a) Coronary venous tree in right anterior oblique (RAO) projection. ALCV, anterolateral cardiac vein; CS, coronary sinus; LCV, lateral cardiac vein; MCV, middle cardiac vein; PCV, posterior cardiac vein. (b) Left anterior oblique (LAO). GCV, great cardiac vein; PLCV, posterolateral. In LAO, it is often easier to separate different lateral vein branches. The RAO projection is most useful for selecting posterior branches. Note, however, that secondary braches from MCV, PCV, LCV, and the ALCV can give rise to suitable pacing sites.

be an excellent site for pacing. In the RAO projection, the AIV is the most anterior vein seen. The middle cardiac vein often abruptly takes off at a 90 degree angle near the CS os or may even have a separate os. This vein courses posteriorly alongside the posterior descending artery and travels toward the apex. On occasion, tributaries of the middle cardiac vein can drain the posterolateral LV.

Oftentimes, the target of LV lead placement will be the posterolateral or left marginal cardiac veins. In AP or RAO, the lateral veins will be seen taking off in between the middle cardiac vein and the AIVs. Usually, the left posterolateral veins take off within 1–2 cm of the CS os. In left anterior oblique (LAO) view, where the lateral border of the heart is seen best, one can see the course of this vein. In the course of implantation of hundreds of LV leads, depending on anatomy, any of these three main coronary veins may be suitable for lead placement. It is important to be flexible and thoughtful in one's approach.

Cannulation of the Coronary Sinus

The CS is most reliably approached by pullback method from the tricuspid valve. The tricuspid valve is located anterior to the CS. Posterior approach from the right atrium (RA) is not advisable because of the Eustachian ridge. Also,

if one comes too inferior, then the Thebesian valve often obstructs the os. Care should be taken in advancing a guide catheter without using a wire as the catheter can cause trauma to tissue and even inadvertently dissect the CS. It is recommended to always advance the guide over a wire.

Often, the most reliable method is to advance the delivery system under fluoroscopic guidance across the tricuspid valve and then slowly pull back, giving 20–30 degrees counterclockwise torque. This maneuver will naturally migrate the catheter posterior and cephalad. It is best to have an assistant to gently advance and retract the wire while doing this until the wire enters into the CS. Confirmation that the wire is indeed in the CS and not in the right ventricular outflow tract (RVOT) can be made by the LAO view, which should show the wire crossing the spine and traveling left. Small puffs of contrast can be used while performing this procedure to confirm when in the CS os. It is recommended that the main operator keep both hands on the catheter for optimal control while an assistant injects 2–4 mL of contrast. Also, the presence of ventricular ectopy when advancing the wire gives the operator clues that the wire is not in the CS; rather, it is in the RVOT. Once the catheter is positioned within the os of the CS, the angiography wire can be advanced slowly inside the CS. Never advance the catheter unless over a wire as the CS can dissect.

Difficulties in Coronary Sinus Access

The CS os can become distorted, especially in patients with right heart failure and dilated right atriums. Usually, the os will become displaced more superiorly, and the likelihood of formation of acute bends of the venous system is higher. Techniques using deflectable catheters, injecting contrast into the vein selector, or coronary angiograms with late venous phase cine imaging can be useful. Creativity and flexibility are often needed, and exchanging for multiple sheaths, guides, and inner catheters will be required. Sheaths with a primary large curve and a smaller secondary curve like the Medtronic 3D allow for negotiation of a prominent Eustachian ridge, as the large curve and the smaller secondary curve naturally bend posteriorly to access the CS. If the CS still cannot be accessed, stiff decapolar catheters can be placed from the femoral vein into the CS, which can help open obstructive Thebesian valves.

In some cases, the guide wire will easily advance into the CS, but the guide catheter, which is considerably stiffer, will not and will push the guide wire out. In these instances, an inner soft-tipped catheter can be placed over the wire, and this acts as a rail from which the guide catheter can easily be advanced. An Amplatz catheter is a very simple inner catheter that can often be used which will easily accommodate the shape of the CS.

Coronary Sinus Venogram

Once guide catheter is into the CS, the inner catheter can be taken out, and preparation for the venogram can begin. A 6 Fr Swan-Ganz catheter is placed through the guide catheter into the proximal CS. Be aware that the Swan-Ganz catheter is much stiffer than traditional guide catheters. Advancing the Swan catheter can dissect the sinus if not carried out with care. One trick is to advance the Swan just up to the leading edge of the guide catheter and then withdraw the catheter, thus freeing the Swan tip. The balloon is inflated to 1.5 mL air to form proximal occlusion of the CS. It is again recommended to have an assistant for the venogram. The main operator should maintain catheter stability, while the assistant injects contrast under cine fluoroscopy. For adequate opacification and visualization of the venous tree, it is recommended to use at least 10 mL of half-strength contrast. It is useful to perform venography with at least two fluoroscopic views (Figure 5.3).

As is the case with coronary anatomy, potential stenosis cannot be appreciated with one simple injection. Also, finding the proper course of the target vessel may be apparent only after careful inspection of multiple views. The cine should run until there is no more contrast visualized. If cine angiography is cut short, collateral vessels may not become apparent, which can lead to suboptimal site selection for LV lead placement.

(a)

(b)

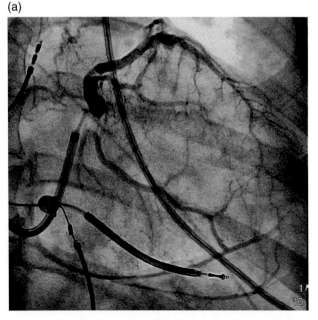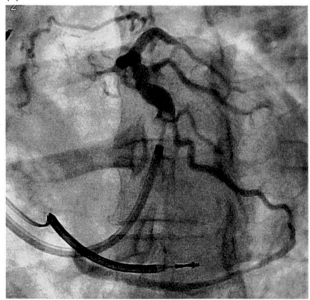

Figure 5.3 (a) RAO venogram. Note the diminutive lateral marginal veins, which is quite common in patients with extensive scarring. There is a prominent posterolateral vein that fills in late, which was chosen as the target site. Also, note the relationship of the coronary sinus (CS) os with the proximal edge of the RV high voltage coil. (b) LAO venogram. There are diminutive lateral veins and the posterolateral vein fills in late because it is proximal to the balloon.

Close to the end of the cine loop, the balloon should be deflated. This will allow proximal vessels to be seen. In patients without an optimal lateral or anterior cardiac target, distal tributaries from the middle cardiac vein can be visualized. Finally, if the balloon is against the ostium of a lateral branch, this will not become apparent until balloon deflation.

In patients with large proximal CS, the standard 1.5 mL of air insufflation into the Swan will be inadequate to occlude the vessel. This can lead to inadequate opacification of the distal venous tree. Double ballooning of the Swan can be performed, but must be carried out very carefully as the risk of vascular trauma increases.

In some patients, target vessels may not be apparent even with multiple occlusive cine angiograms. This can be because of severe stenosis, diminution, or lack of good lateral veins, or the course of the vessel cannot be delineated soon after take off. In all cases, distal venograms may be required. Distal vessels are often too small to perform occlusive venograms safely. When good lateral veins are not seen, one must look to secondary and tertiary tributaries of the middle and the great cardiac vein because these often will form collaterals to drain the lateral myocardium. In this case, a 5 Fr soft-tipped vein selector can be used. With the vein selector in the guide sheath, the inner catheter is advanced over a wire. The type of wire used will depend upon the situation and, as is the case with this entire procedure, having a varied toolkit will help. Hydrophilic-coated wires, such as Whisper, Cougar, or PT-Graphic, can maneuver through mildly stenotic or tortuous segments. Stiffer wires, such as the Mailman, can be used to straighten out bends in the vein. The main drawback to using stiffer wires is that they are difficult to manipulate, thus necessitating the use of a torqueing device similar to those used in interventional coronary procedures. Stiffer wires, such as Amplatz 0.035 cm, can also be used, but with more tortuosity these wires will have the same problems as the catheters.

Lead Placement

The ultimate goal of implantation of an LV lead system is to have the following:

1) The lead advanced into the target vein of choice, no matter how small, tortuous, or distal.
2) The lowest pacing threshold possible without evidence of phrenic nerve capture but having excellently timed biventricular pacing.
3) The smallest possible risk for lead dislodgment.

As no two patients are alike, it is impossible to develop one lead that will fit all three of these stipulations. Thus, there are many types of leads available on the market,

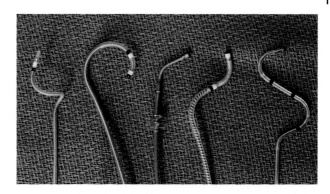

Figure 5.4 Left ventricular lead types. From left to right: Boston Scientific Acuity Spiral Lead. This is one of the smaller leads on the market. The lead tip tapes down to 2.6 Fr. This lead can be useful for very small target veins. Due to its small size, it is only a unipolar lead. Boston Scientific Acuity Steerable Lead. For target veins that have acute take offs, this lead can be deflectable via a stiff inner stylet. With the stylet out, the lead naturally forms a "J" shape, which will help oppose the vein, allowing stability. Medtronic StarFix lead. This is a unique active fixation lead that is excellent for very large target veins. The lobes expand the lead to 24 F size. Biotronik Corox Lead. This lead is either stylet or over the wire driven. There are two acute curves at the distal end of the lead, which allow good contact and stability. St. Jude Quartet Quadripolar Lead. Allows for 10 pacing configurations, allowing much more flexibility on target vessel placement.

and with the advent of international standard lead designs, almost any LV lead can be placed into any pulse generator (Figure 5.4).

As the venogram is completed, the operator will have a sense of how large the target vessel is, what curves the lead system will have to navigate, and how distal the lead will need to go. At the advent of coronary resynchronization therapy (CRT), most LV leads were stylet driven. For the electrophysiologist, stylet-driven LV pacing was familiar to implantation of RV and RA leads. Advantages of using a stylet-driven lead is that in vessels that are very tortuous, the stiffness of the stylet can help straighten the vein, thus allowing for easier passage of the lead. Stylet-driven leads are also larger and may be better in patients who have larger, more proximal target vessels. As with RV and RA leads, stylets can be preformed to assist in navigating angles. Compared with over-the-wire leads, more acute angles are much more difficult for stylet-driven leads to advance. Also, as the stylet is advanced all the way into the lead, the lead tip becomes very stiff, so great care must be taken to ensure the lead tip is always free under fluoroscopy and never advanced when meeting resistance. In using stylets, never bend the stylet once inserted into the LV lead because this can cause damage to the lead and insulation. Over-the-wire techniques have been adopted from the field of interventional cardiology. Nowadays, many leads offer this method of deployment. A standard

(a) (b)

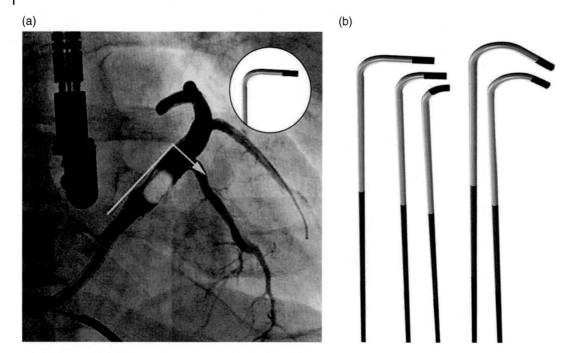

Figure 5.5 (a) LAO occlusive venogram, showing a posterolateral vein branch at a 90 degree angle from CS. A Medtronic™ Select II Extended 90 degree catheter was used to subselect the vein to allow easy passage of lead into target vein. Courtesy of Medtronic. (b) From left to right: Medtronic ™ Select II 90 degree extended; Select II 90 degree standard; Select II 90 degree short; Select II 130 degree Extended; Select II 130 degree Standard catheters. Courtesy of Medtronic.

0.014 inch hydrophilic angiography wire (Whisper, PT Graphic) can be used with a torque device to navigate acute angles. These wires can often be front or back loaded, depending on the LV lead being used.

Often, based on the take off of the target vessel, an inner vein selector catheter may need to be used to deploy the lead. When target vessels come off the main venous trunk at acute angles, vein selectors can telescope through the outer guide for easier lead delivery. Figure 5.5 shows a venogram where the target vein comes off at a 90 degree bend. There are many brands and varieties of inner catheters that can accommodate different angles. In this instance, a catheter with a distal 90 degree bend was used.

In the beginning days of CRT, only unipolar LV leads were available. Unipolar leads paced from the LV lead tip to the RV ring. With better lead design, most LV leads nowadays offer bipolar LV leads. There may be instances when a very distal or small vein will be selected in which case a unipolar LV lead will be chosen because these tend to be smaller. If using a bipolar LV lead, it is important to know the distance between the two poles. There are advantages of having pacing poles widely spaced. In cases of large veins that will not properly secure a lead, the lead may need to be placed into small distal apical branches, but if the proximal lead is spaced further apart, basal pacing is still possible. Having smaller spaced leads can also be useful in cases where the target site for the distal end of the lead is also

the optimal pacing site. The final LV lead position should be in a basal posterolateral location for optimal resynchronization therapy (Figure 5.6).

Once the LV lead is in its desired location, the stylet or wire is withdrawn from the lead. It is hooked up with alligator clips to the pacing system to assess threshold. Even during low output pacing, it is important to be mindful of detecting phrenic nerve capture and diaphragmatic stimulation. Phrenic nerve capture is evident in 3–26% of patients undergoing CRT and often is the cause for revisional procedures or even turning off CRT [1]. Different pacing configurations should be attempted if there is evidence of phrenic nerve capture or a high pacing threshold. If a St. Jude Quartet lead is used, up to 10 pacing configurations can be tested. If there are still unsatisfactory results, the pacing site must be revised.

LV leads have a high rate of dislodgment. There are numerous novel strategies that companies have developed to fix the lead against the vessel wall. The lead is directly against a blood vessel and not muscle, so it cannot be screwed in. Many leads have unique preformed curves, such as a J, corkscrew, or helical shape. With large proximal veins, added stability can be achieved with proximal curves. When a wire or stylet is inserted into the lead, the curve will straighten out and then will form once the stylet is taken out. Therefore it is important to check pacing thresholds once the stylet is withdrawn because pacing characteristics can change with changes

(a)

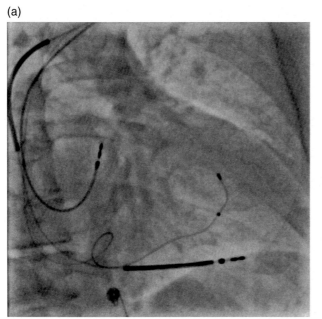

(b)

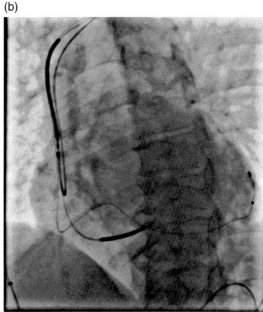

Figure 5.6 (a) RAO cine of final LV lead placement. The LV lead is more posterior than the RV lead tip, which is best appreciated in RAO. (b) LAO cine of final LV lead placement. Notice the very lateral location of LV lead.

in the lead shape. Some leads have tines that will protrude near the distal end of the lead, which help to oppose the lead to the vein. The Medtronic Starfix lead has multiple protruding radio opaque segments that flare out at a 90 degree angle from the lead. These oppose to the vessel wall and often will have tissue growth over them, allowing for excellent stability. However, this comes at a cost in the event that the lead needs to be extracted or revised (Table 5.3).

Removal of Delivery Platform

After all the hard work of locating the CS and placing the lead in a good position, the last step may be the most critical of all – removal of the delivery system. Especially in the early days of CRT before better techniques and tools were developed, lead dislodgement during the final step happened often. Most outer guide catheters are removed with a slicing tool, with the exception of the Pressure Products Worley Catheters. For an example of a cutting tool loaded on to a lead and delivery system see Figure 5.7. To ensure that the pacing lead does not move, the lead is loaded on to the guide cutter. With one hand (usually the right) firmly locked in place over the cutter, the other hand pulls back on the guide catheter with constant pressure. It is important to make sure the direction of force is coaxial with the natural direction of the catheter as it enters the body. If this is not the case, there can be untoward

Table 5.3 Left ventricular leads for coronary sinus anatomy.

Target vessel	LV lead
Small	Boston Sci: Acuity Spiral™ 2.6 Fr lead tip, unipolar St. Jude QuickFlex μ.™ 4 Fr lead tip, steerable Medtronic: Attain Ability 4396™; bipolar with tined fixation Biotronic: Corox OTW-S BP; silicone thread facilitates fixation
Tortuous	Medtronic: Attain Ability 4196™/4296; vein sub-selector catheter compatible Boston Scientific: Acuity™ Steerable LV lead St. Jude: QuickFlex™ u LV Lead: 4.0 Fr lead tip, S-shaped end Biotronic: Corox OTW-S BP. Steerable
Large	St. Jude: Quartet™ LV Lead; 10 different pacing configurations Medtronic: Attain StarFix™; large side lobes, expands to 24 Fr size Boston Scientific: Acuity™ Steerable LV lead Biotronic: Corox OTW-L BP; additional curve allows for more contact

torque that builds up in the catheter which may cause lead dislodgment. As the catheter is pulled back, it will be cut. It is recommended that a second operator watches as the guide exits the pocket, and the LV lead is immediately grabbed to ensure it does not move.

There are two major problems to be cognizant about with removal of the guide. The first is to have an

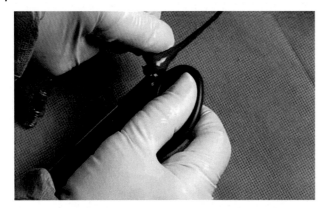

Figure 5.7 The LV lead is loaded on to the cutting tool and with the right hand firmly locked in position, the left hand drags the guide catheter across the blade, cutting the sheath. Courtesy of Boston Scientific.

appreciation of the potential stored torque on the catheter. If the guide catheter is deeply seeded into the CS or there was tortuosity, which the catheter needed to navigate, then as the guide is pulled out of the CS, this can cause the lead to move or even dislodge completely. Catheters are being developed to combat this issue, such as the Biotronik Selectra. As the catheter is cut, the torque immediately dissipates as a result of the enmeshed inner braided core. The other, more common problem is when there is not constant pressure on the catheter as it is pulled back into the slicer. This is because the proximal portion of the guide near the hemostatic valve has higher resistance than the distal portion. When there is changing of resistance to cutting, this can often cause the catheter to slip from the cutting mechanism, which can cause leads to dislodge or, worse, the lead may accidentally be cut by the slicing tool. Companies are working to develop valve portions with the lowest resistance possible and to develop a guide with the least coefficient of resistance possible.

Complications of CRT

It is important to be aware of the many complications that LV leads can pose to manage the expectations of patients. Understanding the complications and their respective occurrence rates will also help in finding ways to best mitigate the risk.

Device infection between pacemaker and implantable cardioverter-defibrillator (ICD) remains around 1%, even despite prophylactic antibiotic usage. For CRT, the risk is slightly higher at 2%. There are several reasons, but the most important factor is often time. The longer a pocket stays open, the more likely is the risk of infection. In cases of difficult-to-access target vessels in CRT,

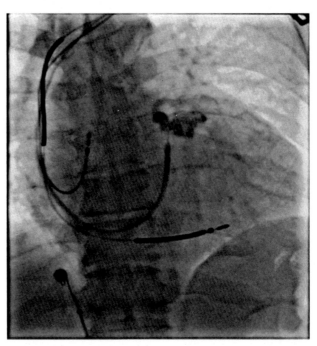

Figure 5.8 Localized rupture of coronary sinus. During implant of LV lead, coronary balloon was not advanced over a wire, resulting in a localized rupture of CS. During contrast injection, there is staining of pericardium just distal to site of rupture. The patient remained hemodynamically stable and following several minutes, successful lead implantation was carried through without any other significant clinical sequelae.

pockets can be exposed for several hours. Continuing to improve on efficiency even for the most seasoned implanting physicians will help to decrease infection rates. Similar to ICDs, pocket hematomas are more common in CRT, occurring in around 2.2%. Hematomas, even if they do not require surgical evacuation, can increase the overall risk of infection so obtaining excellent hemostasis prior to pocket closure should always be practiced.

As with any device implantation, there is a risk of pneumothorax. There is very little added risk of pneumothorax in adding a CS lead when compared with a dual chamber device. Several large registries and meta-analyses have shown the risk is 0.51–1.2% [2]. The risk of pneumothorax is increased in patients with chronic obstructive pulmonary disease (COPD), very thin and very obese patients, and also in the elderly. Strategies to decrease the risk would be to avoid blind vascular access, using a venogram prior, retaining wires, and using cephalic cut-downs.

LV lead dislodgement, similar to other types of devices, has a much higher incidence in the immediate post-implant period than in the long term. The incidence varies among studies but is in the range of 2.9–10.6%, compared with less than 1% for single and dual chamber devices. Given that the CS lead is not screwed in and is also subject to increased torque from navigating several bends, these higher rates are not surprising. Therefore, it is very important that the final CS lead is in a stable position during initial implant. The lead should be in a small enough venous branch to lie opposed to the vessel wall.

Finally, coronary veins are thin-walled epicardial structures that can be subject to trauma from catheter, wire, balloon, or lead manipulation. The incidence of causing perforation or dissection is 2%. Although there is a risk of causing significant pericardial tamponade, it is much less than during coronary artery interventions. Blood tends to flow from areas of high to low pressure, and in coronary veins there is usually very low pressure, meaning that if a perforation were to occur, fluid would flow from the pericardium back into the coronary vein. In instances of large perforation, or severely elevated venous pressure, tamponade or significantly large pericardial effusions are more likely to occur. The published incidence of requiring pericardial evacuation is around 1% (Figure 5.8) [2]. Always use fluoroscopy when inflating balloons, and always advance catheters over a wire. Especially when using a stylet-driven LV lead, careful and deliberate advancement is required because these have a much higher propensity to cause vascular trauma.

References

1 Huizar JF, Kaszala K, Koneru JN, Thacker LR, Ellenbogen KA. Comparison of different pacing strategies to minimize phrenic nerve stimulation in cardiac resynchronization therapy. J Cardiovasc Electrophysiol 2013;24(9):1008–1014.

2 van Rees JB, de Bie MK, Thijssen J, Borleffs CJW, Schalij MJ, van Erven L. Implantation-related complications of implantable cardioverter-defibrillators and cardiac resynchronization therapy devices: a systematic review of randomized clinical trials. J Am Coll Cardiol 2011;58(10):995–1000.

6

How to Place a Lead in the Azygos Vein

Jason S. Bradfield[1], Daniel H. Cooper[2], Noel G. Boyle[1], and Kalyanam Shivkumar[1]

[1] UCLA Cardiac Arrhythmia Center, Ronald Reagan UCLA Medical Center, Los Angeles, CA, USA
[2] Cardiovascular Division, Department of Medicine, Barnes-Jewish Hospital, Washington University School of Medicine, St. Louis, MO, USA

Failed defibrillation during defibrillation threshold (DFT) testing of an implantable cardioverter-defibrillator (ICD) occurs rarely with modern defibrillator systems. Indeed, failure has become so uncommon that DFT testing, which was once a standard component of ICD implantation, is no longer routinely undertaken for primary prevention implantations in many centers. The low defibrillation failure rate is largely thanks to advances in transvenous ICD technology over the past three decades.

Over this time period, there has been a progression from comprehensive DFT testing with multiple ventricular fibrillation (VF) inductions, to "safety-margin" testing with limited VF inductions, and ultimately to the current state where many physicians defer DFT testing altogether because of concerns that the risks of recurrent VF induction may outweigh the benefits. Further, the correlation between acute intra-procedural DFT testing results and real-world defibrillation success is not known. Intra-procedural DFT testing results can be influenced by a number of factors including prolonged operative times, use of general anesthesia, and recurrent VF inductions.

Regardless of this clinical trend, clinicians are still faced with occasional patients, either at the time of implant or after appropriate therapy for ventricular tachycardia (VT)/VF, who have documented unsuccessful defibrillation. Failed defibrillation is more common in young, overweight patients with a non-ischemic etiology for their cardiomyopathy. When failed defibrillation occurs (Figure 6.1), knowledge of techniques to increase the likelihood of defibrillation success is essential. Implanting physicians must have the tools and skills necessary to intervene in these now rare situations to provide optimal protection for their patients from life-threatening arrhythmias.

Initial options for failed defibrillation include programming optimization such as changing the shocking vector (programming out the proximal coil, reversing polarity, "cold-can") and programming the tilt of the biphasic waveform. If initial programming changes are not successful, the original ICD lead position can be reassessed and consideration can be given to right ventricular (RV) lead revision. Moving the lead to a more apical position may improve the shocking vector. Additionally, the ICD generator can be placed in a submuscular position to modify the shocking impedance.

Early data suggested a benefit of dual coil ICD leads over single coil leads, with regards to DFTs. However, with advances in ICD technology this benefit is no longer clear and in patients with severely enlarged hearts the proximal coil is often positioned within the atrial chamber, which potentially could increase DFTs as a result of shunting of energy to the atrial blood pool. Further, in the age of laser lead extraction there has been a movement away from dual coil leads in many centers. This is especially true in younger patients, as dual coil leads pose a significantly increased risk at the time of extraction, because of the risk of superior vena cava–right atrial junction laceration.

Additional available options include subcutaneous array or epicardial patch implantation. However, these techniques either involve a cardiac surgical approach (epicardial patches) or additional incisions and blunt dissection (subcutaneous array implant) which may require a second procedure for surgical access to the required region. An additional tool, a single coil lead without fixation mechanism, was initially designed for use in the superior vena cava (SVC; in patients with single coil RV leads) or the coronary sinus (CS) to alter the shocking vector. However, placement in the CS raises concerns

How-to Manual for Pacemaker and ICD Devices: Procedures and Programming, First Edition. Edited by Amin Al-Ahmad, Andrea Natale, Paul J. Wang, James P. Daubert, and Luigi Padeletti.
© 2018 John Wiley & Sons, Inc. Published 2018 by John Wiley & Sons, Inc.
Companion website: www.wiley.com/go/al-ahmad/pacemakers_and_icds

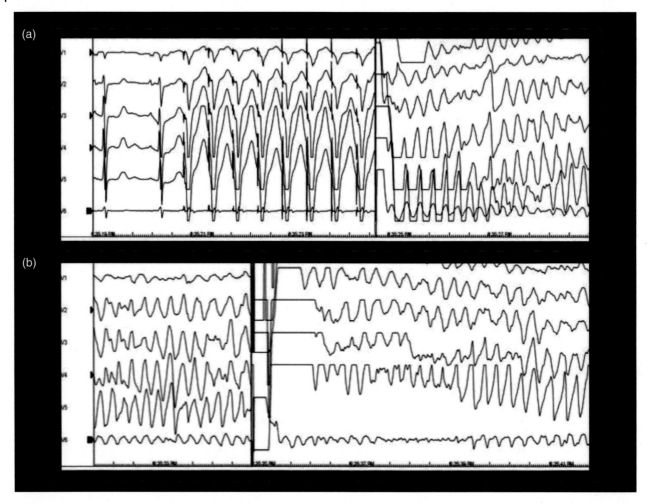

Figure 6.1 Failed defibrillation. (a) Precordial ECG leads of induction of VF and (b) subsequent failed defibrillation at 41 J in a 26-year-old morbidly obese patient with non-ischemic cardiomyopathy.

regarding stability and dislodgement, while limiting the implanting physician's ability to place a CS lead for cardiac resynchronization therapy.

Azygos vein coil implantation has recently been described as an alternative technique to optimize DFTs. The original description of an azygos vein lead implantation with a single coil lead was reported by our group in 2004 [1], and in subsequent case reports and series [2–4]. Placement of a lead in the azygos vein (posterior to the left ventricle) allows for an improved shocking vector that includes more of the left ventricular myocardium.

Azygos Vein Anatomy

The azygos vein arises at the level of the first lumbar or 12th thoracic vertebral body and receives venous drainage from the renal and lumbar veins. It runs rightward of the spine and inserts into the SVC after arching over the

right main-stem bronchus. Azygos means "unpaired" based on its Greek roots, as it is on the right side of the body and does not have a counterpart on the left side. However, the hemizygos vein is a tributary of the azygos on the left side and depending on anatomic variations and relative branch size can be utilized for this technique. A pre-procedure chest computed tomography scan can be considered to assess venous size and relative location to the left ventricle (LV); however, this has not been necessary in our experience.

Implant Technique

Venous access is obtained as per institutional physician preference to either the axillary or subclavian vein via a modified Seldinger technique. A 9 Fr long (25–40 cm) peel-away sheath is advanced to the junction of the SVC and the right atrium over a 0.035 inch 150 cm Terumo glide

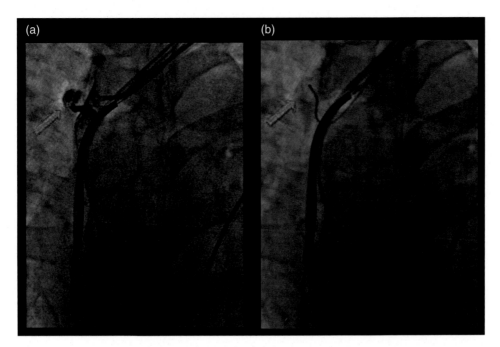

Figure 6.2 Long sheath at superior vena cava–right atrium (SVC–RA) junction. (a) Contrast injected posteriorly into the azygos (orange arrow). (b) Wire advanced into the azygos with previous contrast injection as a guide.

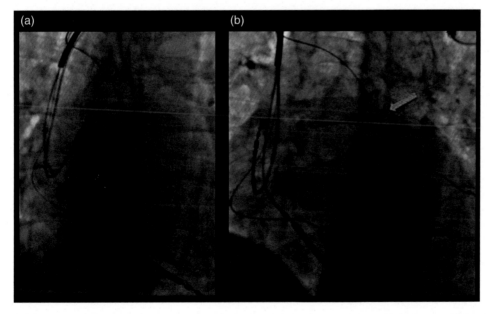

Figure 6.3 Image of wire engagement of azygos. The anteroposterior (AP) (a) and left anterior oblique (LAO) projections (b) are the most helpful views. The LAO view in particular is useful to demonstrate the wire is leftward and not in the right heart.

wire (Terumo Medical Corporation, Somerset, NJ, USA) or a Wholey guide wire (Covidien, Mansfield, MA, USA) (Figure 6.2). The sheath is pulled back and an initial pass is made with the wire to engage the azygos vein. The 30 degree right anterior oblique (RAO) angiographic view is useful for ensuring the posterior direction of the wire. If unsuccessful, a 5 or 6 Fr JR4 coronary diagnostic catheter is advanced through the outer sheath over the wire. The JR4 angiographic catheter is directed posteriorly and the wire is advanced into the azygos vein. If the wire is not easily passed, contrast can be injected through the JR4 to locate the ostium of the azygos and illustrate the tortuosity of the initial portion of the vein. The anteroposterior (AP) and left anterior oblique (LAO) views will demonstrate that the wire is leftward relative to the ICD lead (Figure 6.3).

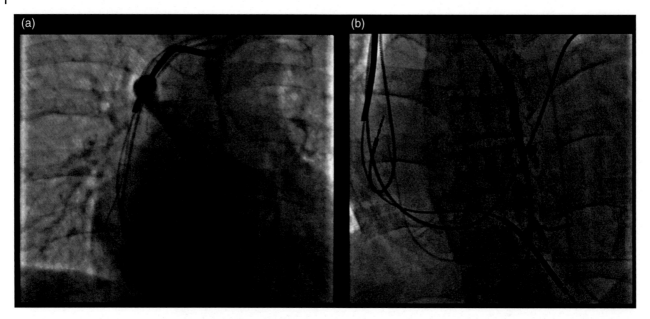

(a) (b)

Figure 6.4 Venography of the azygos vein prior to lead implantation in two patients. (a) A relatively large vein; (b) a more diminutive vessel.

The wire should be advanced distally below the diaphragm for support and the JR4 catheter can then be advanced over the wire into the azygos vein and the outer sheath advanced over the JR4 (used as a rail). If an inner catheter was not used, a second wire can be advanced through the outer sheath to provide additional support to advance the sheath. However, if an inner sheath is not used, care must be taken to only advance the sheath to the ostium of the azygos as aggressive advancement of the sheath around the tortuous entrance to the azygos could cause venous dissection or perforation. We advise the use of an inner sheath to allow distal advancement of the outer sheath into the azygos. This is important, as if the outer sheath is only at the ostium of the azygos, the ability to manipulate the lead within the vein can be limited. Once access is achieved, a venogram can then be obtained to assess azygos anatomy (Figure 6.4), which can be somewhat variable.

A passive fixation defibrillation lead or specially designed lead without fixation can then be advanced to the inferior heart border through the outer sheath after the JR4 catheter and wire are removed (Figure 6.5). The lead most commonly used is a Medtronic 6937A lead (58 or 65 cm length) which was initially marketed for SVC or CS placement, but has been adapted for azygos vein implantation. However, the use of standard passive fixation single coil ICD leads has also been described. It is best to advance the lead as distally as possible, as when the peelaway sheath is removed the lead may retract slightly as it is not actively fixated. If implanted distally, the lead can be easily withdrawn if located too distally to provide an optimal shocking vector, but if placed too proximally it may be difficult to advance the lead after the sheath support is removed. Major movement of the lead after implant is rare, though alternative fixation techniques have been described for those rare cases [5].

The azygos lead can then be attached to the ICD generator at the SVC port in a standard DF1 device. If a dual coil RV lead was used the SVC coil should be capped. Repeat DFT testing can then be performed. Depending on the device company either a RV coil to azygos and can, reverse polarity with the same configuration, can to azygos with RV coil programmed out of the circuit, or a "cold can" configuration can be used (Figure 6.6).

Variation For Right-Sided Implants

The risk of elevated DFTs is higher for right-sided ICD implants as a result of a less optimal shocking vector involving the ICD generator, with less LV mass included in the shocking vector. Therefore, this technique has even more theoretical benefit for right-sided systems. When azygos lead implantation is considered from the right side, a shorter version (25 cm) of the long 9 Fr sheath in combination with a JR4 coronary diagnostic catheter can be used to minimize the amount of catheter outside of the body.

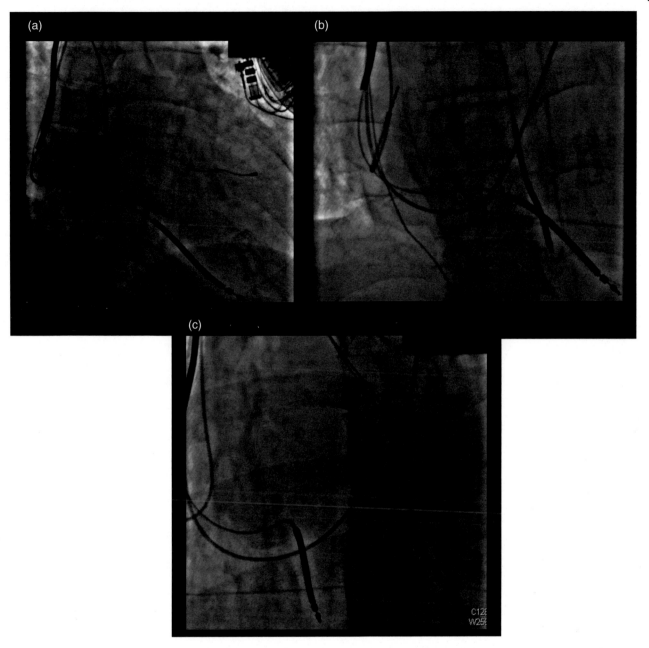

Figure 6.5 (a) Right anterior oblique (RAO), (b) AP, and (c) LAO views of azygos lead final placement. The LAO view demonstrates that an azygos lead is leftward of the left ventricle (LV), but the RAO and AP views demonstrate the lead remains more posterior then would be desired for an ideal shocking vector.

Case Example

A 55-year-old woman with a history of non-ischemic cardiomyopathy, ejection fraction 10%, status-post biventricular ICD implantation was admitted for recurrent ICD therapies secondary to monomorphic VT, with evidence of intermittent failed defibrillation at maximum device output (36 J). She underwent DFT testing, but despite testing in multiple configurations including reversal of polarity, cold can technique and waveform tuning, the DFT remained elevated requiring multiple external shocks. The patient underwent RV lead revision to a more apical position, which did not positively affect the DFT. Therefore, an azygos coil was implanted, resulting in a decrease in her DFT from >35 to 15 J.

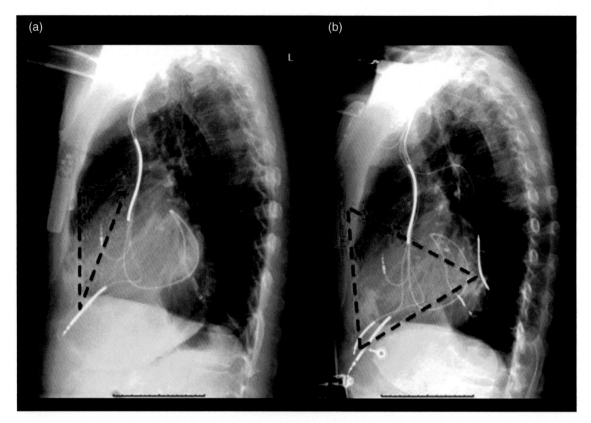

Figure 6.6 Improvement in shocking vector after implantation of an azygos coil. (a) A standard vector incorporating the right ventricle (RV) and SVC coils and implantable cardioverter-defibrillator (ICD) generator. In this configuration minimal left ventricular myocardium is incorporated into the shocking vector. (b) The improved shocking vector with substantial left ventricular myocardium incorporated into the shocking vector (blue triangles).

Equipment Required:
0.035-in, 145 cm long wire
    Wholey guide wire or
    Terumo glide wire
9-Fr long, hemostatic peel-
    away sheath
5 or 6 Fr Judkins-Right 4 (JR4)
Medtronic 6937A lead
    58–65 cm length
If necessary:
Medtronic 5019 HV splitter
IV Contrast

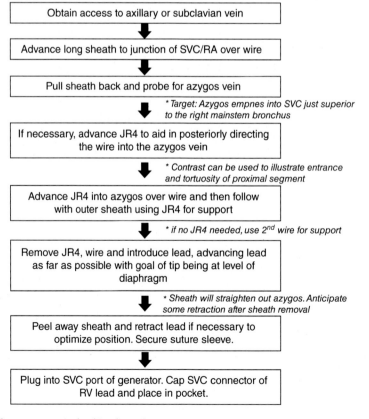

Obtain access to axillary or subclavian vein

↓

Advance long sheath to junction of SVC/RA over wire

↓

Pull sheath back and probe for azygos vein

↓ *Target: Azygos empnes into SVC just superior to the right mainstem bronchus*

If necessary, advance JR4 to aid in posteriorly directing the wire into the azygos vein

↓ *Contrast can be used to illustrate entrance and tortuosity of proximal segment*

Advance JR4 into azygos over wire and then follow with outer sheath using JR4 for support

↓ *if no JR4 needed, use 2nd wire for support*

Remove JR4, wire and introduce lead, advancing lead as far as possible with goal of tip being at level of diaphragm

↓ *Sheath will straighten out azygos. Anticipate some retraction after sheath removal*

Peel away sheath and retract lead if necessary to optimize position. Secure suture sleeve.

↓

Plug into SVC port of generator. Cap SVC connector of RV lead and place in pocket.

Figure 6.7 Schematic diagram of steps to azygos lead implantation.

Limitations

The published case experience with azygos lead implantation for elevated DFTs is limited. Clinical experience at our center and others has been positive, but not all patients will have a decrease in DFT. The azygos vein, while a posterior structure, remains rightward of the bulk of LV mass and therefore this technique may not be successful in all cases. While DFTs were lower in the case series noted [1–3], larger studies are needed to verify these findings.

In the event of endocarditis or a systemic infection requiring ICD lead extraction, the addition of an azygos lead adds an additional lead and coil that must be removed and potentially increases the risks associated with extraction. The risk of vascular damage and bleeding is presumably similar to a lead or coil in the innominate vein. However, limited data exist on extraction of these leads.

The option of implanting an azygos coil or lead and attaching the lead to the SVC port of an ICD generator is not feasible with newer ICD lead technology which has the RV with or without SVC coils integrated into a single proximal component with the pace/sense lead using an "in line" configuration (DF4). With this new lead technology, the option of adding an azygos lead is not possible as there is no SVC port to be used. Until recently, if a DF4 lead was used, RV lead revision to a DF1 lead would be required

prior to adding the azygos lead. However, a new adaptor that will facilitate azygos addition to a DF4 lead has been released [5]. The adaptor (Medtronic 5019 HV adaptor) has a Y-configuration with a DF4 connector on the single end that excludes the SVC coil and two separate connections on the other end for the DF4 lead and the azygos (via a conventional DF1 connector).

Conclusions

The addition of an azygos lead to an already existing ICD system or to a new system at the time of implant is a valuable tool for implanting physicians when DFTs are found to be elevated. Unlike subcutaneous arrays or epicardial patches, azygos lead implantation provides the ability to consistently reduce DFT without the need for additional tools or prep for subcutaneous array placement or surgical access to the pericardium. In addition, there is a risk of additional postoperative discomfort and perioperative infection associated with the alternative procedures, whereas the additional risks are minimal with azygos coil implantation.

Azygos lead addition is a safe, effective, and relatively easy means to lower DFTs in patients with documented high thresholds (Figure 6.7; Video 6.1).

References

1 Cesario D, Bhargava M, Valderrabano M, Fonarow GC, Wilkoff B, Shivkumar K. Azygos vein lead implantation: a novel adjunctive technique for implantable cardioverter defibrillator placement. J Cardiovasc Electrophysiol 2004;15:780–783.

2 Cooper JA, Latacha MP, Soto GE, Garmany RG, Gleva MJ, Chen J, et al. The azygos defibrillator lead for elevated defibrillation thresholds: implant technique, lead stability, and patient series. Pacing Clin Electrophysiol 2008;31:1405–1410.

3 Seow SC, Tolentino CS, Zhao J, Lim TW. Azygous vein coil lowers defibrillation threshold in patients with high defibrillation threshold. Europace 2011;13:825–828.

4 Bar-Cohen Y, Takao CM, Wells WJ, Saxon LA, Cesario DA, Silka MJ. Novel use of a vascular plug to anchor an azygous vein icd lead. J Cardiovasc Electrophysiol 2010;21:99–102.

5 Lim HS. Overcoming the limitations of the DF-4 defibrillator connector. Innovations Cardiac Rhythm Manage 2013;4:1205–1207.

 To watch the videos, please log in to the Companion Website:
www.wiley.com/go/al-ahmad/pacemakers_and_icds

Video 6.1 **How to place a lead in the azygos vein.**

7

Alternative Site Pacing: A Guide to Implantation Techniques

Michael C. Giudici

University of Iowa Hospitals, Iowa City, IA, USA

The first transvenous pacing leads had no active fixation mechanism. The leads were placed at the right ventricular apex (RVA) out of necessity. Patients were restricted in their activity until it was felt sufficient time had passed such that scar tissue would have formed around the lead to hold it in place. Dislodgements were common even with the subsequent addition of tines to the lead tips.

The first atrial leads had a preformed J and small tines. These leads, again by necessity and design, were usually put in the right atrial appendage (RAA). Dislodgements were even more common in the atrium than the ventricle.

With the development of positive fixation leads in the late 1980s, not only did the rate of lead dislodgement markedly decrease, but implanters were no longer restricted to only the RVA and RAA as implant sites.

Electrophysiology in the 1980s and 1990s was an era of programmed stimulation for ventricular tachyarrhythmias. Temporary pacing catheters were placed in the RVA and right ventricular outflow tract (RVOT) and stimulation was performed to try to induce ventricular tachycardia.

In 1991, Dr. Carel DeCock, from the Netherlands, decided to bring an echocardiography unit into the electrophysiology lab and evaluate hemodynamics while pacing the RVA and RVOT. He found a 17% improvement in cardiac index with RVOT pacing compared with the RVA [1]. This led to further studies with permanent leads by numerous investigators which continue to the present time.

In addition to RVOT pacing, the 1990s saw trials with biatrial pacing [2], Bachmann's bundle pacing, His bundle pacing [3], and coronary sinus ostial pacing [4]. Biventricular pacing, or cardiac resynchronization therapy (CRT), appeared in the late 1990s and its impact dwarfed that of other alternative site pacing for a time.

As research has continued, more benefits of pacing the RVOT, now referred to as right ventricular septal (RVS) pacing have been discovered. This chapter looks at techniques for implantation of permanent leads in Bachmann's bundle, His bundle, and the right ventricular septum and discuss the potential advantages to the patient for each site.

Bachmann's Bundle Pacing

Bachmann's bundle (BB) is the anterior of the three connecting fibers between the sinoatrial (SA) and atrioventricular nodes [5]. It courses across the anterior aspect of the roof of the intra-atrial septum before it turns posteriorly and decends towards the AV node (Figures 7.1 and 7.2). The SA node is the only major part of the conduction system that is not near the septum. This leads to asymmetric activation of the atria (right before left) which becomes more of an issue with aging and atrial fibrosis and may contribute to the propagation of atrial fibrillation.

Pacing at BB results in a faster, more symmetric atrial activation resulting in a shorter P-wave duration. A multicenter trial showed a significant decrease in atrial fibrillation burden in patients paced from BB compared with those paced from the RAA [6]. In addition, BB pacing has been shown to improve the contractile coupling between the left atrium and left ventricle during CRT [7].

Technique

Pacing BB is accomplished by using either a fixed-helix or extendable-retractable lead. The lead is advanced to the atrium where the straight stylet is exchanged for a "J" stylet. Depending on the size of the atrium, a shorter

How-to Manual for Pacemaker and ICD Devices: Procedures and Programming, First Edition. Edited by Amin Al-Ahmad, Andrea Natale, Paul J. Wang, James P. Daubert, and Luigi Padeletti.

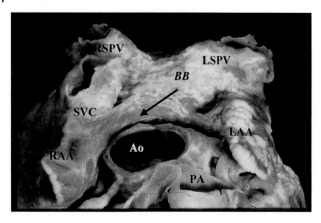

Figure 7.1 Pathologic specimen of the superior aspect of the heart. Ao, aorta; BB, Bachmann's bundle; LAA, left atrial appendage; LSPV, left superior pulmonary vein; PA, pulmonary artery; RAA, right atrial appendage; RSPV, right superior pulmonary vein; SVC, superior vena cava.

curve may be preferred to a longer curve. Putting a small curvature on the tip of the stylet to direct the lead medially into the septum is also helpful (Figure 7.3). If the atrium is cavernous, simply rotate the lead and stylet counterclockwise and bring it up the intra-atrial septum

and fixate the lead with the tip in the anterior aspect of the roof of the septum (Figure 7.4). If the atrium is smaller, it may be helpful to advance the lead across the tricuspid valve and withdraw it back into the atrium while keeping counterclockwise torque as the lead tracks up the septum to the anterior roof or the atrium. I usually perform these implants in the anteriorposterior (AP) view on fluoroscopy and then move the fluoroscopy to a 45 degree left anterior oblique (LAO) view which should show the lead pointing rightward into the high atrial septum.

Some implanting physicians may find that the extendable-retractable leads are difficult to keep directed along the septum for fixation as they have a tendency to slide over into the RAA. If this is the case, the options include: extending one or two turns of the helix to make the lead grip the tissue, extending the entire helix and using it as a fixed-helix lead, changing out to a fixed-helix lead, or using a guide catheter directed lead.

A caveat to keep in mind is that many patients have a probe-patent foramen ovale and the pacing lead can cross into the left atrium as it is dragged up the septum (Figure 7.5). If this is not caught on fluoroscopy, the lead will prop open the foramen and create an ongoing shunt.

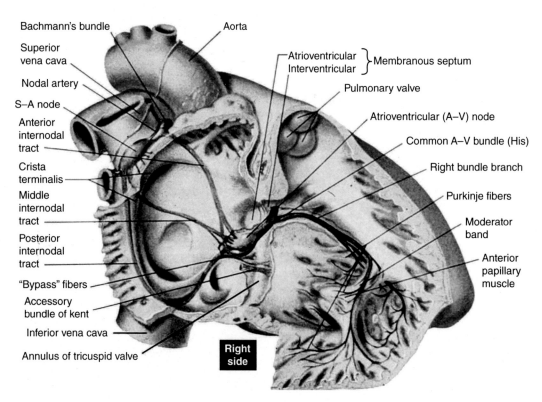

Figure 7.2 Cutaway illustration of the cardiac conduction system.

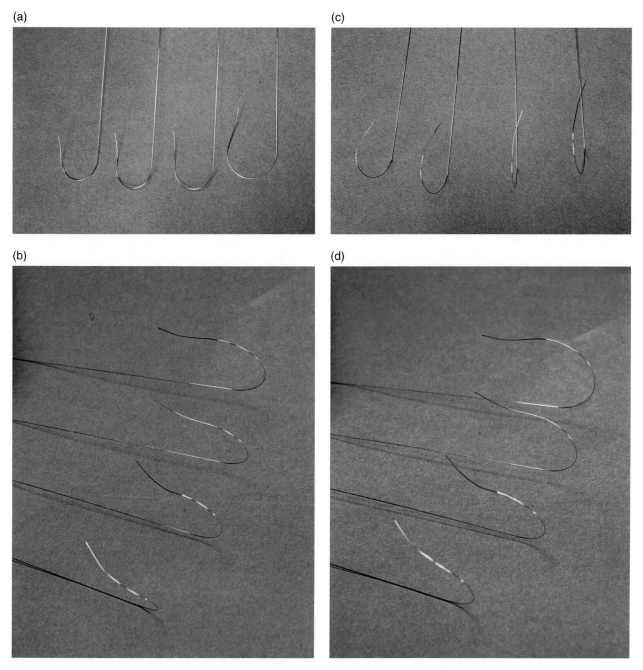

Figure 7.3 Stylets used for accessing Bachmann's bundle in the atrium: various views. Note the curve at the distal tip directing the lead towards the intra-atrial septum.

His Bundle Pacing

His bundle pacing results in normal synchronous left ventricular activation with a narrow QRS complex in patients with intact conduction. Compared with other ventricular pacing sites such as the apex or septum, His pacing is a much more exact, and therefore time-consuming procedure. In the original studies of Deshmukh *et al.* [3], mean procedure duration for a single-chamber pacemaker (including AV nodal ablation in 10 of 12 patients) was 3.7 ± 1.6 hours.

Technique

The procedure consists of placing a His bundle catheter from a femoral or subclavian approach and finely mapping that region to identify the largest His potential. The permanent pacing lead is usually positioned by shaping

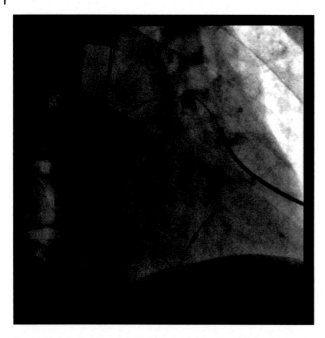

Figure 7.4 Pacing leads in Bachmann's bundle and the mid-septum.

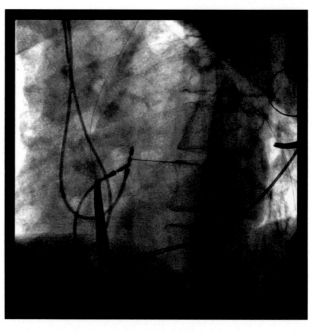

Figure 7.5 Pacing lead across a patent foramen ovale. Note that it is perpendicular to the screen in the LAO view.

the stylet with a secondary curve orthogonal to the first and aiming medially. The pacing lead is then directed into the membranous interventricular septum just above the tricuspid valve at the site of the largest His spike (Figures 7.6 and 7.7). As with BB pacing, a fixed helix lead may be advantageous as it will be less likely to slide out of place prior to fixation. This is a procedure where a millimeter or two makes a difference in whether a narrow QRS will be achieved – or not. The success rate in achieving true His pacing and a normal, narrow QRS is improved with either adding more turns during lead fixation to penetrate farther into the tissue, or using a lead with a longer helix.

There have been issues with high pacing thresholds and lead dislodgement with His bundle pacing. Some implanting physicians will implant a second ventricular lead in either the septum or apex for safety and use a dual chamber device with the His lead in the atrial port and the RV lead in the ventricular port. The device is then programmed DDIR and the RV lead only stimulates if needed.

Right Ventricular Outflow Tract (Septal) Pacing

Since the early studies of de Cock, there has been a great deal of interest in RVS pacing. There have been numerous small studies showing increased cardiac output [1, 8–10], a narrower QRS complex [9, 11], less

mitral and tricuspid valular insufficiency [11, 12], less progression to atrial fibrillation [13], and better long-term preservation of LV function [14]. One study [15] even suggested that pacing the RVS improves the performance of a pacemaker ventricular rate regulation algorithm in patients with rapid conduction of atrial fibrillation.

As a result of these and many similar studies, many implanting physicians have adopted RVS pacing as their standard approach. There are currently larger, randomized trials in progress that will shed further light on the optimal RV pacing site [16].

Technique

The most common technique for RVS pacing is to advance an active-fixation pacing lead through the tricuspid valve, either by pulling the stylet back and prolapsing the lead across the valve or putting sufficient curve on the lead stylet to direct the lead into the right ventricle. Once across the tricuspid valve, the lead is advanced into the RVOT and out into the pulmonary artery (PA) (Figure 7.8). Once in the PA, a specifically shaped stylet (Figure 7.9) is advanced to the lead tip and the lead is brought down the septum with small back and forth, withdrawl and advance, movements until the lead drops just below the Moderator Band where it is advanced and fixated (Figure 7.10). The stylet is shaped with a large curve to keep the lead from dropping down to the apex and a secondary curve at the tip to direct the

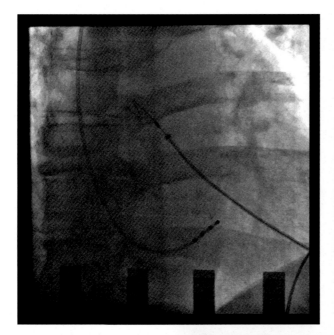
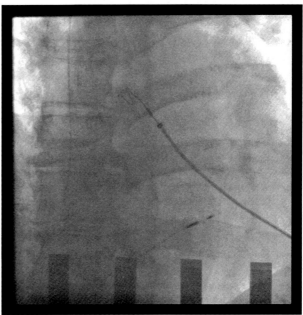
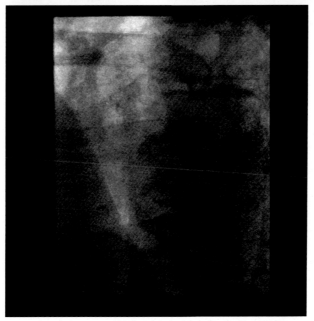

Figure 7.6 Right anterior oblique fluoroscopic projection demonstrating final position of His bundle pacing electrode. AbL-cath, ablation catheter; Hx-map, His bundle mapping catheter; PPM-L, permanent pacemaker lead. (Image courtesy of P. Deshmukh, MD.)

lead tip towards the septum. I prefer to monitor the positioning of the lead in a shallow (20–30 degrees) right anterior oblique (RAO) position. This lays out the right ventricle well and one can easily see the lead dropping over the Moderator Band (Figure 7.11). To confirm septal placement rather than the RV free wall, move fluoroscopy to the 45 degree LAO position and the lead should be coming towards the screen and turning right into the septum (Figure 7.4).

As with BB and His pacing, some implanters will prefer a fixed-helix lead as it will more easily drop down the septum in small increments rather than dropping lower than desired which may require several attempts at optimal positioning and reshaping lead stylets.

These techniques are also appropriate for implantable cardioverter-defibrillator (ICD) leads. Studies have shown RVS placement of ICD leads to be safe [17, 18] and have acceptable sensing and defibrillation thresholds [19, 20].

(a)

(b)

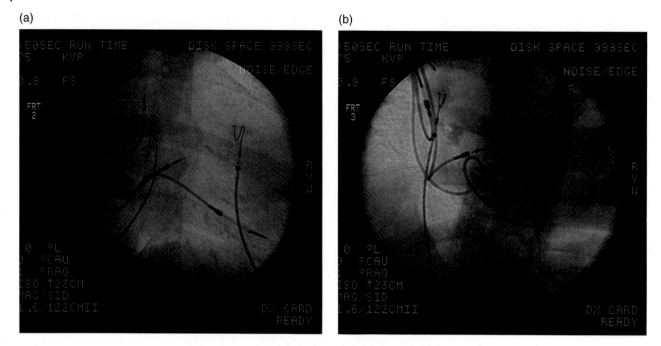

Figure 7.7 (a) Right anterior oblique, and (b) left anterior oblique views of permanent His bundle lead placement. (Images courtesy of R. Hoyt, MD.)

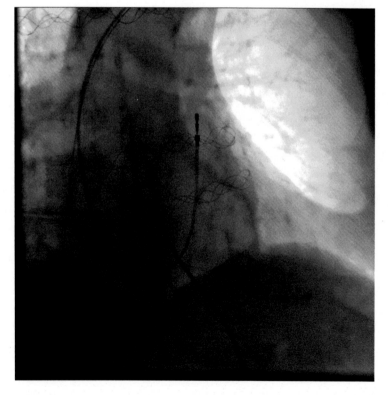

Figure 7.8 Right anterior oblique view of pacing lead in the pulmonary artery.

(a)

(b)

(c)

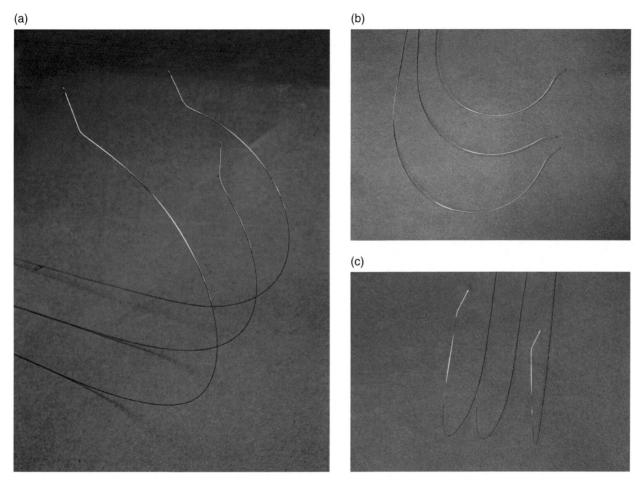

Figure 7.9 Stylets used for mid-septal lead placement: various views. Note the curve at the distal tip directing the lead towards the right ventricular septum.

(a)

(b)

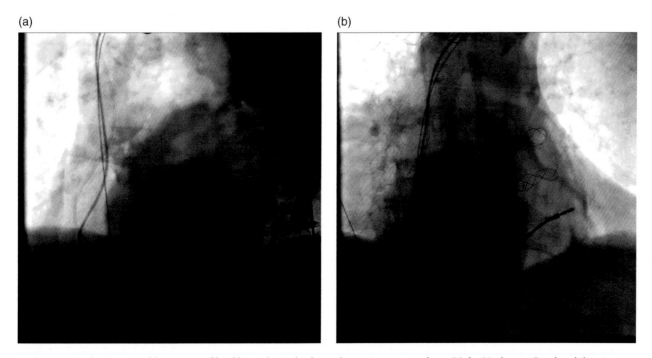

Figure 7.10 Right anterior oblique view of lead being brought down the septum to just above (a) the Moderator Band and then just below (b) where it is fixed to the septum.

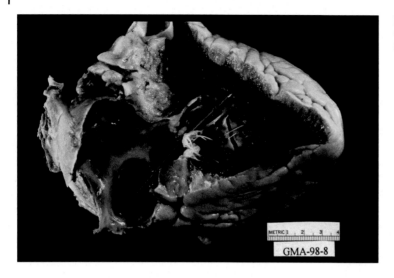

Figure 7.11 Pathologic specimen showing right ventricular septal pacing lead just below the Moderator Band.

Conclusions

Alternative site pacing, like most things we do, has a small learning curve. By taking the initial time to learn these techniques in the atrium, you will very quickly be achieving shorter P wave durations and less intra-atrial conduction delay, helping suppress atrial fibrillation, and seeing better LA–LV synchrony with CRT. In the ventricle, you will normalize the QRS axis, narrow the QRS, preserve the LV ejection fraction, and decrease the incidence of perfusion defects on nuclear scans.

References

1 de Cock CC, Meyer A, Kamp O, Visser CA. Hemodynamic benefits of right ventricular outflow tract pacing: comparison with right ventricular apex pacing. Pacing Clin Electrophysiol 1998;21(3):536–541.

2 Saksena S, Prakash A, Ziegler P, Hummel JD, Friedman P, Plumb VJ, *et al.* Improved suppression of recurrent atrial fibrillation with dual-site right atrial pacing and antiarrhythmic drug therapy. J Am Coll Cardiol 2002;40(6):1140–1150; discussion 1151–1152.

3 Deshmukh P, Casavant DA, Romanyshyn M, Anderson K. Permanent, direct His-bundle pacing: a novel approach to cardiac pacing in patients with normal His-Purkinje activation. Circulation 2000;101(8):869–877.

4 Delfaut P, Saksena S, Prakash A, Krol RB. Long-term outcome of patients with drug-refractory atrial flutter and fibrillation after single- and dual-site right atrial pacing for arrhythmia prevention. J Am Coll Cardiol 1998;32(7):1900–1908.

5 de Micheli Serra A, Iturralde Torres P, Aranda Fraustro A. About the specialized myocardial conducting tissue. Arch Cardiol Mex 2013;83(4):278–281.

6 Bailin SJ, Adler S, Giudici M. Prevention of chronic atrial fibrillation by pacing in the region of Bachmann's bundle: results of a multicenter randomized trial. J Cardiovasc Electrophysiol 2001;12(8):912–917.

7 Suzuki T, Osaka T, Kuroda Y, Hasebe H, Yokoyama E, Kamiya K, *et al.* Potential benefit of Bachmann's bundle pacing on left ventricular performance in patients with cardiac resynchronized therapy. Circ J 2012;76(12):2799–2806.

8 Giudici MC, Thornburg GA, Buck DL, Coyne EP, Walton MC, Paul DL, *et al.* Comparison of right ventricular outflow tract and apical lead permanent pacing on cardiac output. Am J Cardiol 1997;79(2):209–212.

9 Mera F, DeLurgio DB, Patterson RE, Merlino JD, Wade ME, León AR. A comparison of ventricular function during high right ventricular septal and apical pacing after His-bundle ablation for refractory atrial fibrillation. Pacing Clin Electrophysiol 1999;22(8):1234–1239.

10 Victor F, Mabo P, Mansour H, Pavin D, Kabalu G, de Place C, *et al.* A randomized comparison of permanent septal versus apical right ventricular pacing: short-term results. J Cardiovasc Electrophysiol 2006;17(3):238–242.

11 Lewicka-Nowak E, Dabrowska-Kugacka A, Tybura S, Krzymińska-Stasiuk E, Wilczek R, Staniewicz J, *et al.* Right ventricular apex versus right ventricular outflow tract pacing: prospective, randomised, long-term clinical and echocardiographic evaluation. Kardiol Pol 2006;64(10):1082–1091; discussion 1092–1093.

12 Hemayat S, Shafiee A, Oraii S, Roshanali F, Alaedini F, Aldoboni AS. Development of mitral and tricuspid regurgitation in right ventricular apex versus right ventricular outflow tract pacing. J Interv Card Electrophysiol 2014;40(1):81–86.

13 Parekh S, Stein KM. Selective site pacing: rationale and practical application. Curr Cardiol Rep 2008;10(5):351–359.

14 Tse HF, Yu C, Wong KK, Tsang V, Leung YL, Ho WY, *et al.* Functional abnormalities in patients with permanent right ventricular pacing: the effect of sites of electrical stimulation. J Am Coll Cardiol 2002;40(8):1451–1458.

15 Tse HF, Siu CW, Lau CP. Impact of right ventricular pacing sites on exercise capacity during ventricular rate regularization in patients with permanent atrial fibrillation. Pacing Clin Electrophysiol 2009;32(12):1536–1542.

16 Da Costa A, Gabriel L, Romeyer-Bouchard C, Géraldine B, Gate-Martinet A, Laurence B, *et al.*

Focus on right ventricular outflow tract septal pacing. Arch Cardiovasc Dis 2013;106(6-7):394–403.

17 Giudici MC, Barold SS, Paul DL, Schrumpf PE, Van Why KJ, Orias DW. Right ventricular outflow tract placement of defibrillation leads: five year experience. Pacing Clin Electrophysiol 2004;27(4):443–446.

18 Lubinski A, Lewicka-Nowak E, Królak T, Kempa M, Bielawska B, Wilczek R, *et al.* Implantation and follow-up of ICD leads implanted in the right ventricular outflow tract. Pacing Clin Electrophysiol 2000;23(11 Pt 2):1996–1998.

19 Mollerus M, Lipinski M, Munger T. A randomized comparison of defibrillation thresholds in the right ventricular outflow tract versus right ventricular apex. J Interv Card Electrophysiol 2008;22(3):221–225.

20 Crossley GH, Boyce K, Roelke M, Evans J, Yousuf D, Syed Z, *et al.* A prospective randomized trial of defibrillation thresholds from the right ventricular outflow tract and the right ventricular apex. Pacing Clin Electrophysiol 2009;32(2):166–171.

8

How to Maximize CRT Response at Implant

Attila Roka[1], Gaurav Upadhyay[2], Jagmeet Singh[3], and E. Kevin Heist[3]

[1] Cardiovascular Institute of the South, Meridian, MS, USA
[2] Heart Rhythm Center, University of Chicago Hospital, Chicago, IL, USA
[3] Cardiac Arrhythmia Service, Massachusetts General Hospital, Boston, MA, USA

Pre-implantation Evaluation

Assessment of heart failure severity, left ventricular ejection fraction (LVEF), and 12-lead ECG is required to establish the indication for cardiac resynchronization therapy (CRT) implantation [1]. To optimize patient selection, potentially reversible factors contributing to heart failure and cardiomyopathy should be addressed (e.g., uncontrolled hypertension, ischemia, suboptimal medical management) prior to the procedure.

Although most patients who undergo CRT implantation have at least moderately severe heart failure, care must be taken to avoid performing the procedure when the patient is unstable. Volume overload and pulmonary congestion may limit the time the patient is able to spend in a flat, supine position, and increases the risk associated with procedure. Most implanting physicians prefer conscious sedation for the procedure, as it has the lowest risk of periprocedural complications. In patients with severe heart failure or comorbidities, however, anesthesia consultation may be required to consider general anesthesia.

Multiple imaging modalities have the capability to evaluate left ventricular dyssynchrony, although the role of mechanical dyssynchrony assessment in the prediction of CRT response is controversial. Echocardiography is the most common modality used to assess LVEF, but it may also be used to assess right ventricular (RV) dysfunction, contribution of valvular pathology, and intra- or interventricular delay. Although these may be helpful to identify a higher risk of non-response, there are insufficient data to withhold therapy from patients who would otherwise be candidates for CRT based on their QRS morphology and LV dysfunction. Cardiac MRI may also be used to assess dyssynchrony and scar burden, which may affect outcome.

Assessment of Coronary Vein Anatomy

Transvenous left ventricular lead positioning is often limited by the anatomy of the coronary veins. Imaging studies of the anatomy of the coronary sinus (CS) may help to determine whether the patient is suitable for transvenous implantation and to plan CS access, although these are not routinely performed.

In particular, delayed images after contrast injection during conventional coronary arteriography can be used to outline the anatomy of the CS and its main branches. Although this technique cannot assess the terminal branches of the CS, the images may be used to identify fluoroscopic markers for CS ostium to guide cannulation and to assess whether larger side branches are present.

Cardiac CT venography provides a detailed view of coronary venous anatomy. Pre-implantation evaluation of the coronary venous anatomy was shown to decrease the procedural time of CRT implantation. Additional uses include identification of the area of latest mechanical activation for targeted LV lead placement and visualization of phrenic nerve course. The CT images can be fused with fluoroscopic images and electroanatomic mapping during the procedure, providing excellent guidance. Contrast allergy or severe renal dysfunction may preclude the use of CT imaging. Fusion of CT and electroanatomic mapping requires special hardware and software capability.

Cardiac MRI can also be utilized to assess the coronary veins. In addition, this technique can describe the area of latest activation, scarred regions, and general scar burden. In ischemic cardiomyopathy, less than 15% of total myocardium infarcted and absence of significant posterolateral scar is associated with better response. Contraindications include severe renal dysfunction, previously implanted non-MRI compatible hardware, long scanning time, and need for patient cooperation.

Although these advanced imaging modalities improved implantation success rate and responder rate in smaller studies, routine utilization may not be cost-effective. Advanced modalities could be reserved for cases where difficult anatomy is anticipated or if the patient had an unsuccessful implantation attempt.

Transvenous LV Lead Implantation

The standard approach to CRT is to implant three endo-vascular leads for cardiac stimulation: RV, RA, and an epicardial LV lead into a coronary vein through the CS (Figures 8.1 and 8.2). Although this is the most commonly used approach, it is dependent on highly variable venous anatomy. The most common reasons for failed LV lead implants are the inability to cannulate the CS or unsuitable venous anatomy. In almost all cases of CRT implants, a venogram is obtained after the CS is cannulated, with the use of an occluder balloon and hand-injected contrast agent. Care must be taken to avoid underfilling of the CS, as side branches otherwise suitable for lead placement can be missed.

Even with a suitable CS, an unstable LV lead position, high pacing threshold, or phrenic nerve stimulation may hinder LV pacing. Implantation success rate is currently above 90% in experienced centers, although some of these implants may involve suboptimal LV lead locations because of the issues described earlier.

Techniques of LV lead implantation are elaborated in Chapter 7. The European Heart Rhythm Association (EHRA) and Heart Rhythm Society (HRS) have published guidelines for the recommended approach for transvenous CRT implantation [1]. The RV lead should typically be placed first as it is less likely to dislodge

Figure 8.1 Coronary sinus (CS) venography with an occluder balloon and manual contrast injection. The CS body is completely occluded by the balloon and the veins, even the smaller branches, are well visualized. The posterior vein, which is proximal to the site of the occlusion, is filling via collaterals.

Figure 8.2 Same patient as in Figure 8.1. The posterolateral vein was selected as the site of the left ventricular (LV) lead implant. A quadripolar lead is placed into a stable wedge position. Stimulation if the basal–mid posterolateral LV segment is achieved via pacing between the proximal electrode pair.

during manipulation of other leads, provides information about the position of the tricuspid valve and right atrial size, and can be utilized for back-up pacing if the right bundle develops mechanical trauma during CS cannulation, which can lead to transient complete AV block in patients with pre-existing left bundle branch block (LBBB).

Most current LV leads are bipolar or quadripolar with a low profile (5 Fr or less) and the lead delivery to the target vein is performed over a guide wire. Alternatively, a stylet can be used to directly advance the lead into the vein. The lead is usually thin and flexible enough to be advanced at least into the basal to mid portion of a coronary vein. Quadripolar CS leads allow multiple pacing configurations, providing options to avoid phrenic nerve stimulation or sites with high threshold. It also enables a more stable distal lead position, while still allowing pacing on the proximal electrodes if desired. Acute echoguided CRT optimization with these leads in a study of 22 patients showed improvement in New York Heart Association (NYHA) and LVEF at 6 month, compared with bipolar controls [2]. Quadripolar leads are also safe – the MORE-CRT study included 1068 heart failure patients scheduled for CRT from 63 centers in 13 countries. Patients were randomized in a 1: 2 ratio to undergo CRT with either a bipolar or a quadripolar lead. At 6 months, compared with bipolar controls, patients with quadripolar leads were significantly more likely to be free from a composite endpoint of both intra- and postoperative LV lead-related complications (85.97% vs. 76.86%). The driver of this benefit was mainly the intraoperative complication rate (5.98% vs. 13.73%).

Quadripolar leads may also enable multipolar LV pacing with a compatible pulse generator. Forty-four patients receiving a CRT implant were randomized to receive biventricular or multipolar pacing. For each patient, an optimal pacing configuration for the assigned pacing mode was programmed based on intraoperative pressure–volume loop measurements. After 3 months, 50% of biventricular paced and 76% of multipolar paced patient were responders (reduction in end-systolic volume (ESV) ≥15%). ESV reduction, ejection fraction increase and NYHA class reduction relative to the baseline was significantly greater in the multipolar group than in the conventional biventricular group.

In patients in whom the target vein is stenotic, balloon angioplasty may be attempted. Angioplasty may also be used as a rescue when dissection of the CS is observed during implantation, which would otherwise preclude further attempts at lead placement. The risk of perforation and tamponade is low. In patients with unfavorable coronary vein anatomy in the target area, dilatation and use of collateral veins may be considered. With access to these interventional techniques, implantation success rate may be as high as 99%. A retrospective single center analysis showed that 3.5% of patients required venoplasty for LV implantation; of these, 77% coronary vein, 13% subclavian vein, 10% valvular structures within the CS or a Marshall vein. The required inflation pressures for ring-like structures were high (16 ± 3 atm), but complications were rare. Mostly, short balloons with 3 mm diameter were used.

High pacing threshold or phrenic nerve stimulation may require achieving an electrode position where traditional fixation mechanisms are not be effective. Stabilizing the lead position with retained stylets is not recommended because of the high risk of late lead failure. Instead, a coronary stent implanted near the distal end of the lead may stabilize the new position. A large single center study of 312 patients with stent fixation of the CS lead showed that the method was safe and effective in the long term to prevent lead dislocation. Ninety-five percent of patients had stenting because of intraoperative lead instability or phrenic nerve stimulation, while 5% required it as a result of previous lead dislocation. Bare metal stents were implanted 5–35 mm proximal to the most proximal electrode. There was no mechanical damage to the lead and no CS perforation was observed. During an average follow-up of 28.4 months, a significant increase in the left ventricular pacing threshold was found in four cases and reoperation was necessary in two patients (0.6%). Phrenic nerve stimulation was observed in 18 patients, endovascular repositioning with an ablation catheter was performed in seven patients. In three patients the leads were removed without complications 3–49 months after the initial implant (because of infection or heart transplant).

Targeting LV Lead Placement

The goal of CRT is to decrease the hemodynamic consequences of intra- and interventricular dyssynchrony. The optimal position for the LV lead is thought to be where biventricular pacing leads to the greatest decrease in ventricular activation time – in absence of significant electromechanical uncoupling/delay, this should lead to decreased mechanical dyssynchrony.

There is a large variability in the ventricular activation pattern and distribution of mechanical dyssynchrony even in patients with LBBB. In clinical practice, detailed mapping during transvenous implantation is not feasible. Lead placement via endocardial and surgical epicardial approach may have more potential for individualized targeted pacing. Targeting methods include electrical, mechanical, and anatomic parameters.

Anatomic positioning is still the most commonly used method to achieve "optimal" lead positions. Targeting "segments" of the LV is a commonly utilized LV lead placement strategy, aiming for the basal–mid posterolateral–lateral area. Apical lead placement was shown to be inferior in 115 patients undergoing CRT who were followed prospectively for 15.1 ± 9.0 months (combined endpoint of heart failure hospitalization, cardiac transplantation, or all-cause mortality). Event-free survival was significantly lower in the apical group: 52% vs. 79%. The apical group also experienced less improvement in NYHA functional class and less LV reverse remodeling. Apically positioned LV leads were associated with worse clinical outcome also in the REVERSE and MADIT-CRT trials. The COMPANION and MADIT-CRT studies showed a comparable response between lateral, anterior, and posterior LV lead locations, while patients in the REVERSE trial benefited from a lateral lead location. The importance of the interlead distance was demonstrated in 51 patients, who underwent CRT; the separation of the LV and RV lead tips was determined on postprocedural anteroposterior and lateral radiographs. The corrected direct LV–RV interlead distance on the lateral radiograph correlated significantly with the delta dP/dt. The corrected horizontal interlead distance on the lateral film was greater in acute hemodynamic responders; other parameters did not correlate with the hemodynamic change.

Aiming for maximum electrical delay is another option to enhance CRT efficacy [3]. Several algorithms based on intracardiac electrograms have been investigated to guide LV lead positioning. Measurement of the LV lead electrical delay (LVLED, Q-LV) may identify areas of late activation in different locations, by moving the LV lead within the coronary veins. In a study of 52 patients, the LVLED was predictive of response to CRT (reduction in LVESV >15% at 6 months; Figure 8.3).

As clinical improvement is expected to be the consequence of improving mechanical function, targeting areas with maximum mechanical delay can also be used to guide CRT. Echo tissue Doppler imaging (TDI) and tagged MRI can be utilized for this purpose. A study evaluating the role of this technique to identify the latest activated LV areas included 244 heart failure patients treated with CRT. On the basis of radial strain–time curves obtained at the mid ventricular short-axis images of the left ventricle, the most frequent latest activated areas were the posterior (36%) and the lateral (33%) regions. Pacing at the site of latest mechanical activation resulted in superior echocardiographic response after 6 months of CRT and better prognosis during long-term follow-up.

Imaging studies may help to select specific sites for left ventricular pacing based on anticipated optimization of electromechanical effects. Echocardiography (TDI or tissue synchronization imaging) may identify LV sites with marked mechanical delay. Pacing these sites may result in greater ventricular remodeling and improved clinical outcomes. Currently, there are not enough data

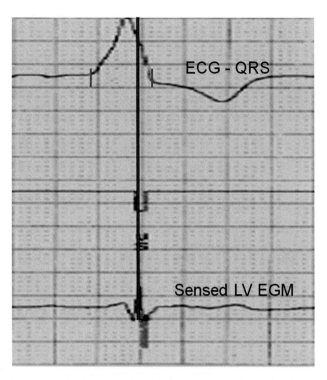

Figure 8.3 Optimizing LV lead placement using electrical delay. The delay between the initiation of the QRS and the sensed LV signal (Q-LV) and the Q-LV: QRS duration ratio (LVLED) can be measured while positioning the lead. The LVLED was shown to correlate with clinical outcome during cardiac resynchronization therapy (CRT).

supporting the role of acute hemodynamic measurements during implantation to target lead implantation.

The randomized TARGET study assessed the impact of targeted LV lead placement on outcomes of CRT [4]. Two hundred and twenty patients had baseline echocardiographic speckle-tracking two-dimensional radial strain imaging and were then randomized 1: 1 into two groups. In the TARGET group, the LV lead was positioned at the latest site of peak contraction with an amplitude of ≥10% to signify freedom from scar. In the control group, patients underwent standard unguided CRT. Patients were classified by the relationship of the LV lead to the optimal site as concordant (at optimal site), adjacent (within 1 segment), or remote (≥2 segments away). The primary endpoint was a ≥15% reduction in LVESV at 6 months. Secondary endpoints were clinical response (≥1 improvement in NYHA functional class), all-cause mortality, and combined all-cause mortality and heart failure-related hospitalization. In the TARGET group, there were a greater proportion of responders at 6 months (70% vs. 55%). Compared with controls, TARGET patients had a higher clinical response (83% vs. 65%) and lower rates of the combined endpoint.

Multisite or multipolar ventricular stimulation (more than one LV lead) may provide even greater benefits with more homogenous ventricular activation. More clinical data will be needed to evaluate whether this is superior to biventricular stimulation.

The randomized TRIP-HF study compared the effects of triple-site versus dual-site biventricular stimulation. It was a multicenter, single-blind, crossover study which enrolled 40 patients with moderate to severe heart failure, a mean LV ejection fraction of 26%, and permanent atrial fibrillation (AF) with slow ventricular rate. A CRT device, connected to one RV and two LV leads, inserted in two separate coronary sinus tributaries, was successfully implanted in 34 patients. After 3 months of biventricular stimulation, the patients were randomly assigned to stimulation for 3 months with either one RV and two LV leads (3-V) or to conventional stimulation with one RV and one LV lead (2-V), then crossed over for 3 months to the alternate configuration. The primary study endpoint was quality of ventricular resynchronization (Z ratio). Secondary endpoints included reverse LV remodeling, quality of life, distance covered during 6-min hall walk, and procedure-related morbidity and mortality. No significant difference in Z ratio, quality of life, and 6-min hall walk was observed between 2-V and 3-V. However, a significantly higher LVEF (27% vs. 35%) and smaller LVESV (157 vs. 134) and diameter (57 vs. 54 mm) were observed with 3-V. The results will need to be verified in a larger CRT population.

Alternative LV Lead Placement Techniques

In the first cases of CRT, the LV lead was surgically placed via thoracotomy. This approach was associated with considerable morbidity, requiring general anesthesia and longer recovery time. Long-term electrical stability of surgically placed electrodes was inferior when compared with transvenous leads. However, this method does not require fluoroscopy, is not constrained by the venous anatomy, allows the visual identification of the segment with latest contraction, and can prevent phrenic nerve stimulation. Most surgical implants can be performed via limited thoracotomy. The surgery is performed using single-lung ventilation on a beating heart. A 2–3 inch incision is made over the 4th or 5th intercostal space anterior to the mid axillary line. The lung is pushed back and the pericardium is opened anterior to the phrenic nerve. The left ventricle is mapped for optimal pacing site and an epicardial lead placement device is used to attach the electrode. The leads are tunneled to the generator site, usually in the left infraclavicular region. This technique is a safe and acceptable option, with benefits comparable to transvenous CRT. In 33 patients, functional

and echocardiographic parameters showed similar improvement, however, with a delayed onset of peak VO2 improvement. Instead of minimal thoracotomy, video-assisted thoracoscopy may also be used for lead placement.

Biventricular pacing with endocardial stimulation may provide more homogenous intraventricular resynchronization than with epicardial stimulation. Trans-septal approach can be utilized to implant a conventional endocardial lead into the LV cavity for endocardial stimulation. The endocardial surface of the LV may be mapped with an EP catheter or the lead itself to localize the site most suitable for lead implantation–electroanatomic mapping may be used to precisely identify the area of latest activation in the LV. The main disadvantage of this technique is the unknown long-term thromboembolic risk, which requires long-term anticoagulation. Over an average 85 month follow-up of six patients in a case series, one patient had LV lead dislodgment at 3 months requiring re-intervention. One patient had a transient ischemic attack, when anticoagulation was accidentally interrupted. These patients require full anticoagulation immediately after the implantation, increasing the risk of periprocedural bleeding complications. Mitral valve damage and endocarditis are rare but serious complications.

Transapical endocardial LV lead placement was also investigated in a case series. This technique combines the minimally invasive surgical approach with the presumed advantages of endocardial pacing in patients in whom extensive epicardial adhesions prohibit access to the pericardial space. After induction of general anesthesia and selective bronchial intubation, the LV apex is localized with transthoracic echocardiography, then a small left thoracotomy is performed. The apex of the left ventricle is punctured and an active fixation lead is inserted into the cavity, using the Seldinger technique. The bleeding is controlled with purse-string sutures. The lead is guided into its final position with a guide, using fluoroscopy. As transapical endocardial lead implantation does not involve the mitral valve, the risk of mitral valve endocarditis is likely less. The lead is subcutaneously tunneled to the pocket to be connected to the generator. Long-term anticoagulation is required. Advantages of this technique are the accessibility of the endocardial segments without limitations of the CS anatomy and absence of phrenic nerve stimulation.

Position of the RV Lead

The optimal position for the right ventricular pacing or pacing/defibrillation lead is not clear. In the 346 patients enrolled in the active (CRT on) arm of the REVERSE study, there were no significant differences between

RV apical and non-apical lead positions in the analyzed endpoints (death and first heart failure hospitalization). Khan et al. [4] also analyzed the effect or RV lead positioning on CRT outcomes. In 131 CRT patients, the LV lead was positioned preferentially in a lateral or posterolateral position. The RV leads were implanted on the septum or RV apex. There were no significant differences in mean reduction of LVESV at 6-month follow-up (RVS vs. RVA: $-23.3 \pm 16\%$ vs. $22.1 \pm 18\%$; $p = 0.70$) or rate of responders (58.2% vs. 57.9%; $p = 0.97$). This study also found that LV lead position correlated with the outcome: if it was placed to pace the segment that contracted the latest (as determined by 2D speckle tracking radial strain imaging), the response rate was higher (76.1% vs. 36.7%; $p < 0.001$). This difference was not affected by RV lead position.

Increased defibrillation threshold is a common concern when placing implantable cardioverter-defibrillator (ICD) leads into non-apical positions. A prospective, randomized study performed on 33 patients by Reynolds et al. [5] found no significant differences in RVOT or RV apical positions (RVA, 9.8 ± 7.3 J; RVOT, 10.8 ± 7.2 J; $p = 0.53$).

Device Optimization at Implant

There has been extensive research on AV and VV echocardiographic optimization after CRT, with variable overall success. The practice of echocardiographic CRT optimization is still highly variable between implanting centers as the optimal method and timing is unknown and the technique is time-consuming. More recently, ECG optimization at the time of implant has been advocated. Methodologies focus on altering LV offset timing in order to minimize paced QRS duration while maintaining evidence of LV pre-excitation (usually confirmed with presence of an R-wave in V1). Early evidence suggests that ECG optimization of VV intervals may be a simple, cost-effective means of improving CRT response. Novel methods, such as automatic CRT optimization, are being investigated as alternatives (RESPOND CRT, FREEDOM).

Atrial Fibrillation

Ablation of the AV node is generally recommended in CRT patients with persistent and/or permanent atrial fibrillation and elevated ventricular rates leading to reduced biventricular pacing [6]. The SPARE II observational, prospective, multicenter study grouped patients by intrinsic rhythm (sinus rhythm vs. AF). For the first 2 months, negative chronotropic drugs were optimized in the AF group. If ventricular pacing was ≤85%, AVJ ablation was recommended. Responders were defined as patients who survived without requiring heart transplant and had a ≥10% reduction in LVESV at 12 months after implantation. Of 202 patients included, 156 (77%) were in sinus rhythm and 46 (23%) had AF. After drug optimization, only 28% of the AF patients required AVJ ablation. 53% were responders in the sinus rhythm group, vs. 48% in the AF group ($p = NS$). Among AF patients, the response was 48% for AF with non-AVJ ablation vs. 46% with AVJ ablation ($p = NS$). The LVESV decreased in all three groups. Mortality was higher in patients with AF compared with sinus rhythm: 21% vs. 5.7% ($p < 0.05$).

Device Upgrades

New guidelines emphasize the role of CRT in certain groups of patients who already have conventional pacemakers, to avoid pacing-induced dyssynchrony and remodeling [1]. Upgrade of an existing device may pose difficulties because of scarring or venous occlusion (Figures 8.4 and 8.5). The perioperative risks in these patients are higher: the 6-month major complication rate was 18.7% in the REPLACE registry in patients undergoing upgrade to a CRT device with addition of a new endocardial LV lead to the existing leads. The risk of subclavian vein thrombosis is related to the number of leads implanted; in CRT patients it can be up to 30%. Subclavian venography with injection through the upper extremity veins is a simple and effective technique to evaluate venous anatomy prior to an upgrade or lead revision. Venoplasty may be performed if ipsilateral implantation is favored, otherwise the lead can be tunneled to the device pocket from the contralateral site.

Peri- and Postoperative Period

The implanting physician should be prepared to address most common complications of CRT implants: failure to implant the LV lead (requiring to pursue an alternative implantation method), pocket hematoma, hemothorax or pneumothorax, CS dissection, cardiac perforation or tamponade, extracardiac stimulation, complete heart block, LV lead dislodgement, congestive heart failure exacerbation, acute renal failure. Overall perioperative complication rates are around 4%, declining from 28% noted in early CRT trials.

Figure 8.4 Revision of a CRT system. The patient with ischemic cardiomyopathy had an earlier system revision, where a CS lead was removed from the lateral vein and a new one was placed into the anterolateral vein. As response was poor, adding a new lead into the lateral vein was planned but hindered by severe stenosis in the proximal segment. Balloon angioplasty was attempted but, despite inflations up to 18 atm, the stenosis did not resolve.

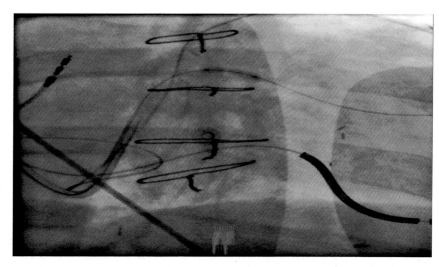

Figure 8.5 Same patient as in Figure 8.4. A right ventricular (RV) lead has been added into the right ventricular outflow tract (RVOT) position to enable "triventricular" pacing with two RV and an LV lead.

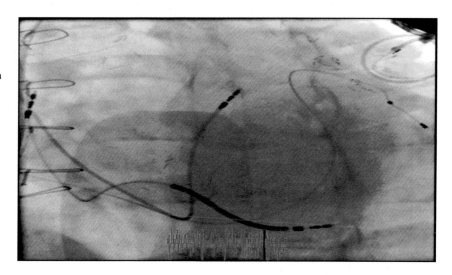

The optimal duration of postprocedural hospitalization is unknown; most centers observe the patient overnight following the implant. Although proarrhythmia from biventricular pacing is extremely rare, it can be a very serious complication leading to ICD shocks or sudden death. Less than optimal biventricular pacing may be recognized (fusion beats, frequent premature beats, atrial tachyarrhythmia with rapid ventricular rate) and corrected before the patient is discharged.

Medications may be adjusted shortly after the implant. Bradycardia should not be a limiting factor during titration of the beta blockers and patients may be able to tolerate angiotensin converting enzyme (ACE) inhibitor with less hypotension. With improvement in heart failure symptoms and congestion, the dosage of diuretics may be decreased, although this may occur over the ensuing months after implant.

Conclusions

Efficacy of CRT is dependent on proper patient selection, optimal lead placement, device programming, and minimizing the risk of peri- and postprocedural complications. Although large randomized trials continue to identify patient groups who may benefit from CRT, there are still a substantial minority of patients who do not respond appropriately. Evidence-based perioperative care and access to alternative implant techniques may improve efficacy of CRT and decrease complication rates.

References

1 European Heart Rhythm Association; European Society of Cardiology; Heart Rhythm Society; Heart Failure Society of America; American Society of Echocardiography; American Heart Association; European Association of Echocardiography; Heart Failure Association, Daubert JC, Saxon L, Adamson PB, Auricchio A, Berger RD, Beshai JF, *et al.* 2012 EHRA/HRS expert consensus statement on cardiac resynchronization therapy in heart failure: implant and follow-up recommendations and management. Heart Rhythm 2012;9(9):1524–1576.

2 Calò L, Martino A, de Ruvo E, Minati M, Fratini S, Rebecchi M, *et al.* Acute echocardiographic optimization of multiple stimulation configurations of cardiac resynchronization therapy through quadripolar left ventricular pacing: a tailored approach. Am Heart J 2014;167(4):546–554.

3 Gold MR, Birgersdotter-Green U, Singh JP, Ellenbogen KA, Yu Y, Meyer TE, *et al.* The relationship between ventricular electrical delay and left ventricular remodelling with cardiac resynchronization therapy. Eur Heart J 2011;32(20):2516–2524.

4 Khan FZ, Virdee MS, Palmer CR, Pugh PJ, O'Halloran D, Elsik M, *et al.* Targeted left ventricular lead placement to guide cardiac resynchronization therapy: the TARGET study – a randomized, controlled trial. J Am Coll Cardiol 2012;59(17):1509–1518.

5 Reynolds CR, Nikolski V, Sturdivant JL, Leman RB, Cuoco FA, Wharton JM, *et al.* Randomized comparison of defibrillation thresholds from the right ventricular apex and outflow tract. Heart Rhythm 2010;7(11):1561–1566.

6 Yin J, Hu H, Wang Y, Xue M, Li X, Cheng W, *et al.* Effects of atrioventricular nodal ablation on permanent atrial fibrillation patients with cardiac resynchronization therapy: a systematic review and meta-analysis. Clin Cardiol 2014;37(11):707–715.

9

How to Perform Sub-pectoral Device Implants

Gurjit Singh and Claudio Schuger

Cardiac Electrophysiology, Henry Ford Hospital, Detroit, MI, USA

Cardiac device generators have slowly scaled up from the abdominal wall to the left pectoral position since the inception of the technology. Pacemakers have traditionally been implanted in the pre-pectoral area because of their smaller sizes and, with the evolution of bipolar pacing and smaller pacemaker generators, interest in submuscular implant diminished further except for pediatric patients. Earlier abdominal internal cardioverter-defibrillator (ICD) implants were frequently positioned in submuscular locations, mainly for aesthetic reasons. With the advent of active ICD cans requiring pectoral implantation, submuscular placement of generators became the mainstream approach given the bulky size of earlier ICD systems. Since then, major advances in defibrillator technology, such as biphasic waveforms, smaller and more efficient battery systems, and marked reduction in capacitor sizes, have made possible much smaller generators, and so the need for submuscular implantation has reduced dramatically. Still, there exists a niche for this surgical technique for patients in whom even the current sized generator poses risks for erosion and skin necrosis, and sometimes for a better aesthetic result.

Various surgical techniques have been advanced in the last century mainly by cardiac surgeons in relation to this field. Use of general anesthesia was necessary in the early days because of the need for extensive dissection and the resultant pain. Implantation of pacemakers and defibrillators can now be safely performed in the electrophysiology laboratory under sedation or under general anesthesia with minimal additional tools. In a study of submuscular implants by Lipscomb *et al.* [1], 12 patients under general anesthesia were compared with 33 patients under local anesthesia which showed no major differences in patient perception or reported pain (Table 9.1).

Venous Access for Lead Placement

Venous access for sub-pectoral implantation is similar to the subcutaneous route. Some implanting physicians recommend obtaining venous access in the same plane as the pocket as there is a concern for increased lead stress while traversing the plane from superficial to deeper submuscular tissue. Typically, a submuscular pocket is created first after making the skin incision followed by venous access in the subcutaneous plane. Access via the subclavian, axillary, or cephalic vein is generally equally successful when using the sub-pectoral approach as with the subcutaneous approach.

Technique

Familiarity with the regional anatomy of the pectoral, clavicular, and axillary regions is essential prior to a device implantation. The implantation can be performed on the left or the right side, although the left-sided approach is preferable because of issues related to defibrillation efficacy. The key superficial areas to be identified at the outset are the clavicle, coracoid process, deltopectoral groove, deltoid muscle, and the pectoralis major muscle.

The pectoral region mainly consists of the pectoralis major and minor muscles in front of the rib cage surrounded inferiorly with the serratus anterior muscle and laterally by the latissimus dorsi muscle (Figure 9.1). The pectoralis major muscle is a fan-shaped muscle collection, which originates from three main regions: the clavicle, sternum, and the aponeurosis of the oblique abdominal muscle. The clavicular head arises from the medial half of the clavicle and fans out laterally into

How-to Manual for Pacemaker and ICD Devices: Procedures and Programming, First Edition. Edited by Amin Al-Ahmad, Andrea Natale, Paul J. Wang, James P. Daubert, and Luigi Padeletti.
© 2018 John Wiley & Sons, Inc. Published 2018 by John Wiley & Sons, Inc.
Companion website: www.wiley.com/go/al-ahmad/pacemakers_and_icds

Table 9.1 Benefits and risks of sub-pectoral device implants.

Indications for sub-pectoral implant
1) Scarce subcutaneous tissue
2) History of prior erosion
3) Cosmetic reasons
4) Pediatric implants
5) Prior infection and significant subcutaneous tissue debridement and contraindication for implant on contralateral site
6) Twiddler's syndrome

Benefits of submuscular implant
1) Enhanced cosmesis
2) Lesser lead dislodgement rate
3) Lesser Twiddler's syndrome
4) Lower erosion rate

Complications or disadvantages of sub-pectoral implant approach
1) Increased bleeding risk and hematoma formation
2) Possible disruption of pectoral muscle function
3) Increased risk of lead fracture
4) Difficulty during generator replacement
5) Issue with lateral migration into the axilla
6) Greater postoperative pain

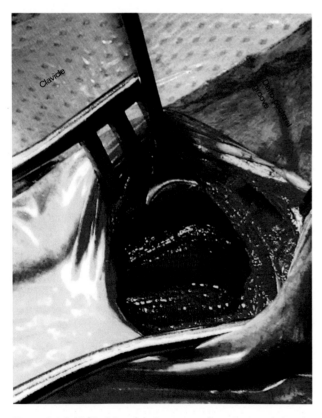

Figure 9.1 Initial incision showing pectoralis major muscle heads and relationship to clavicle, deltopectoral groove, and sternum in a left side implant.

the lamina of a two-layered tendon. The sternocostal bundle arises from sternum and upper six costal cartilages which runs laterally to form the rounded anterior axillary fold. All these muscle bundles eventually conglomerate toward the axilla to insert into the bicipital groove of the humerus. There is a clear plane between the sternal head and clavicular head which can be separated to create a pocket. The clavipectoral fascia is a layer of fascial tissue lying under the pectoralis major muscle. In its superior margin, it splits to enclose the subclavius muscle and laterally it forms a thick bundle to join the coracoid process of the scapula. When traced inferiorly, it splits to enclose the pectoralis minor muscle. The axillary artery and brachial plexus run deep in the axilla underneath the clavipectoral fascia. The anterior wall of the axilla is formed by the clavipectoral fascia and the pectoralis muscle. Underneath the pectoralis major muscle lies the smaller pectoralis minor muscle, originating from the third, fourth, and fifth rib surface and inserting into the coracoid process of the scapula. The cephalic vein, throacoacromial artery, and the lateral pectoral nerve emerge from the clavipectoral fascia between the clavicle and upper border of pectoralis minor muscle. Pectoral muscles obtain their nerve supply from medial and lateral pectoral nerves which arise from the medal and lateral chords of the brachial plexus. The medial pectoral nerve travels inferiorly under the clavicle and under the pectoralis minor muscle. A distal branch of this nerve pierces through the pectoralis minor muscle and supplies the lower portion of the pectoralis major muscle. The lateral pectoral nerve arising from the lateral chord of brachial plexus runs under the pectoral major muscle inferiorly and innervates the majority of the pectoralis major muscle. Damage to the lateral pectoral or medial pectoral nerve can result in complete atrophy of the pectoralis muscle group.

The plane between the pectoralis major and minor muscle provides an excellent entry point to create the submuscular pocket using various incision techniques, including anterior sub-pectoral, lateral, anterior axillary, and infra-mammary approaches.

Anterior Sub-pectoral Approach

This is the most widely accepted and straightforward technique. The patient is draped and prepped as for the subcutaneous approach. The arm on the side of implant is kept by the side without any abduction. A straight incision is made 3 cm below the clavicle starting in the mid clavicular line and extended laterally to end in the deltopectoral groove. Dissection is carried out using electrocautery and blunt methods with the subcutaneous tissue being held taut by a Weitlaner retractor. The subcutaneous tissue and fat is dissected until the pre-pectoral fascia is visualized. Then the fascia is dissected to expose the pectoralis major muscle where

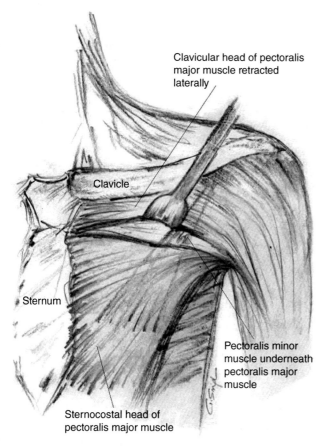

Figure 9.2 Anterior sub-pectoral approach. The clavicular head of pectoralis major is retracted up and laterally to expose the pectoralis minor muscle and a pocket is created medially underneath the pectoralis major.

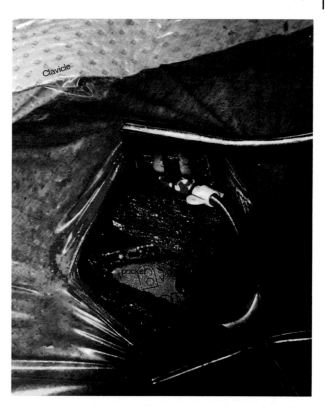

Figure 9.3 Pacemaker implant in sub-pectoral pocket using anterior approach underneath the two muscle heads of pectoralis major muscle.

a fibrofatty band is visualized demarcating the sternal and clavicular portions of the muscle (Figure 9.2). The two portions of the pectoralis major muscle can then be separated using blunt dissection with the aid of Metzenbaum scissors or curved artery forceps. At this point, gentle separation of the two heads can be continued by inserting a finger and running from side to side in an arc fashion. Extreme caution should be exercised while handling the muscle tissue as the bleeders are sometimes hard to control despite using cautery with resultant risk of hematoma formation. Creating a pocket between the two heads is usually straightforward as there is no major resistance, unlike creating a pocket in a subcutaneous fashion. The clavicular head usually overlaps the sternal head for few centimeters and initial dissection requires an upward sweep under the clavicular head to create a plane. Thereafter, the plane can be extended under the sternal portion of the muscle by flexing the fingers in the inferior direction. Again, extreme care must be taken not to damage the thoracoacromial neurovascular bundle which lies in front of the pectoralis minor muscle. The leads are connected to the pulse generator and the generator is

housed in the pocket after performing an antibiotic wash. It is recommended that the pulse generator is secured to underlying tissues with a non-absorbable No. 0 suture. Once the generator is placed in the pocket, the two muscle heads are apposed to each other using interrupted vicryl sutures (Figure 9.3). The wound is then closed using the standard three-layer technique.

Lateral Sub-pectoral Approach

This technique is similar to the anterior sub-pectoral approach except for the initial skin incision and retraction of the clavicular head of the pectoralis major muscle. The initial skin incision is made in the deltopectoral groove a few centimeters below the clavicle. With a Weitlaner retractor and electrocautery, the incision is deepened until the pectoralis major muscle is visualized. The pectoral fascia is then incised and the pectoralis major and deltoid relationship is explored. At this point, the lateral border of the clavicular portion of the pectoralis major muscle is retracted in an inferomedial direction and a submuscular plane is created by blunt dissection using the fingers (Figure 9.4). The pocket is created in the inferomedial direction and usually requires more dissection medially to avoid lateral migration and interference of the pulse generator in the axilla.

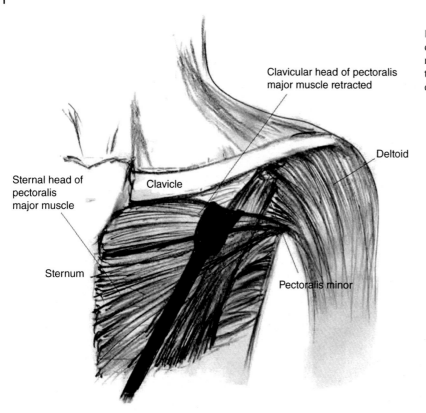

Figure 9.4 Lateral sub-pectoral approach. The clavicular head of pectoralis major muscle is retracted medially and downwards to expose the pectoralis minor muscle and dissection is carried out under the pectoralis major.

Lateral Anterior Axillary Approach

This technique can be further divided into single and double incision techniques.

Single Incision Technique

The patient is prepped and draped in a supine position with the arm abducted away. Careful and meticulous sterile preparation of the axilla is required for the axillary approach. After infiltrating the skin with local anesthetic, an incision is made more or less vertically in the anterior axillary line along the lateral border of pectoralis major muscle. The incision is deepened until the muscle is visualized and dissection is carried out behind the pectoralis major muscle in the axilla. The lateral border of pectoralis major muscle is retracted medially to visualize the structures underneath (Figure 9.5). A plane is created between the pectoralis major and minor muscle and blunt dissection is carried out medially to create a pocket. Careful attention should be paid to control muscle bleeders as perforating arteries typically run under the pectoralis major belly. Contrast venography is typically recommended for this technique as venous access is in the same plane under the pectoralis major muscle. The axillary or subclavian vein access is obtained using an extra-long needle. After the pulse generator is placed

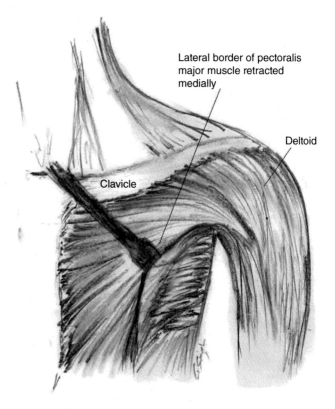

Figure 9.5 Anterior axillary approach. The lateral border of pectoralis major muscle is retracted medially and a dissection plane is created in the anterior axillary fold.

in the pocket, the lateral ends of the anterior axillary soft tissue are approximated to the pectoralis major muscle using interrupted sutures. Care should be taken to prevent suturing of the pectoralis major and minor muscle together, which will otherwise limit upper extremity movements.

Another single incision sub-pectoral technique has been described by Hammel *et al.* [2], where the initial skin incision is made parallel and medial to the deltopectral groove. Venous access is obtained as per usual in the pre-pectoral plane then the submuscular pocket is created by dividing the pectoralis major muscle fibers along the fiber direction 2–3 cm below the deltopectoral sulcus. Using blunt dissection, a plane is created between the pectoralis major muscle and the chest wall to create the submuscular pocket.

Double Incision Technique

This technique, as first described by Foster [3], requires two separate incisions for venous access and the subpectoral pocket. The patient is positioned supine in the usual fashion with arm abducted. A small 2–3 cm incision is first made parallel and inferior to the clavicle at the junction of the medial and lateral third of the clavicle. The incision is deepened by dissection until prepectoral fascia is visualized. Access to the subclavian or axillary vein is then obtained by the usual technique and leads are advanced into the respective chambers under fluoroscopy. The leads are anchored to the underlying fascia and muscle using non-absorbable sutures. A vertical 5–7 cm incision is made along the anterior axillary line behind the lateral end of the pectoralis major muscle. Dissection is carried deep until the pectoralis major muscle is visualized. Then an attempt to locate the plane between the pectoralis major and minor muscle is made and a pocket created by blunt dissection.

Another method of dividing the posterior attachments of the serratus anterior muscle to the ribs (lateral to the pectoralis major muscle border) has been proposed as this allows excellent approximation of the fascial layer of the serratus to the pectoralis major to avoid generator migration into the axilla. After division of the serratus muscle, the anterior surface of the intercostal fascia is followed into the subpectoral space. After the pocket is created, the leads are tunneled into this pocket using various tunneling methods. The wounds are then closed in the usual fashion. Again, it is recommended to anchor the pulse generator to the underlying tissue to prevent migration and leads should not be coiled under the generator to avoid can abrasions against the bony rib cage. The benefit of axillary incision is the possibility it affords of placing a subcutaneous patch or coil in case of elevated defibrillation thresholds should the need arise.

Infra-mammary Implantation

The infra-mammary approach usually requires two incisions, one for the venous access for lead placement and other one for the generator. A 5–7 cm skin incision is made 5 cm inferior to the areolar complex in males and in the breast fold crease in females. The incision is extended down to the pre-pectoral fascia. The inferolateral margin of the pectoralis major muscle is identified and retracted medially to define the plane between the major and minor muscle. Sometimes, muscle dissection using electrocautery is required to dissect the lateral attachments of pectoralis major and serratus anterior muscle. A pocket is then formed to accommodate the device can. The leads are tunneled into the pocket using a 24 Fr chest tube as a tunneling device.

Another technique using a 20 cm pericardiocentesis needle has been proposed by Roelke *et al.* where the needle is directed towards the superior subclavicular incision. A J guide wire is passed and the needle is removed. Using the retained guide wire technique, two 10 Fr introducer dilators are positioned through which the leads are brought into the submuscular pocket.

Comparison of Subcutaneous and Sub-pectoral Implants

The largest study to date assessing the complication rates between subcutaneous and sub-pectoral implants came from the Worldwide Jewel Investigators in which 604 subcutaneous implants were compared with 396 subpectoral implants. The investigators found shorter procedure times and more lead dislodgements for the subcutaneous approach but, interestingly, more pocket erosions with the submusclar approach. Erosions in the submuscular group was a surprising finding and the authors explained it as a likely selection bias with patients weighing less and having smaller body surface area. Overall, there were no major differences in the cumulative freedom from complications between the two groups (4.1% vs. 2.5%; p = 0.1836) [4].

There is a theoretical concern about increased lead stress using the submuscular approach as the lead usually bends around the muscle and then courses deep across the muscles which can cause issues by repeated stress imposed by muscle contraction. In a study by Bernstein *et al.* [5] analyzing the predictors of failure for Medtronic Sprint Fidelis leads, submuscular implantation was a significant predictor on both univariate and multivariate analysis, raising the risk of lead fracture by 14-fold.

Defibrillation Threshold and Efficacy

The impact of submuscular versus subcutaneous position of pulse generator using "active" can configuration has been studied by Iskos *et al.* [6] when they compared 20 patients who underwent sub-pectoral implant with 46 patients with subcutaneous implants. They found a small 3–4 ohm impedance difference in the high voltage defibrillation pathway among the two groups (higher impedance in the subcutaneous group). No major differences in the energy required for successful defibrillation were noted based on the anatomic location of the active can (9.9 ± 3.8 vs. 7.4 ± 3.3 J; $p = 0.057$) [6].

Generator Replacement

Because of the submuscular nature of the generator, generator replacement can pose significant impediment requiring extensive dissection and electrocautery to relieve the generator. Moreover, there is always a concern for significant muscle bleeding during dissection if proper attention to detail is not practiced. Similar attention should be paid during dissection to avoid damage to the lateral pectoral nerve and arterial structures. No major study has compared the outcomes after generator replacement in the submuscular position with the subcutaneous location. Experience with sub-pectoral implants has been published by Kistler *et al.* [7] in which no major issues were encountered during generator replacements for pacemakers in the sub-pectoral position.

Conclusions

Implantation of cardiac devices has become a routine procedure in cardiac electrophysiology laboratories predominantly utilizing a subcutaneous pre-pectoral approach. Miniaturization of generator cans has led to a decline in the use of the sub-pectoral approach, but occasionally one will encounter a situation where lack of significant subcutaneous tissue or need for better cosmesis will require sub-pectoral implantation. Device implantation in the submuscular position can be accomplished in several ways, with the anterior approach being the easiest and most straightforward. Overall, no significant long-term issues have been reported with submuscular techniques except for a requirement for significant dissection during generator replacement.

References

1 Lipscomb KJ, Linker NJ, Fitzpatrick AP. Subpectoral implantation of a cardioverter defibrillator under local anaesthesia. Heart 1998;79(3):253–255.

2 Hammel D, Block M, Geiger A, Bocker D, Stadlbauer T, Breithardt G, *et al.* Single-incision implantation of cardioverter defibrillators using nonthoracotomy lead systems. Ann Thorac Surg 1994;58(6):1614–1616.

3 Foster AH. Technique for implantation of cardioverter defibrillators in the subpectoral position. Ann Thorac Surg 1995;59(3):764–767.

4 Gold MR, Peters RW, Johnson JW, Shorofsky SR. Complications associated with pectoral cardioverter-defibrillator implantation: comparison of subcutaneous and submuscular approaches. Worldwide Jewel Investigators. J Am Coll Cardiol 1996;28(5):1278–1282.

5 Bernstein NE, Karam ET, Aizer A, Wong BC, Holmes DS, Bernstein SA, *et al.* Right-sided implantation and subpectoral position are predisposing factors for fracture of a 6.6 French ICD lead. Pacing Clin Electrophysiol 2012;35(6):659–664.

6 Iskos D, Lock K, Lurie KG, Fahy GJ, Petersen-Stejskal S, Benditt DG. Submuscular versus subcutaneous pectoral implantation of cardioverter-defibrillators: effect on high voltage pathway impedance and defibrillation efficacy. J Interv Card Electrophysiol 1998;2(1):47–52.

7 Kistler PM, Fynn SP, Mond HG, Eizenberg N. The subpectoral pacemaker implant: it isn't what it seems! Pacing Clin Electrophysiol 2004;27(3):361–364.

10

Device Extractions

Sean D. Pokorney[1], Donald D. Hegland[1], and Patrick M. Hranitzky[2,3]

[1] *Duke University Medical Center, Durham, NC, USA*
[2] *Texas Cardiac Arrhythmia, Austin, TX, USA*
[3] *WakeMed Heart and Vascular Center, Raleigh, NC, USA*

Background

Implantation rates of pacemakers and implantable cardioverter-defibrillators (ICDs) have increased over time [1]. Unfortunately, the infection rate with cardiovascular implantable electronic devices (CIEDs) has also increased over time because of device implantation in older patients with more comorbidities. The incidence of device related infections is approximately 2–3% [1,2]. The combination of more devices implanted with higher infection rates has driven an increased need for lead removal.

Scar tissue can develop around the lead over time based on a patient's fibrotic response to the lead. Leads that are removed with simple traction and without advanced techniques are known as lead explants, and these are most typically leads with a dwell time of less than 1 year [3]. Leads with dwell times of greater than 1 year or leads with more extensive scar tissue even within 1 year of implantation may require advanced extraction techniques with the use of locking stylets, femoral snares, cutting tools, telescoping sheaths, and laser sheaths for extraction; these techniques constitute lead extraction [3]. Locking stylet and laser extraction sheath assisted procedures result in high complete procedural success rates of 90–97%; the intra-procedural mortality is as low as 0.3%, although risk of in-hospital mortality may be as high as 2.2% with an approximately 2% risk of major complications [4–7]. At high volume centers, lead extraction safety has improved over time, and the procedure has even been shown to be safe in patients over the age of 80 [6,8,9].

The decision to pursue lead removal must be individualized. The Telectronics Accufix fixed atrial J lead was associated with a risk of lead fracture that could cause atrial laceration, but periprocedural mortality with extraction was 0.4%, so widespread extraction of the lead likely increased mortality relative to a strategy of no extraction [10]. In the case of lead failure, the alternative to lead extraction is taking a "cap and abandon" strategy by placing a lead end-cap cover over the end of the lead, securing the lead end-cap with non-absorbable suture, and implanting a new lead to be connected to the generator to take over the function of the capped and abandoned lead. The quantitative risk of capping a lead is difficult to determine, but extraction has been shown to result in lower rates of long-term device infections, relative to capping and abandoning [11]. Patient-specific factors and individual patient wishes are important for lead mangement decision-making. The REPLACE registry evaluated the procedural complication rates associated with pacemaker or ICD replacement procedures with the addition of a new lead, and reported an 11% major complication rate among patients who underwent a revision of a non-cardiac resynchronization system [12].

The numbers of major adverse events in published analyses of lead extraction are relatively small. In the Lead Extraction in the Contemporary Setting (LExICon) Study, there were only 20 major adverse events, and body mass index of less than $25\,kg/m^2$ was the only patient characteristic that was associated with higher major adverse event rates [6]. A separate study with 32 major adverse events identified female sex as the only patient characteristic associated with higher major adverse event rates [5]. One study of 2176 extracted ICD leads (82% dual coil) showed that extractions of dual coil ICD leads were associated with a higher risk of major complications than single coil leads [13]. Another extraction study of 1385 ICD leads (67% dual coil) found that dual coil, relative to single coil, ICD leads were associated

How-to Manual for Pacemaker and ICD Devices: Procedures and Programming, First Edition. Edited by Amin Al-Ahmad, Andrea Natale, Paul J. Wang, James P. Daubert, and Luigi Padeletti.
© 2018 John Wiley & Sons, Inc. Published 2018 by John Wiley & Sons, Inc.
Companion website: www.wiley.com/go/al-ahmad/pacemakers_and_icds

with higher 30-day all-cause mortality (approximately 4% vs. 2%, adjusted odds ratio [OR] 2.7; 95% confidence interval [CI] 1.6–4.5; p < 0.001) [7]. This retrospective analysis had 54 major adverse events and a multivariable model identified the following characteristics as being associated with major adverse events: history of cerebrovascular disease (adjusted OR 2.2; 95% CI 1.1–4.4), ejection fraction of 15% or less (adjusted OR 2.0; 95% CI 1.1–5.0), lower platelet count with a mean in patients with an event versus no event of 178 000 versus 197 000 (adjusted OR 1.7; 95% CI 1.0–2.5), international normalized ratio (INR) ≥1.2 (adjusted OR 2.7; 95% CI 1.2–5.7), and the use of mechanical (dilator or telescoping sheaths: adjusted OR 3.4; 95% CI 1.9–6.2) or powered sheaths (Excimer Laser Sheath, Spectranetics, Colorado Springs, CO; Evolution Mechanical Dilator Sheath, Cook Medical, Bloomington, IN;, and Perfecta Electrosurgical Dissection Sheath: adjusted OR 2.3; 95% CI 1.1–4.9) [7]. However, the sample size is too low to develop a predictive model of major adverse events with all of the relevant variables in the setting of these low event rates. For example, older age is associated with higher adverse event rates, and a history of prior sternotomy is associated with lower risk of extraction-related major adverse events.

Indications

Pocket infection, infective endocarditis, and occult gram-positive bacteremia are all class I indications for complete device and lead removal (Table 10.1) [3]. Patients with bacteremia or infective endocarditis should have imaging performed to assess for the presence and size of a lead-related vegetation. Given that vegetations can embolize during percutaneous lead removal causing septic emboli, there has been some consideration for open lead removal in patients with lead-related vegetations >2 cm [14]. That said, both an AHA Scientific Statement and a HRS Consensus Statement report that decisions to percutaneously remove leads with vegetations >2 cm should be individualized, as there is no specific size cutoff rule mandating open surgical removal, and in many circumstances the risks associated with thoracotomy or sternotomy may be greater than the risks associated with septic emboli during percutaneous extraction in a patient with active endocarditis [2,3].

Device infections are the most common reason for lead removal, while the second most common reason is lead failure. Non-functioning leads are a class IIa indication for removal (Table 10.1). Reports of ICD lead failure rates vary, but have been reported to be as high as 10% at 2 years, 15% at 5 years, and 40% at 8 years, although these failure rates have declined substantially in most currently utilized ICD

Table 10.1 Indications for lead extraction.

Indication for extraction	Class	Level of evidence
Infection		
Infective endocarditis	I	B
Pocket infection	I	B
Occult gram-positive bacteremia	I	B
Persistent occult gram-negative bacteremia	IIa	B
Superficial or incision infection	III	C
Non-CIED source bacteremia and plan for suppressive antibiotics	III	C
Refractory chronic pain	IIa	C
Thrombus/venous stasis		
Lead thrombus and clinically significant thromboembolic events	I	C
Planned stent procedure that would entrap a lead	I	C
SVC stenosis with symptoms	I	C
Need for additional lead, venous occlusion, and contraindication to contralateral vein access	I	C
Bilateral subclavian or SVC occlusion	I	C
Need for additional lead, venous occlusion, and no contraindication to contralateral vein access	IIa	C
Lead-related indications		
Life-threatening arrhythmia or immediate threat from a lead	I	B
Lead interferes with the function of the CIED	I	B
Leads that interfere with malignancy treatment	IIa	C
Abandoned functional lead may interfere with CIED	II*	C
Leads not being used or that are potential future threats	II*	C
Non-functioning lead with >4 leads on 1 side or >5 through SVC	IIa	IIa
To facilitate access to MRI	IIb	C
Non-functioning leads at time of other CIED procedure	IIb	C
Anomalous placement of leads	III	C
Functional, redundant leads with <1 year life expectancy	III	C

CIED, cardiac implantable electronic device; SVC, superior vena cava.
* IIa for non-functional leads and IIb for functional leads.

lead designs [15]. Historically, 56% of lead failures have been caused by insulation defects, but lead failure as a result of the conductor component of the ICD lead has also been problematic, as was the case with the Medtronic Sprint Fidelis 6949 lead [15]. Classically, insulation failure presents as a drop in lead impedance. Exposed conductor elements that result from insulation failure are at increased risk of electrical failure, which can manifest as over-sensing, under-sensing, elevated pacing thresholds, increased pacing impedance, or creation of an electrical short circuit that prevents the delivery of high voltage tachytherapy. Leads with higher than expected rates of lead failure may be placed under a lead advisory, and advisory leads are a cause of concern for patients and have a negative impact on patients' quality of life even if they are not among those experiencing direct morbidity or mortality from the advisory lead's performance. Extraction of an electrically normal ICD or pacemaker lead that is under advisory has a class IIb indication for removing these functioning leads that are at risk for causing future harm.

Qualifications

To be qualified to extract ICD or pacemaker leads, the HRS Consensus Statement from 2009 recommends that the extracting physician be the primary extraction operator for at least 40 leads under the supervision of a physician who has performed at least 75 extractions [3]. After the initial 40 leads, extracting physicians should perform at least 20 extractions per year in order to maintain their skillset. Transesophageal echocardiography needs to be available during the extraction procedure. The extraction procedures can be performed in an operating room or in the electrophysiology laboratory, as long as high quality fluoroscopy is available and a cardiothoracic surgeon, perfusionist, and a cardiopulmonary bypass machine are available to allow a patient to rapidly undergo emergent sternotomy with cardiopulmonary bypass in the event of a complication such as a tear of the superior vena cava, cardiac avulsion, or cardiac perforation. The cardiothoracic surgeon should be familiar with the patient and the type of complication injuries that are seen in lead extraction, as well as the necessary repair for these injuries.

Preparation for Device Extraction

As with any procedure, history, physical exam, and informed consent are all important. Given that there is variation in adverse events by center and device extraction volume, it is important to quote your hospital's procedural outcomes, including sternotomy risk, procedure-related mortality and 30-day mortality rates, risk of cardiac or vascular injury requiring surgical repair, and alternatives to lead extraction (capping and abandon with lead failure, suppressive antibiotics for infection, and open surgical extraction). The cardiothoracic surgeon and the anesthesia team should also perform a history and physical exam, including exploration of vascular access options (exclude the presence of vascular access ports, dialysis grafts, dialysis fistulas, or dialysis access catheters), so that the entire procedural team knows that patient's characteristics in the event of a complication. A pre-procedure device interrogation is also critical to understand whether the patient is pacemaker dependent and will require a temporary pacemaker at the time of the procedure.

Likewise, a pre-procedure chest X-ray is important to exclude the presence of abandoned hardware that may otherwise have been unknown to the extracting physician and to rapidly identify lead characteristics to confirm that they match with the reported model numbers in the patient medical record (e.g., active fixation versus passive fixation mechanisms and single coil versus dual coil ICD leads). The pre-procedure postero-anterior and lateral chest X-rays will also be useful in: (i) clarifying lead position (including exclusion of an inadvertent arterial lead placement, providing insight on vascular access angles and approaches used at implant, and following the course of the leads to exclude anomalous vasculature such as a persistent left superior vena cava); (ii) evaluating for conductor fracture; (iii) assessing for conductor cable externalization; and (iv) evaluating for evidence of previous failed extraction attempts that might increase the difficulty of the currently planned procedure (e.g., identifying an abandoned lead that appears pulled or stretched out of position, identifying high voltage coils that have separated because of a previous attempt at pulling on the lead that was unsuccessful in removing the lead).

An important part of the history and device interrogation is identification of the number of leads, characteristics of leads, and dwell time of all leads in situ, including abandoned leads. These characteristics need to be known for all leads, not just leads being targeted for extraction, as sometimes a non-targeted lead may be inadvertently disrupted during the extraction procedure and may need to be removed and replaced, or a non-targeted lead may need to be removed to allow for removal of the targeted lead. Once the lead vendor and model numbers have been identified, there are several resources to help describe the lead fixation mechanism, the lead diameter, the number of coils, the coating or backfilling around the coils, and the recommended laser sheath size [16].

Pre-procedure laboratory tests should include a complete blood count, complete metabolic panel, prothrombin time (PT)/INR, and partial thromboplastin time (PTT). Patients should have an active type and cross in place, and consideration should be given to having packed red blood cells in the procedure room, available for immediate transfusion. Oral anticoagulants and anti-platelet agents such as P2Y12 inhibitors should be held prior to the procedure for a period of time sufficient to allow the effect of that medication to dissipate (e.g., holding clopidogrel for 5 days, holding factor Xa inhibitors for at least 2 days, and holding warfarin until the INR is <1.5).

An electrocardiogram is needed prior the procedure. If the patient has an underlying left bundle branch block, there is a chance that right bundle branch conduction may be interrupted by mechanical contact force during the extraction of a right ventricular lead, so the operator may consider placing a temporary pacing wire at the start of the procedure or have a temporary wire accessible in the event of complete heart block during extraction.

An echocardiogram is needed before the procedure to determine the presence of valvular lesions, tricuspid regurgitation, a baseline pericardial effusion, right heart function and pulmonary pressures, exclusion of a high burden of thrombus on the lead, exclusion of a patent foramen ovale or atrial septal defect that could result in paradoxical embolism during lead extraction, and ejection fraction. Transthoracic and transesophageal echocardiograms may be useful to identify and charac-terize vegetations in bacteremia or endocarditis. The use of pre-extraction chest computed tomography (CT) may help to identify patients with lead perforations and lead adherence to venous or cardiac structures (Figure 10.1), as there are data to indicate that these patients have longer procedure times and are at higher risk for compli-cations [17]. In patients at risk for underlying coronary artery disease, it is reasonable to consider pre-procedure coronary angiography by either cardiac catheterization or coronary CT angiography, so that the cardiothoracic surgeon knows the coronary anatomy and/or previous coronary artery bypass anatomy (such as the status of vein grafts and the left internal mammary artery) in case the patient has to undergo sternotomy. These modalities of pre-procedural imaging assist with anticipating diffi-culties, procedural planning, and assessing risks of the procedure, risks of sedation, and risks and challenges of possible sternotomy rescue if needed.

Lead Extraction Procedure

Before starting the procedure, desired brady pacing parameters can be chosen (e.g., VVI 40 for a patient with no pacing indication or DOO 70 for a patient who is pacemaker dependent) and tachytherapies disabled to prevent inappropriate shocks resulting from noise from electroacautery. Confirm that all of the necessary supplies

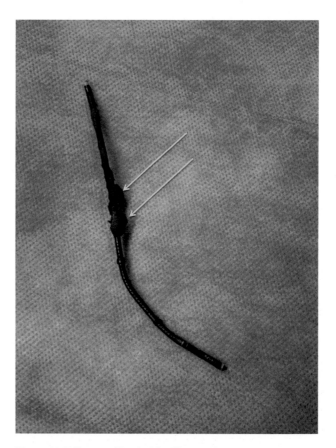

Figure 10.1 Extracted lead with adherent tissue.

are in place and readily available for the procedure itself, as well as for sternotomy in the event of a complication. Patients will need to be clipped and prepped from bilat-eral femoral regions to the bilateral clavicles to allow femoral vascular access, device pocket access, and allow sternotomy if needed for rescue. Although the cardio-thoracic anesthesiologist may elect to place an internal jugular triple lumen vascular access catheter in addition to a radial arterial line and Foley catheter, there should also be consideration of placing femoral venous access for the purpose of delivering blood in the event of a supe-rior vena cava (SVC) laceration, or for placement of a temporary pacing wire, snare, or SVC occlusion balloon as a bridge to SVC repair if needed, as well as femoral arterial access for the purpose of peripheral bypass in the event of any difficulty with median sternotomy. For example, this may be of particular importance for patients with a history of prior sternotomy. Femoral vas-cular access can be minimized (e.g., utilizing 4 Fr "micro-puncture" sheaths for the femoral vein and femoral artery) in hopes of minimizing the risks of vascular access and decreasing sheath pull times, but these small sheaths still facilitate rapid upsizing for peripheral bypass cannulas. Femoral cut-down with direct visualization for placement of peripheral bypass cannulas can also be used. The approach to femoral vascular access should be individualized for the patient's and cardiothoracic surgeon's needs. An arterial line is needed for accurate hemodynamic monitoring during the procedure. Packed red blood cells (4 units) should be rapidly available if not in the room in case of a complication and cell saver technology should be immediately available. It may be useful to cine the heart borders and costophrenic angles prior to starting the case, and these images can serve as a reference during the case to evaluate for pericardial effusion and hemothorax, respectively.

When accessing the pacemaker or ICD pocket, it is important to make the incision long enough (remembering scar tissue contracts and therefore the extraction incision will usually need to be longer than the scar from the device implant) and high enough to provide an angle of approach parallel to (or slightly above) the access of the axillary/subclavian vein but still close enough to the device generator to allow its retrieval, as well as access to the sewing rings. Extracting from below the venotomy site makes it difficult to remain coaxial with the extraction tools. When approaching the device and leads with electrocautery, consideration may be given to dissection along the plane of the capsule to removed the entire generator and leads as a unit and to facilitate performance of a full capsulectomy. The degree of scar tissue and calcification in the pocket can be instructive, as to the burden and composition of scar and adhesions around the leads.

At the point where the leads enter the pectoralis muscle, it is often helpful to place slight traction on the lead to be extracted and advance the electrocautery in "coagulation" mode along the lead to free it through the pectoralis muscle. A prevascular fat-pad can be seen once the dissection plane is through the pectoralis muscle, prior to approaching the central venous vasculature. With creation of this dissection plane using electrocautery, the index finger can also be advanced over the lead to bluntly dissect in this region. The idea is to create open space to prevent the need for the extraction sheath to follow any unnecessary contours when these points can be opened with pectoral dissection.

In preparing the leads, it is important to carry out the procedure in the same way in every case, so that all steps are performed in the proper order and without skipping steps. First, leads need to be dissected and freed down to their sewing rings. Caution should be used to minimize lead traction that might disrupt the integrity of the leads targeted for extraction, as well as minimizing electrocautery and traction over leads that are to be retained. This is especially the case for left ventricular leads, which are often the most fragile and most difficult to replace. It is important to remember that electrocautery can melt the silicone, polyurethane-like compounds can split, and simple traction can dislodge leads.

After cutting and removing the sutures over the sewing rings on leads to be extracted, the sewing rings should be withdrawn to the maximal extent outside the pocket, so that the sewing rings removed when the leads are cut and not at risk for being forgotten and pushed into the central venous vasculature by the extraction sheath (remember there may be more than one sewing ring on some leads). Next, insert the clearing stylet in an attempt to clear any debris in the lumen of the lead. If the clearing stylet will not advance, attempt to place the lead under gentle traction, while withdrawing and advancing the clearing stylet in an attempt to bypass the obstruction. If the lead lumen cannot be cleared as a result of blood or infectious material in the lumen, wipe the clearing stylet with a wet saline gauze, reattempt inserting the clearing stylet as close to the tip of the lead as possible.

If the lead is an active fixation lead, use the fixation screw clip or hemostat to attempt to retract the screw. Leave the clearing stylet in place when attempting to retract the fixation screw, as this improves the delivery of torque to the fixation screw and helps to maintain the luminal integrity. Fluoroscopy may be helpful in determining whether the fixation screw retracts. It is important not to over-retract the fixation mechanism to the point that the mechanism breaks, as this may compromise lead integrity. Most modern ICD and pacemaker leads can have their rotation mechanism turned counterclockwise approximately 15–20 rotations without breaking. If there is spin-back on the pin with removal of the rotation tool, then the fixation mechanism is likely still intact, but if there is no spin-back, then the fixation mechanism is likely fractured.

After the clearing stylet is removed, the lead can then be cut with heavy scissors below the region of the connection portion of the lead, making sure to leave at least 5 cm of lead beyond the point where the lead enters the pectoral muscle. Approximately 2–3 cm of outer insulation should be removed from the cut end of the lead by cutting circumferentially with a No. 15 blade and applying manual traction on the outer insulation. For pacing leads, conductor cables beyond those wrapping the central lumen can be unwound and cut off with heavy scissors. For ICD leads, the high voltage cables can be knotted together. Next, the locking stylet can be placed in position. Confirm with fluoroscopy that the locking stylet is advanced all the way to the lead tip. If the locking stylet does not advance to the lead tip, apply gentle traction to the lead with alternating advancement and retraction to get the locking stylet as close to the lead tip as possible. The locking stylet should at least be able advance to the furthest point achieved by the clearing stylet. If the locking stylet cannot be advanced to the tip of the lead, consideration can be given to using a different, usually smaller, locking stylet to try to get to the lead tip. In general, it is better to have a less robust locking stylet get all the way to the tip than a more "heavy duty" locking stylet that cannot reach the lead tip. When the locking stylet is in the best achievable position, the locking stylet fixation mechanism should be deployed. For locking stylets with the ability to be retracted, assure familiarity with the retraction process so that the locking stylet is not inadvertently retracted during the extraction procedure.

If the lead is active fixation and the screw did not retract initially, a hemostat can be placed over the central conducting cables with a locking stylet in place and about 5–7 counterclockwise turns can be attempted under fluoroscopy in order to determine whether the fixation screw retracts. Rotating beyond 5–7 turns could result in compromising lead integrity and/or introducing kinks and twists into the lead.

After deploying the locking stylet fixation mechanism, a high tensile strength suture, such as Ticron, can be tied over the outer insulation about 1–2 cm from where the outer insulation was cut. The knot should be tight enough to see indentation into the outer insulation, but excess bulk to the knot should be minimized to avoid difficulty in passing the extraction sheath over the knot. Next, place three half hitches over the outer insulation between the knot and the location of the cut insulation. If the lead is a high voltage lead, an additional high tensile strength suture can be placed between the knotted high voltage cables; the suture can be tied approximately 1 cm from the knot of voltage cables with three half hitches placed between the suture knot and the knot in the high voltage cables.

Alternative lead preparations include using: (i) a fixation device called a Bulldog™ or (ii) a locking stylet only with no fixation over the outer insulation. Although many leads can be extracted without the time and effort it takes to secure the outer insulation and/or the high voltage cables, the operator must decide, based on their approach and patient characteristics, what lead preparation measures are needed. In the event of an externalized conductor, such as with a Riata lead (Figure 10.2), the high voltage cables can be tested with traction individually under fluoroscopy to identify which cable is externalized. High voltage cables that are externalized can be knotted together and secured with a high tensile strength tie that is separate from the other secured components of the lead.

There are several tools that can be used to facilitate safe extraction (Table 10.2). When using a laser sheath or a mechanical sheath, the operator's body position and weight balance are important in order to avoid unwanted forward movement of the extraction sheaths. Fluoroscopy angles should be varied as needed to ensure that the extraction sheaths are remaining coaxial. There needs to be adequate traction (pull) on the leads along with the

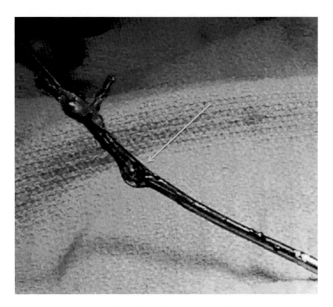

Figure 10.2 Riata lead with conductor externalization.

countertraction (push) forward of the sheaths in order to allow the extraction sheath to follow the "rail" that is created by the traction on the lead. If an appropriate amount of traction on the lead and push on the extraction device repeatedly does not result in advancement of the sheath over the locking stylet, then consider the possible reasons:

- Not coaxial
- "Snowplowing"
- Ineffective deliver of force because of binding or friction under the clavicle
- Calcification.

Use fluoroscopy to watch for movement of surrounding structures when operating the laser extraction sheath. If there is insulation snowplow or lead on lead binding, the outer sheath may be advanced over the laser sheath to break up these binding sites or create space for the laser to advance. If this is unsuccessful, the laser sheath may need to be upsized or if entering a region of high risk, such as the SVC, then a switch to the more flexible TightRail may be helpful. If there is calcification, a mechanical cutting sheath or TightRail may be needed. It is important to avoid getting the extraction sheath stuck on the lead or creating a situation in which excessive forward force begins to create a channel through the visceral structure rather than staying along the course of the lead. In either case, it is important to retract the extraction sheath frequently and confirm that the extraction sheath is not stuck on the lead when pulling back and tracking the lead well when pushing forward.

Femoral snares may be helpful to maintain traction during laser use or to retract a severed lead. In the event that there are lead fragments (Figure 10.3), the femoral

Table 10.2 Extraction tools.

Tool	Description
Standard, non-locking stylet	Used for support with simple traction
Fixation screw retraction clip	Counterclockwise rotation may retract the active fixation mechanism
Locking stylet	Allows the extractor to pull from the distal tip of the lead instead of the proximal lead
Snare (gooseneck snare, needle's eye snare, ensnare, and bioptome)	Can be used through a femoral workstation, with or without a deflectable sheath to direct the snare to the targeted lead or lead fragment
Mechanical sheath	Frequently composed of metal, Teflon, or polypropylene, providing stiffness and stability
Rotational cutting sheath	Beneficial in patients with calcified scar tissue, such as end stage renal disease or older leads in younger patients
Laser sheaths	Excimer laser that cuts through endothelialization and fibrotic scar tissue but does not cut through calcium
Electrosurgical sheaths	Radiofrequency energy emitted between two electrodes at the sheath tip
Telescoping sheaths	Any extraction sheath that can be paired with a second sheath, allowing the flexibility of the inner sheath but the support of the outer sheath, as needed to facilitate lead extraction
Angiovac	22 Fr cannula for the removal of thrombus or vegetation adherent to leads or tricuspid valvular tissue
TightRail/TightRail Mini	Flexible extraction tools particularly useful for extraction around points of curvature, rotational cutting mechanism useful for regions of adherent calcification with alternating directionality of rotational cutting to avoid building up unwanted torque on in situ leads during extraction
Bridge Balloon	Low pressure compliant balloon (80mm × 20mm; 60cc) designed to conform to the SVC to occlude bleeding while obtaining access for surgical repair

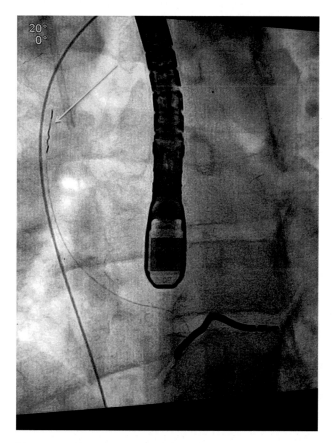

Figure 10.3 Fluoroscopy image of a broken lead.

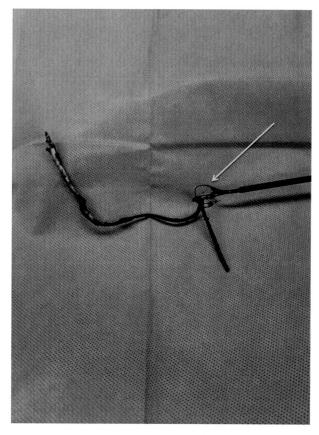

Figure 10.4 Needle's eye snare holding an extracted lead.

snares can also be used to retrieve those fragments (Figure 10.4). Snares can be put through deflectable sheaths or guide catheters for better maneuverability. Extraction through the right internal jugular vein is another, although infrequently used, alternative [18]. The femoral workstation is a 16 Fr venous access (alternatively, there are 18 Fr and 20 Fr femoral workstations); although this may present hemostasis challenges, the large access allows for multiple techniques, including:

- Needles eye snare to entrap an in tact of lead or portion of lead
- Goose neck snare or ensnare passed over the end of an exposed lead tip or lead fragment
- Use of a deflectable sheath to direct the snare to the targeted lead
- Large enough inner lumen to allow passage of a doubled over ICD lead without binding in the sheath.

In the case of device infections, a complete capsulectomy for pocket debridement may be performed. The pocket must be fully debrided with pocket tissue sent for gram stain, culture, and sensitivity. If there is not substantial infectious tissue, the pocket can be debrided and closed primarily with a high tensile strength absorbable suture (such as Vicryl 2-0, Vicryl 3-0) and staples with placement of a JP or Blake drain. If there is substantial infectious tissue, a wound vacuum can be applied primarily; however, great care must be taken to assure adequate hemostasis prior to its application. If there is any question about hemostasis, it is best to pack the wound with Kerlex or NuGauze soaked in saline or bacitracin and re-consider wound vacuum placement on the following day.

Complications

As mentioned in the preparation section of the chapter, patients with left bundle branch blocks are at risk for complete heart block during the extraction procedure, in the event that the right bundle branch block secondary to catheter manipulation is encountered. Patients who are pacemaker dependent and have a temporary pacing wire in place may have their temporary wire dislodged during the extraction procedure, resulting in asystole. In both of these cases, a temporary pacing wire from the femoral vein should be placed prophylactically or be easily accessible for use in the case of complete heart block and asystole.

During the procedure, it is important to use constant and steady traction (sustained traction) on the leads whenever the extraction sheath is being advanced. Scar may form within venous structures, in the atria, on tricuspid valve leaflets, or in the right ventricle, and the sus-

tained traction will allow time for tissue release, while sudden pulling carries a greater risk of tearing apart larger amounts of adherent tissue during lead removal. This is particularly important when an extraction sheath approaches the tip of the lead in the right atrium or right ventricle, because use of the laser or mechanical extraction sheaths at the lead–myocardium interface could result in damage to that myocardial chamber. As the lead tip is approached, it is important to be patient with the use of traction and countertraction to provide the necessary support for the laser sheath around the lead, allowing the tissue to release with minimal removal of the surrounding myocardium. In some instances of active fixation leads with screws that do not retract, counterclockwise torque of the lead and laser sheath as a unit may help the fixation screw disengage from the myocardium.

One of the reasons that active fixation leads are preferable to passive fixation leads for purposes of extractability is that fixation screws that do not retract usually straighten with traction forces used routinely in lead extraction cases. Although straightening of the fixation screw may help the lead release from the myocardium, additional care must be taken to retract the lead into the extraction sheath before removal of the lead from the central circulation in order to avoid potential risk of vascular laceration with the sharp tip of the exposed fixation screw.

Also during the procedure, the right ventricular lead may be adherent to the tricuspid valve. If the lead is adherent to the tricuspid valve, less damage may be done to the tricuspid valve by using a laser to separate the lead from the tricuspid valve leaflet instead of ripping the lead off the tricuspid valve. Worsening tricuspid regurgitation after lead extraction is relatively common and has been reported in as many as 4–9% of cases [3,19]. However, flail tricuspid leaflet after extraction requiring surgical repair or replacement was rare at less than 0.5% [7].

Transesophageal echocardiography to evaluate the status of the tricuspid valve and evaluate for pericardial effusion at any point during the case where there is suspicion of cardiac or vascular compromise and at the end of the case is useful. Also, fluoroscopy images can be compared with the baseline cine image of the heart to monitor for pericardial effusion, as well as to detect blood in the costophrenic angle, which may indicate hemothorax resulting from compromise of the SVC. Intracardiac echocardiography (ICE) is another tool that can be used to assess lead adherence characteristics and to evaluate procedural complications during lead extraction, but this tool adds meaningful cost to the extraction procedure. The ICE can help differentiate true tamponade from pseudo-tamponade, which can be seen when there is right ventricular eversion [20].

Larger extraction sheaths have a greater chance of leading to bleeding complications, so it may be helpful to consider purse string sutures at the entrance site of the extraction sheath to assist with hemostasis. Purse string sutures to assist with hemostasis may be particularly important in patients with coagulopathy, dialysis patients with an ipsilateral AV graft or shunt, patients with high right-sided pressures, or patients being considered for placement of a wound vacuum immediately after device extraction. In the event that a patient becomes acutely hypoxic during the procedure, consider a pulmonary embolism, air embolism, or septic embolism from a lead-related thrombus or vegetation. If patients develop upper extremity swelling after the procedure, consider an upper extremity ultrasound or other imaging to evaluate for vein thrombosis.

In conclusion, there are many infectious and non-infectious indications for lead removal. Given that a greater number of devices with an increased number of leads are being implanted in younger patients who have more years to live with and experience complications from in situ pacing and defibrillator leads, lead extraction is an important procedure to be available for patients beyond indications of removal for infection. Lead extraction can be carried out safely and effectively, but it is important for the procedure to be performed by operators with sufficient experience and at centers with the necessary facilities and cardiothoracic surgery back-up, as serious complications and death can occur.

Acknowledgments

The authors would like to thank Ruth Ann Greenfield, Jonathan Piccini, Roger Carrillo, and Scott Beaver.

References

1 Greenspon AJ, Patel JD, Lau E, Ochoa JA, Frisch DR, Ho RT, *et al.* Trends in permanent pacemaker implantation in the United States from 1993 to 2009: increasing complexity of patients and procedures. J Am Coll Cardiol 2012;60:1540–1545.

2 Baddour LM, Epstein AE, Erickson CC, Knight BP, Levison ME, Lockhart PB, *et al.* American Heart Association. Update on cardiovascular implantable electronic device infections and their management: a scientific statement from the American Heart Association. Circulation 2010;121:458–477.

3 Heart Rhythm 2017 Sep 15. pii: S1547–5271(17)31080–9. doi: 10.1016/j.hrthm.2017.09.001. [Epub ahead of print] 2017 HRS expert consensus statement on cardiovascular implantable electronic device lead management and extraction.

4 Wilkoff BL, Byrd CL, Love CJ, Hayes DL, Sellers TD, Schaerf R, *et al.* Pacemaker lead extraction with the laser sheath: results of the pacing lead extraction with the excimer sheath (PLEXES) trial. J Am Coll Cardiol 1999;33:1671–1676.

5 Byrd CL, Wilkoff BL, Love CJ, Sellers TD, Reiser C. Clinical study of the laser sheath for lead extraction: the total experience in the United States. Pacing Clin Electrophysiol 2002;25:804–808.

6 Wazni O, Epstein LM, Carrillo RG, Love C, Adler SW, Riggio DW, *et al.* Lead extraction in the contemporary setting: the LExICon study – an observational retrospective study of consecutive laser lead extractions. J Am Coll Cardiol 2010;55:579–586.

7 Brunner MP, Cronin EM, Duarte VE, Yu C, Tarakji KG, Martin DO, *et al.* Clinical predictors of adverse patient outcomes in an experience of more than 5000 chronic endovascular pacemaker and defibrillator lead extractions. Heart Rhythm 2014;11:799–805.

8 Rodriguez Y, Garisto JD, Carrillo RG. Laser lead extraction in the octogenarian patient. Circ Arrhythm Electrophysiol 2011;4:719–723.

9 Brunner MP, Cronin EM, Jacob J, Duarte VE, Tarakji KG, Martin DO, *et al.* Transvenous extraction of implantable cardioverter-defibrillator leads under advisory: a comparison of Riata, Sprint Fidelis, and non-recalled implantable cardioverter-defibrillator leads. Heart Rhythm 2013;10:1444–1450.

10 Kay GN, Brinker JA, Kawanishi DT, Love CJ, Lloyd MA, Reeves RC, *et al.* Risks of spontaneous injury and extraction of an active fixation pacemaker lead: report of the Accufix Multicenter Clinical Study and Worldwide Registry. Circulation 1999;100: 2344–2352.

11 Pokorney SD, Mi X, Lewis RK, Greiner M, Epstein LM, Carillo RG, et al. Outcomes Associated with Extraction Versus Capping and Abandoning Pacing and Defibrillator Leads. Circulation 2017;136:1387–1395.

12 Poole JE, Gleva MJ, Mela T, Chung MK, Uslan DZ, Borge R, *et al.* Complication rates associated with pacemaker or implantable cardioverter-defibrillator generator replacements and upgrade procedures: results from the REPLACE registry. Circulation 2010;122:1553–1561.

13 Epstein LM, Love CJ, Wilkoff BL, Chung MK, Hackler JW, Bongiorni MG, *et al.* Superior vena cava defibrillator coils make transvenous lead extraction more challenging and riskier. J Am Coll Cardiol 2013;61:987–989.

14 Smith MC, Love CJ. Extraction of transvenous pacing and ICD leads. Pacing Clin Electrophysiol 2008;31:736–752.

15 Kleemann T, Becker T, Doenges K, Vater M, Senges J, Schneider S, *et al.* Annual rate of transvenous defibrillation lead defects in implantable cardioverter-defibrillators over a period of >10 years. Circulation 2007;115:2474–2480.

16 Spectranetics Website. http://www.spectranetics.com/resources/lead-lookup/. Accessed August 14, 2017.

17 Lewis RK, Pokorney SD, Greenfield RA, Hranitzky PM, Hegland DD, Schroder JN, *et al.* Preprocedural ECG-gated computed tomography for prevention of complications during lead extraction. Pacing Clin Electrophysiol 2014;37:1297–1305.

18 Bongiorni MG, Soldati E, Zucchelli G, Di Cori A, Segreti L, De Lucia R, *et al.* Transvenous removal of pacing and implantable cardiac defibrillating leads using single sheath mechanical dilatation and multiple venous approaches: high success rate and safety in more than 2000 leads. Eur Heart J 2008;29:2886–2893.

19 Glover BM, Watkins S, Mariani JA, Yap S, Asta J, Cusimano RJ, *et al.* Prevalence of tricuspid regurgitation and pericardial effusions following pacemaker and defibrillator lead extraction. Int J Cardiol 2010;145:593–594.

20 Sadek MM, Epstein AE, Cheung AT, Schaller RD. Pseudo-tamponade during transvenous lead extraction. Heart Rhythm 2015;12:849–850.

11

How to Extract Pacemaker and Defibrillator Leads from the Femoral Approach

Leenhapong Navaravong and Roger A. Freedman

Division of Cardiovascular Medicine, University of Utah Health Sciences Center, Salt Lake City, UT, USA

It is estimated that 10 000–15 000 pacemaker and defibrillator leads are extracted worldwide per year, and the numbers of extracted leads and lead extraction procedures are growing. This growth is fueled by the growing base of patients with implanted pacemakers and defibrillators, the increasing complexity of the implanted systems, increasing rates of infection, and recently marketed lead models with high rates of mechanical failure. Whereas 20 years ago lead extraction was an infrequently performed procedure, lead extraction programs have emerged as integral components of comprehensive cardiac arrhythmia centers. Fellows in clinical cardiac electrophysiology training programs increasingly value training in lead extraction as a high priority.

As the frequency of lead extraction procedures has increased, so have the numbers of approaches and tools available to perform the technique. Most of the available tools are focused on manipulating the leads as they enter the venous system from the subclavian, cephalic, or axillary veins. Approaching leads from their entry point into the venous system has obvious appeal in that the proximal portion of the lead is in hand and, but for loosening adhesions of the lead to endovascular and endocardial structures, the lead can be removed with direct traction. Conversely, any approach to the lead not via the implanted vein – such as the femoral or jugular approach – necessitates securely snaring the lead from a distance within a vein or the heart and, at some point in the procedure, abandoning control of the lead from the implanted vein. Nevertheless, these alternate approaches have been durable components of the lead extraction armamentarium for decades and even today represent arguably equally safe and effective alternatives to more commonly utilized extraction techniques. Indeed, it is not uncommon to encounter leads that have been partially extracted or severed at the vein entry site, or leads where the central lumen will no longer accept a stylet, and in these cases there is no option for extraction but to snare the leads within a vein or the heart.

Femoral Lead Extraction Approach Within the Larger Context of the Lead Extraction Procedure

With the exception of rare cases, the femoral approach to lead extraction is performed within the context of a superior surgical approach (i.e., from within the generator pocket and via the implanted vein). At a minimum, the necessary steps performed from within the pacemaker or defibrillator pocket include mobilizing the generator, disconnecting leads from the generator, freeing the leads of their subcutaneous adhesions, cutting the sutures on the suture sleeve, mobilizing the suture sleeves, and attempting to retract extendable–retractable distal fixation helices.

Beyond these basic steps performed within the generator pocket, it is discretionary how much additional work will be carried out from the surgical approach before "converting" to the femoral approach. Here are several examples that highlight the range of options:

- A single 2-year-old active-fixation pacemaker lead is to be extracted. It is likely that the lead can be extracted from a superior approach with relatively few tools and minimal risk. The extracting physician may plan on an expeditious superior extraction and resort to the femoral approach only if unexpected difficulty is encountered.
- A 16-year-old non-backfilled dual coil defibrillator lead, with the proximal coil located in the brachiocephalic vein, is to be extracted. A reasonable strategy

How-to Manual for Pacemaker and ICD Devices: Procedures and Programming, First Edition. Edited by Amin Al-Ahmad, Andrea Natale, Paul J. Wang, James P. Daubert, and Luigi Padeletti.

would be to advance a powered or mechanical sheath from above until the distal end of the proximal coil has been reached but no further, and then convert to femoral approach. This would serve to mobilize the proximal coil from above but avoid the risk of superior vena cava tear.

- Several leads all implanted for longer than 15 years are to be extracted. Some of these leads have relatively little slack in the right atrium where they would typically be snared from below. In this case, a reasonable approach would be to avoid locking stylets and any traction or sheaths from above, and convert to femoral approach immediately after the basic pocket steps are completed. The advantages of this strategy are: (i) saving time, avoiding additional fluoroscopy, and conserving supplies if there is a very high likelihood of resorting to femoral approach; and (ii) avoiding losing available lead slack in the right atrium to make snaring from below easier.

Choosing the balance between superior and femoral approaches depends on the experience, skill, and available tools of the extracting physician. Some relatively high volume extraction centers have little or no experience with femoral extraction, do not have femoral tools in stock, and rely almost exclusively on their expertise in superior extraction. Obviously, such a center would rarely resort to the femoral approach. Other centers have more balanced expertise and can select the best strategy on a case-by-case basis.

Tools for Femoral Extraction

Femoral extraction requires two basic categories of tools.

1) *Outer femoral sheath.* This is the introducer that is placed in the femoral vein through which the snare is placed and leads removed. The outer sheath can usually be left in place as multiple leads are snared and removed. The most commonly used outer sheath is a 16 Fr hemostatic introducer that extends from the femoral area to the right atrium (Femoral Introducer Sheath, Cook Medical). It is available in both straight and curved shapes (Figure 11.1) and comes with a dilator.

2) *Snares.* There are several snares that can be used through the outer femoral sheath:

- Dotter basket (Cook Medical) and deflectable tip wire (Figure 11.2). The deflectable tip wire can be looped over a lead segment and then snared in the Dotter basket. This technique does not require a free end of lead for snaring.
- Amplatz gooseneck snare (Covidien). An Amplatz snare can be used to "lasso" an accessible free end of the lead. Alternatively, it can be used to snare a tip deflecting wire which is looped over a lead segment and then snared with the Amplatz snare (Figure 11.3).
- Needle's Eye Snare (Cook Medical; Figure 11.4). The Needle's Eye Snare is the most commonly used snare for lead extraction and forms the focus of this chapter. The Needle's Eye Snare can be used to snare a segment of lead or a free end of lead. The snare consists of a loop or "cobra head" which is draped over the lead segment and the Needle's Eye or "tongue" which is extended through the "cobra

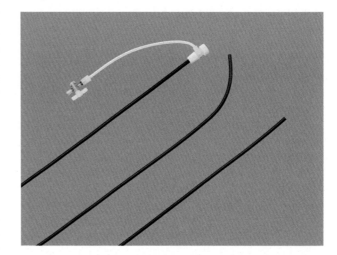

Figure 11.1 Outer sheaths utilized for femoral approach to lead extraction. The sheath is placed percutaneously in the femoral vein and the distal end advanced to the right atrium. Top: Proximal end of 16 Fr sheath with hemostatic valve and side arm. Middle: Distal end of curved outer sheath. Bottom: Distal end of straight outer sheath. *Source*: Reproduced with permission of Cook Medical Incorporated.

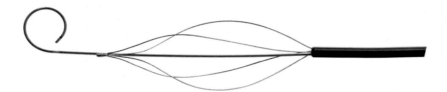

Figure 11.2 Dotter basket with deflectable tip wire, used together to snare pacemaker defibrillator leads in the right atrium or great veins. *Source*: Reproduced with permission of Cook Medical Incorporated.

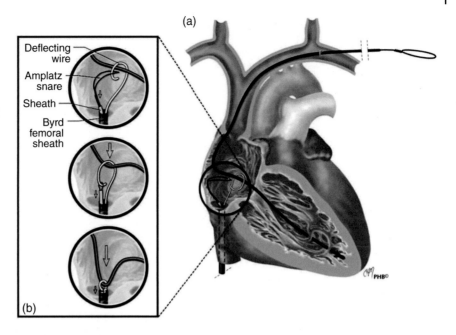

Figure 11.3 Deflectable tip wire used with Amplatz gooseneck snare to snare pacemaker lead. (a) Wire and snare deployed in the right atrium around the lead. (b) Demonstrating snaring end of deflectable wire and pulling the lead within the femoral sheath. *Source*: Belott (1998) [2]. Reproduced with permission of Futura Publishing.

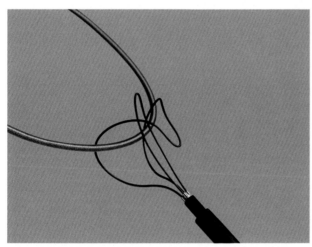

Figure 11.4 Needle's Eye Snare with "cobra head" and "tongue" surrounding the lead. The 16 Fr outer femoral sheath and 12 Fr inner femoral sheath are also visible. *Source*: Reproduced with permission of Cook Medical Incorporated.

head," thus encircling the lead segment. An inner femoral sheath (12 Fr) is used to cinch the snare (Figure 11.4). Snares are available with 13 or 20 mm "cobra head" diameters. The inner sheath is supplied in both straight and curved shapes.

Using the Tools

Practical Tips for Inserting Outer Femoral Sheath

The 16 Fr outer sheath has an outer diameter of 5.3 mm, which is larger than typical catheters familiar to cardiologists. There is a tendency to undersize the length

of the skin nick in the femoral area – doing so will impede entry of the catheter. When the sheath reaches the femoral vein, there is another area of resistance which requires additional force. A palpable "pop" signals entry of the catheter into the vein. The outer sheath should be advanced over the supplied guidewire to the inferior right atrium.

Deploying the Needle's Eye Snare

The snare and the inner sheath containing it are advanced into the right atrium. Pacemaker and defibrillator leads, be they right ventricular, right atrial, or coronary sinus, are usually snared in the right atrium. Less commonly, leads can be snared in the superior vena cava, brachiocephalic vein, or inferior vena cava. The Needle's Eye Snare should not be advanced to or beyond the tricuspid valve, as deployment of the snare near the tricuspid valve is likely to cause severe damage to the valve and/or its supporting structures.

Once in the right atrium, the snare, inner sheath, and femoral outer sheath should be rotated to see if one or more of leads targeted for extraction are "bumped." Bumping a lead signifies that it can be snared with the snare and sheaths being used. Failure to bump a lead, even as the snare is moved from the superior vena cava down to the inferior vena cava, suggests that a different snare size or sheath curve may be needed.

The next step is to drape the "cobra head" over the lead segment (Figure 11.5). The goal is position the lead segment as far back in the lobes of the "cobra head." It is important not to torque the "cobra head" against resistance so much as to distort its geometry. Angulated fluoroscopic views can be useful to confirm positioning of the

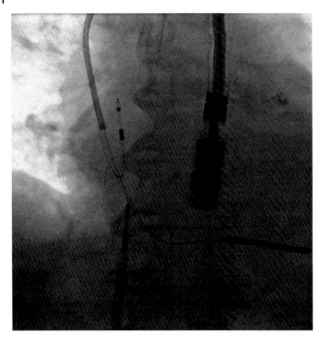

Figure 11.5 "Cobra head" of Needle's Eye Snare draped over atrial lead in the right atrium.

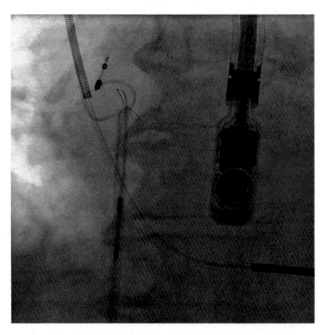

Figure 11.7 Inner sheath advanced up to atrial lead, cinching it between the "cobra head" and "tongue" portions of the Needle's Eye Snare.

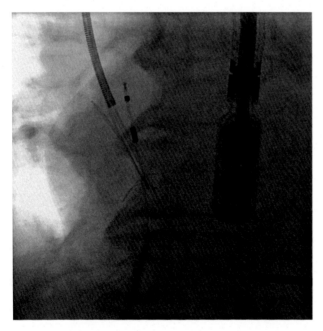

Figure 11.6 "Tongue" portion of Needle's Eye Snare extended through the "cobra head," thus surrounding the atrial lead.

snare over the lead, although commonly sticking to a single fixed fluoroscopic view is most expeditious.

Once the "cobra head" is draped over the lead segment, the tongue is extended by advancing a plunger on the proximal end of the snare apparatus (Figure 11.6). Importantly, for effective snaring the targeted lead segment must be bracketed between the lobes of the "cobra head" and the tongue. In a single fluoroscopic view it is not always possible to determine if that is the case. Very commonly, the extended tongue will end up behind the lead and the lead will not be effectively snared. In addition to taking angulated fluoroscopic views, ways to test for effective snaring are to check to see if the lead segment rotates when the snare is rotated and to advance the inner sheath.

After extending the tongue, the inner sheath is then advanced over the snare towards the lead. If the lead is effectively snared, the inner sheath will abut the lead (Figure 11.7), cinching it between the tongue and "cobra head." If the lead is not effectively snared, however, the inner sheath will be advanced past the lead, and this is the sign to the operator that it is time to redeploy the snare and try again.

As mentioned above, one of the steps of lead extraction performed from the pocket area is to attempt to unscrew the distal helices of active fixation leads by manipulating leads from their proximal end. For extendable–retractable helices, this involves counterclockwise rotation of the proximal electrode pin. For fixed helices, this involves counterclockwise rotation of the entire lead. However, it is not uncommon for these maneuvers to be unsuccessful. Most likely the reason is failure to transmit sufficient counterclockwise torque to the distal end of the lead from rotation at the proximal end. Snaring leads from below, much closer to the endocardial attachment site, allows for torqueing of the leads much closer to the location of the helix. When unscrewing leads from their proximal end fails, it is almost always possible to unscrew them from below by counterclockwise torqueing of the snare after the lead is well cinched into the snare (Video 11.1). Once the helix is unscrewed from the endocardium, any residual coiling of the lead near the snare should be relieved by rotating the snare clockwise; this will permit easier advancement of the outer sheath over the doubled over lead.

Delivering the Lead

After the lead has been firmly cinched by the snare and inner sheath, and if active fixation it has been unscrewed from the endocardium, the snared lead is doubled over inside the outer femoral sheath. This is accomplished in one of two ways. If the lead is free of the endocardium, it can be simply pulled down into the outer sheath (Video 11.2). If the lead is still attached to the endocardium, the outer sheath is advanced forward over the doubled over lead while tension is held on the lead from the snare below. Ideally, the outer sheath is advanced all the way to the endocardium to stabilize the heart as the distal end of the lead is detached. Frequently, however, the distal end of the lead will pull free of its attachment during the process of advancing the outer sheath, especially when a ventricular lead is being extracted. Failure to advance the femoral outer sheath all the way to the endocardium is particularly common in the case of larger diameter defibrillator leads which cannot be readily doubled over within the outer sheath.

As the lead is pulled into the femoral outer sheath, the proximal portion of the lead should be cut at the vein entry site in the pectoral area. Often, a locking stylet will have been inserted into the lumen of the lead and frequently it is not possible to remove the locking stylet at this point in time, so it too is cut along with lead. Fortunately, although the locking stylet certainly adds rigidity to the lead, its presence does not appear to impair removal of the lead via the outer femoral sheath.

Once the lead is delivered the lead via the outer femoral sheath, fluoroscopy of the chest and abdomen is performed to confirm no retained lead fragments. It is prudent to image the outer sheath (still in the femoral vein) as well to make sure no fragments are retained in its lumen. The outer sheath should be aspirated forcefully and flushed as thrombi can be retained in the sheath.

The inner sheath and snare can be re-advanced into the femoral outer sheath to snare additional leads. Once all leads are extracted, the outer sheath is pulled from the vein and hemostasis is obtained. A 20-minute manual groin hold and 6 hours bedrest is recommended.

Special Situations

Need for Temporary Pacemaker

When temporary pacing is needed during lead extraction, our practice in most patients has been to place the temporary pacemaker via the left femoral vein, reserving the right femoral vein for the extraction tools. To the degree possible the right atrial "heel" of the temporary pacemaker should be positioned away from the target segments of the leads to be extracted.

Retaining or Creating Subclavian and Brachiocephalic Access During Femoral Extraction

Occasionally, leads are extracted from patients whose ipsilateral subclavian or brachiocephalic veins are stenosed or occluded, and it is desirable to reimplant new leads via those veins after the extraction. The method of accomplishing this using the femoral extraction approach is to make a 2 mm nick in the insulation of one (or more) of the leads to be extracted and then to insert the straight end of a 0.035 inch guidewire between the insulation and the outer conductor for a distance of 3–4 mm, far enough so it will withstand gentle traction. (A standard vein lifter can facilitate inserting the guide wire under the insulation.) After the lead is snared from below and is being pulled through the femoral outer sheath, the guide wire is gently fed along into the vasculature. Once the leading end of the guide wire is beyond the area of vascular occlusion or stenosis, a quick tug is exerted on its proximal end to free it from the lead. If a tug is not sufficient, then a dilator can be advanced over the guide wire to free it from the lead.

Retaining Femoral Access When Extracting Larger Defibrillator Leads

Most leads can be delivered by doubling them over within the femoral outer sheath and without removing the femoral outer sheath from the femoral vein, as described in the previous section. Notable exceptions are larger diameter defibrillator leads (those requiring 9 Fr introducers or larger for insertion), which are too thick to readily double over within the femoral outer sheath. For these leads, the snared portion is brought back to the distal and of the outer sheath and pulled within it for as far as possible, which may be up to several centimeters. Once the lead cannot be pulled any further into the outer sheath, the outer sheath along with lead are removed together from the femoral vein.

When a larger defibrillator lead is one of multiple leads to extract, one strategy is to remove that lead last so that losing groin access is not a concern. However, when that strategy does not work (i.e., if there are multiple larger defibrillator leads to extract or if it is not possible to snare the larger defibrillator lead first), it will be necessary to regain femoral vein access. Generally, this can be done on the original femoral vein used, although a groin hold will first be necessary to achieve hemostasis. When it is anticipated that access to the femoral vein will be lost, it is advisable to place in advance a "spare" guide wire from the access site adjacent to the femoral outer sheath up to the inferior vena cava. This is accomplished by inserting two long guide wires through an introducer in the femoral vein earlier in the case, and then advancing the femoral outer sheath over one of them, saving the other as the "spare."

Calcified or Heavily Fibrosed Leads

Whereas calcified or heavily fibrosed leads present a major challenge for extraction using superior techniques, they are readily removed using the femoral approach. Figure 11.8 shows the non-backfilled, non-coated proximal shocking coil of a defibrillator lead extracted 17 years after implantation. After extraction, the proximal shocking coil was found to have a rigid sheath of calcium about 1.5 mm in thickness surrounding it, which was cracked in two for illustrative purposes after extraction (Figure 11.8). Despite the calcific sheath, the lead was extracted femorally with little force and no difficulty.

Previous Extraction Using Femoral Approach

Patients who have a prior extraction from a femoral venous approach may have excessive scar tissue in the area of that vein resulting from the prior extraction. The scar tissue may impede placement of the femoral outer sheath or of pulling leads through the femoral area, especially in cases when leads cannot be pulled out through the outer sheath, such as larger defibrillator leads. In such cases, the leads can be wedged into the scar tissue and if excessive force is used can break with potential embolization back to the heart or pulmonary artery. Therefore it is recommended to consider utilizing the left femoral vein in patients who have had prior extraction from the right femoral vein. A similar recommendation would apply to patients known to have excessive scar tissue in the right femoral area from repeated vascular instrumentation of any nature.

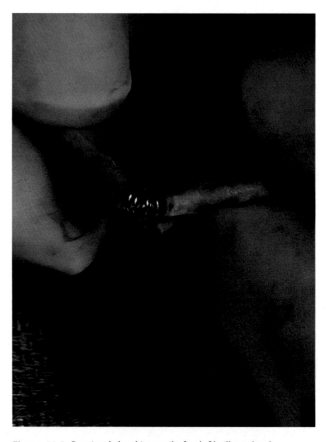

Figure 11.8 Proximal shocking coil of a defibrillator lead extracted using femoral approach 17 years after implantation. The lead was a Guidant model 0125 which has no backfill or coating to prevent tissue ingrowth into shocking coils. After extraction, the proximal shocking coil was found to have an intact rigid sheath of calcium about 1.5 mm in thickness surrounding it, which is shown cracked in half after extraction for illustrative purposes. Despite the calcific sheath, the lead was extracted femorally with little force and no difficulty.

Precautionary Measures

The same precautionary measures that are typically taken with lead extractions using the superior approach are advised for the femoral approach. The precautionary measures that we employ are as follows:

- General anesthesia, ideally with a cardiac anesthesiologist.
- Entire chest, abdomen, and groin areas prepped and draped as a single field.
- Defibrillation pads placed, typically in right scapular area and left mid axillary line.
- Arterial catheter for continuous blood pressure monitoring. Generally, the arterial line will be placed in a radial artery. When it is placed in a femoral artery, it is advised to place it contralateral to the femoral vein used for extraction.

- Transesophageal echocardiography with continuous monitoring for complications.
- Cardiac surgery standby back-up with appropriate surgical supplies and equipment available.
- Withholding of warfarin (goal INR ≤1.2) and other oral anticoagulants, heparin, and thienopyridines (e.g., clopidogrel, prasugrel). Aspirin can be continued if there is a firm medical indication for its use.
- 4 units paced red blood cells in the procedure room. If there is any question of INR not being at goal of ≤1.2, then plasma should also be available.

An additional precaution not generally utilized with the superior approach is sequential compression devices on the lower extremities to lower the risk of deep venous thrombosis following extraction.

Complications

The complication profile of femoral extraction differs somewhat from that of superior extraction. Table 11.1 lists the complications of the femoral approach.

The most common life-threatening complication of lead extraction from the femoral approach is myocardial perforation resulting from avulsion or tear with resulting hemopericardium and cardiac tamponade. A published series comparing femoral with superior extraction approaches reported two myocardial perforations among 189 femoral extractions (1.1%) and two among 268 superior extractions (0.7%) [1]. It is extremely helpful to have continuous transesophageal echocardiography monitoring in place for early detection of pericardial effusion. In the event of pericardial effusion, transthoracic echocardiography is helpful to

Table 11.1 Complications of pacemaker and defibrillator lead extraction utilizing the femoral approach.

Myocardial perforation with hemopericardium and cardiac tamponade

Superior vena cava tear rarely seen
Tricuspid valve damage
Damage or dislodgement of companion leads
Fragmentation of leads, possibly with embolization
Vascular complications

- Hematoma
- Femoral artery pseudo-aneurysm
- A-V fistula
- Deep venous thrombosis/pulmonary embolism
- Inability to pull leads out of femoral vein – require cut-down and venotomy

Dislodgement of temporary pacemaker
Radiation exposure

direct pericardiocentesis. A pericardiocentesis tray and a physician with expertise in the technique of pericardiocentesis should be immediately available. Occasionally, percutaneous pericardiocentesis is not adequate to control bleeding and a limited thoracotomy is required for repair of the myocardial defect.

Vascular complications occur occasionally, generally involving the femoral venous access site and include hematoma, femoral artery pseudoaneurysm, arteriovenous fistula, deep venous thrombosis, and pulmonary embolism. Rarely, pacemaker or defibrillator leads will get wedged into a scarred femoral area and require cut-down and venotomy for removal.

As with the superior approach, leads can fragment during a femoral extraction procedure and potentially embolize. If lead fragments remain in the right atrium or the great veins, then it is usually possible to snare them and extract them. A deflectable catheter, such as an ablation catheter, is occasionally useful to insert in the inner femoral extraction sheath to advance it into less easily accessible veins such as the brachiocephalic veins; once the inner sheath is positioned the deflectable catheter is replaced with the Needle's Eye Snare. Under no circumstances should the Needle's Eye Snare be advanced through the tricuspid valve. Attempting to snare a lead within the right ventricle carries a high risk of severe damage to the tricuspid valve. Lead fragments that have embolized to the proximal pulmonary artery can often be snared with Amplatz goose neck snare or other snares familiar to vascular surgeons and interventional radiologists. The Needle's Eye Snare is too rigid to allow for safe deployment within a pulmonary artery.

Damage to companion leads (i.e., implanted leads that are not specifically targeted for extraction) can occur during a femoral lead extraction procedure, but this complication is probably less common using the femoral approach than with the superior approach. The reason is that with the superior approach, leads are often adhered together in the subclavian vein, brachiocephalic vein, and/or the superior vena cava, and the process of advancing powered sheaths over the lead being extracted is at significant risk for damaging companion leads. It is much less common for leads to be adhered in the right atrium and when they are the adhesions tend to be focal and relatively easy to lyse with simple traction. Therefore, when target leads are snared in the right atrium using the femoral approach, they can almost always be freed from adhesions to companion leads in the right atrium with moderate traction. Furthermore, when snared from below, target leads can generally be freed with minimal traction from adjacent leads in the superior vena cava, brachiocephalic vein, and subclavian vein.

When damage to companion leads does occur during the femoral approach, it is usually because the companion lead interferes with successful snaring of the target lead and therefore the companion lead is intentionally extracted to allow for snaring of the target lead. Dislodgement of companion leads may occur when they are repeatedly contacted by the snare; this complication is generally limited to newly implanted companion leads or leads placed within the coronary sinus tree.

Tear of the superior vena cava as a complication of the femoral approach to lead extraction is extremely rare. We are aware of only one report of superior vena cava tear resulting from a femoral lead extraction [1]. We have never experienced a superior vena cava tear using the femoral approach to lead extraction, and a search of the FDA Manufacturer and User Facility Device Experience (MAUDE) database for fatal tears of the superior vena cava with the Needle's Eye Snare yielded no reports.

In a comparison of femoral with laser superior approaches to lead extraction, total fluoroscopy time was found to be higher (21 min) for the femoral approach than the laser superior approach (7 min) [1]. In that study, patients undergoing extraction by the femoral approach had locking stylets inserted from above and also attempts were made to detach the distal end of the lead from the endocardium by pulling from above. It is arguable that these maneuvers are not necessary for a femoral approach

lead extraction, and that the fluoroscopy time for these patients would have been shorter had they not been performed. Furthermore, pulling on leads from above generally eliminates any slack the leads would have had in the right atrium and therefore makes snaring from below more challenging and time consuming.

Why is Less Force Required to Extract Leads from Femoral Approach than Superior Approach?

Physicians who have experience extracting leads from both the femoral and superior approaches are struck by the significant difference in required force to extricate and remove leads between the two techniques, with less force required for the femoral than the superior approach. The explanation for this discrepancy is unclear. One possibility is that with pulling from above, especially using locking stylets that exert upward traction from the distal end of the lead, the leads may shorten and "bunch up," leading to slight increase in their effective diameter and impeding their passage through tight adhesions. Conversely, when leads are pulled from below, they

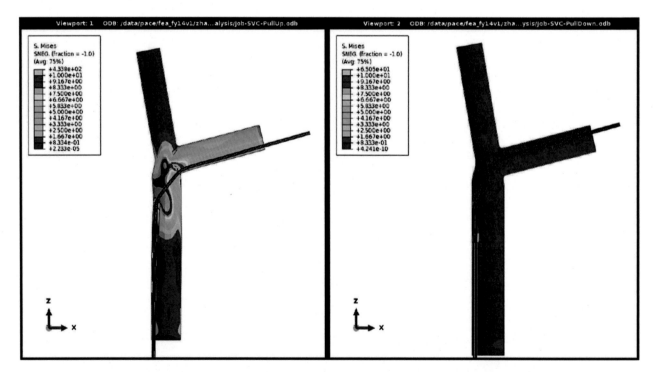

Figure 11.9 Wall stress in superior vena cava when shear force is exerted on an adhered lead from superior approach (left) compared with force exerted from femoral approach (right). Wall stress is sixfold higher from the superior approach than from the femoral approach.

stretch slightly and their diameter decreases or "neck," and this eases their passage through tight adhesions (Mark T. Marshall, personal communication). Another possibility for the discrepancy in required force is that adhesions have a "barb" effect such that they impair passage of leads in one direction more than the other.

A related question is why tear of the superior vena cava is so much less common when leads are extracted from the femoral approach than the superior approach. A recent study of a computer model of the effect of shear forces exerted by traction on a lead adhered to the superior vena cava showed sixfold higher stress in the wall of the superior vena cava when shear force is exerted by traction from the superior direction than equal shear force exerted from the inferior direction (Figure 11.9).

Conclusions

The femoral approach to pacemaker and defibrillator lead extraction is an alternative and complementary approach to the more commonly practiced superior approach. Tools and methodology for the femoral approach have been developed after years of refinement. Reported head-to-head comparisons of the femoral and superior approaches are sparse, but available evidence suggests similar rates of procedural success and complications between the two approaches. The incidence of various procedural complications differs between the two methods, and in particular tear of the superior vena cava with resulting hemothorax appears to be much less common with the femoral than with the superior approach.

References

1 Bordachar P, Defaye P, Peyrouse E, Boveda S, Mokrani B, Marquié C, *et al.* Extraction of old pacemaker or cardioverter-defibrillator leads by laser sheath versus femoral approach. Circ Arrhythm Electrophysiol 2010;2:319–323.

2 Belott PH. Endocardial Lead Extraction: A Videotape and Manual. Futura Publishing; Armonk, NY, 1998.

 To watch the videos, please log in to the Companion Website: www.wiley.com/go/al-ahmad/pacemakers_and_icds

Video 11.1 Unscrewing atrial lead with counterclockwise rotation of femoral snare. Snared active fixation atrial lead is unscrewed from endocardium with counterclockwise rotation of Needle's Eye Snare inserted via femoral approach.

Video 11.2 Pulling snared atrial lead down the outer femoral sheath. After being unscrewed from atrial endocardium, the snared atrial lead is pulled down the outer femoral sheath. The outer femoral sheath will stay in place if needed to extract other leads.

12

How to Extract Leads from the Jugular Approach

Maria Grazia Bongiorni, Andrea Di Cori, Luca Segreti, Giulio Zucchelli, Ezio Soldati, Stefano Viani, and Luca Paperini

Second Division of Cardiovascular Diseases, Cardiac-Thoracic and Vascular Department, Azienda Ospedaliero Universitaria Pisana, Pisa, Italy

The advent of implantable devices has produced the subsequent need for removal of these devices. Malfunction, erosion, pocket infection, endocarditis, and other unique device-related issues are common reasons for removal. Removal of the subcutaneous or sub-muscular pulse generator alone is a fairly uncomplicated procedure. However, removal of the chronically implanted transvenous lead system can be a significantly complex procedure [1–5].

Over the years of lead development, the early, large diameter, solidly built wires have been replaced by smaller, more delicate, and structurally complex leads. The major barrier to removal of these leads is fibrosis that progressively grows around the lead body and electrode tip, securing leads to the venous endothelium and to the myocardium. The goal is to free the lead from these binding sites safely.

Standard surgical techniques through a midline sternotomy, lateral thoracotomy, or limited atriotomy were developed as solutions for lead removal. However, they remain an option of last resort given their invasiveness, morbidity, and longer recovery time, with a reported mortality rate of 0–12.5% [6,7]. The desire for safe extraction techniques, performed via the implant vein and compatible with the pectoral pocket transvenous implant method, led to the development of transvenous techniques [5,6]. By using telescoping sheaths made of polymer and/or steel material which slide over the lead body, a countering force is applied to the intravascular fibrotic overgrowth that resists the traction force applied to the lead. This technique of intravascular counterpressure localizes shear stress on the fibrotic tissue and aids in blunt dissection or dilation of the tissue away from the lead circumference. Many tools, techniques, and approaches may be used and combined in order to remove cardiac leads. This chapter focuses on the incremental role of a transjugular approach in the field of percutaneous lead extraction.

Background

Definition of Terms

According to the North American Society of Pacing and Electrophysiology (NASPE) Policy Statement [8] and Heart Rhythm Society (HRS) Expert consensus [9] on transvenous lead extraction, "lead removal" is defined as the removal of pacing and defibrillating lead using any technique. Within the general category of lead removal, distinctions must be made between:

1) *Lead explant:* simple procedures that can be performed via the implant vein without specialized tools; and
2) *Lead extraction:* removal of leads involving more complex procedures and specialized tools.

Extraction Tools

Extraction tools are all the potential items used to accomplish lead removal. The following tools can be used for lead removal:

- *Implant tools:* tools typically supplied for lead implant, allowing manipulation of the lead so that the lead exits the vasculature via the implant vein. These tools include such items as standard stylets (non-locking) and fixation screw retraction clips.

How-to Manual for Pacemaker and ICD Devices: Procedures and Programming, First Edition. Edited by Amin Al-Ahmad, Andrea Natale, Paul J. Wang, James P. Daubert, and Luigi Padeletti.
© 2018 John Wiley & Sons, Inc. Published 2018 by John Wiley & Sons, Inc.
Companion website: www.wiley.com/go/al-ahmad/pacemakers_and_icds

- *Traction devices:* specialized locking stylets, snares, sutures, grasping, or other devices used to engage or entrap and remove the lead or lead fragments.
- *Sheaths:* dilatators used to disrupt fibrotic adherences across the leads. These may be "mechanical" (composed of metal, Teflon, or polypropylene and requiring manual advancement over the lead and rely on the mechanical properties of the sheath to disrupt fibrotic attachments) or "powered" (using laser, radiofrequency, or rotational technology to dissect binding sites).

Extraction Techniques

Techniques for lead removal include all practical methods or arts applied to extract leads from the body. The major obstacle to lead removal is the body's response to an intravascular foreign body. A few months after the implant, the leads are fixed at binding sites along their course and at the tip, mainly by the growth of fibrous tissue including the lead itself [10]. Usually, leads implanted for 1 year or more are not likely to be removed by simple traction, particularly in the presence of implantable cardioverter-defibrillator (ICD) leads, where the defibrillating coils are usually responsible for significant growth of fibrous adherences. The sites where binding sites are most likely to be present are the site of insertion into the subclavian vein, the junction between innominate vein and superior vena cava (SVC) and right atrium, the tip of the lead and, in the case of ventricular leads, the tricuspid valve [11–13]. The key point in order to remove a lead is to free the lead by these binding sites, from the venous entry to the tip. Most of the currently available techniques combine traction with the dissection of the binding sites, and the most important difference between them is the energy used to dissect the binding sites.

Any technique used for extraction should have good lead control. The aim of lead control is to allow traction force application uniformly over the entire length of the lead. Lead control is important for improving success rates and reducing complications. First, lead control is obtained by securing the inner coil with a stylet. Secondly, a suture is used as an additional traction device. Finally, once the lead is prepared, lead control is obtained by assessing constantly the tensile properties of the lead during traction application. Changes in the tensile response may be a result of detachment of the stylet from the lead, freeing of the lead from binding sites, unravelling of the inner conductor, or rupture of the outer insulation.

Lead traction, counterpressure and countertraction, progressive dissection and mechanical dislodgement represent the techniques for lead extraction [14–18].

Lead Traction

Simple traction is the most primitive method of lead removal. It was the only method of extracting leads during the early years of pacing, when leads to be removed had large and strong bodies, no effective fixation mechanisms, and short implant duration [18]. Traction was performed for minutes to days manually using various weights or elastic bands [19]. Later, fibrous encapsulation along the lead–vascular wall–myocardium interface developed, making simple traction ineffective and potentially risky. Although standard or locking stylets have considerably improved the effectiveness of direct traction, the success rate remains pretty low, requiring the use of additional tools like dilating sheaths with the related techniques (i.e., counterpressure and countertraction).

Counterpressure and Countertraction

Counterpressure is performed by applying simultaneously a forward pressure on the sheath and traction to the lead. Pressure describes the pushing force applied to the sheaths that is directed towards the heart, and its objective is to overcome binding sites between the lead and vascular system. The goal of counterpressure is to counterbalance the advancement force (pressure) with the retraction force (traction). An imbalance between these two forces can cause the procedure to fail or lead to complications.

Countertraction is performed when the sheath has been progressed to the lead tip–myocardial surface. The traction applied on the lead is counterbalanced by the pressure obtained by pushing the outer sheath to support the myocardium; in other words, the force is applied perpendicular and in opposition to the heart wall. This allows centering and limiting the traction force to the binding sites surrounding the lead tip, minimizing the risk of myocardial invagination or tear.

No single technique for transvenous lead removal should be considered "standard" and applicable in all cases. The different tools and approaches must be tailored to each individual case [20].

Extraction Approaches

Cardiac leads are usually removed via the implant vein. The implant vein is the venous access by which the lead was inserted. Sometimes, however, alternative venous access is required from a non-implant vein. Examples of alternative approaches to subclavian vein include femoral and jugular veins. There are three approaches for transvenous lead extraction (Figure 12.1) [21]:

1) Venous entry approach (VEA), also known as the superior approach;
2) Transfemoral approach, also known as the inferior approach; and
3) Internal transjugular approach.

1. Venous entry approach (VEA)

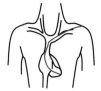

2. Transfemoral approach (TFA)

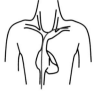

3. Internal transjugular approach (ITA)

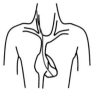

Figure 12.1 Summary of transvenous extraction approaches.

Most operators begin with a VEA using the implant vein and switch to a transfemoral approach if necessary. Moreover, when leads are broken or flee-floating, the transfemoral approach is historically performed [22].

Different venous approaches using the mechanical dilatation technique represent the personal contribution to transvenous removal, using the internal jugular vein (IJV) in patients with free-floating leads or difficult exposed leads [20].

Internal Transjugular Approach

Rationale

We introduced the internal transjugular approach (ITA) to approach two complex clinical scenarios: difficult lead extraction from VEA and free-floating leads. Although the described success rate is 90% for standard approaches, extraction may be risky or impossible in some cases. The introduction of ITA allows us to shorten the road from the skin to lead tip and to change the dilatation angle, overcoming difficulties and increasing the success rate from 91.1% to 98.5% [22,23].

Difficult conditions for the removal of leads exposed at the implant site are damage of the lead (fracture, loss of insulation), hard turns in the course of the lead (the energy of dilatation may be applied to venous wall, increasing the risk of venous tears), very thin costo-calvicular space (avoiding the use of large dilation sheaths), and the presence of very tight binding sites (sometimes calcified) where dilatation is not effective.

Gross Anatomy

The IJV is the major venous return from the brain, upper face, and neck. It is formed by the union of inferior petrosal and sigmoid dural venous sinuses in or just distal to the jugular foramen (forming the jugular bulb). It descends in the carotid sheath with the internal carotid artery. The vagus nerve (cranial nerve X) lies between the two. After receiving tributaries from the face and neck, it continues to descend into the thorax, usually between the heads of the sternocleidomastoid muscle, before uniting with the subclavian vein to form the brachiocephalic vein [24,25]. The IJV is surrounded by accompanying lymph nodes. Main relations are with the following structures (Figure 12.2):

1) Relation to internal carotid artery:
   - C2 – posteriorly
   - C3 – posterolaterally
   - C4 – laterally.
2) Vagus nerve (CN X) always situated between the ICA and IJV.
3) Anteriorly (i.e., is crossed by these structures):
   - Upper third – spinal root of accessory nerve (CN XI)
   - Middle third – lower root of ansa cervicalis
   - Lower third – sternocleidomastoid muscle, tendon of omohyoid muscle.
4) Posteriorly (from superior to inferior as the IJV descends in the neck):
   - Lateral mass of C1 (atlas)
   - Middle scalene muscle
   - Anterior scalene muscle
   - Pleura of lung apices.

The jugular veins are relatively superficial and not protected by tissues such as bone or cartilage. As the IJV is large, central, and relatively superficial, it is often used to place venous lines. Because the IJV rarely varies in its location, it is easier to find than other veins. This procedure has no absolute contraindications. Relative contraindications include the following:

- Severe coagulopathy
- Physical status unfit for anesthesia
- Unavailability of a suitable access site
- Thrombosed veins
- Overlying skin infection.

Equipment

The following material is necessary for cannulation:

- Sterile gloves
- Antiseptic solution with skin swab
- Sterile drapes or towels
- Sterile gown

(a)

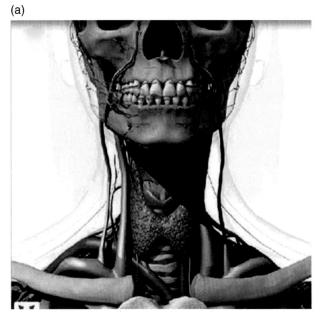

(b)

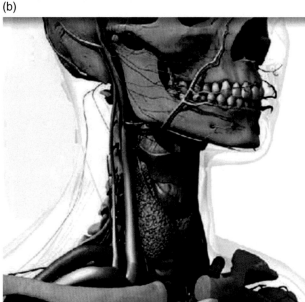

Figure 12.2 Frontal (a) and right oblique (b) anterior view of the right internal jugular vein.

- Sterile saline flush, approximately 30 mL
- Lidocaine 1%
- Gauze
- Dressing
- Scalpel, No. 11
- Needle driver
- Prolene suture 4/0
- Introducer 11 Fr.

Skin cleansing with 2% chlorhexidine in alcohol is recommended for skin antisepsis, as this has been shown to be superior to povidone-iodine or 70% alcohol. Expose the neck from the angle of the jaw superiorly, to the nipples inferiorly, to the midaxillary line laterally, and to the sternum medially. Surround the exposed area with sterile drape or towels.

Catheterization Technique

The patient is placed in the Trendelenburg position with his or her head turned to the contralateral side. The physician stands above the patient on the contralateral side, and a large skin wheal is raised with local anesthetic over the junction of the sternal and clavicular divisions of the sternocleidomastoid muscle. The IJV is located between the clavicular heads of sternomastoid muscle. It is accessed best at the apex of the triangle the muscle heads make with the clavicle (Figure 12.3).

While the medially located carotid artery (which courses under the sternal division) is palpated, a 2 cm, 22-gauge needle and syringe are used to locate the IJV

which lies lateral to the carotid artery, immediately beneath the medial border of the clavicular division. The needle should enter the skin at a 30–450 angle directed laterally toward the mid-clavicle, thereby avoiding possible puncture of the carotid artery. On entering the vein, the syringe is disengaged but the needle is not removed; it remains in the vein to serve as a direct visual guide to the underlying vein. After ensuring that the needle is within the lumen of the vein, the J guide wire is passed through the needle and the tip is positioned in the uppermost inferior vena cava (IVC). Fluoroscopy is used to confirm the position of the guide wire tip. After confirming that the guide wire is positioned correctly, withdraw the needle and introduce a 11 Fr dilator sheath with the aid of an image intensifier to monitor correct travel of the sheath into the vein. Remove the dilator sheath and, using a screwing motion, pass a peel-off sheath, ideally into the uppermost IVC or into the right atrium. Remove the guide wire and trocar of the dilator sheath, and aspirate blood from the side arm to confirm positioning within the vein. Flush the sheath with saline.

ITA for Lead Extraction

Free-Floating Leads

Free-floating leads are defined as leads previously cut and abandoned intravascularly. A VEA approach is impossible. The femoral approach is technically possible but challenging, considering the required tools (transfemoral station, snares) and the suboptimal angle to

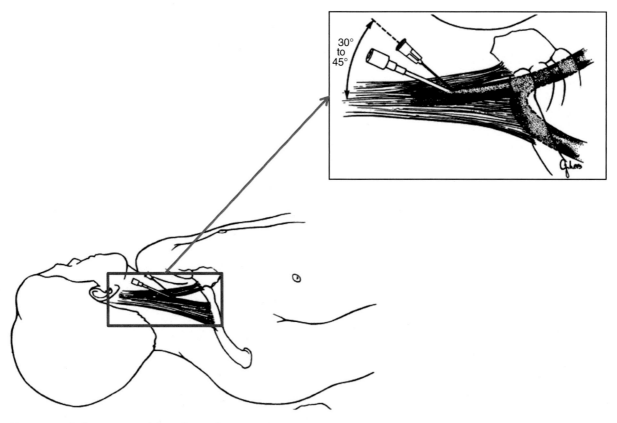

Figure 12.3 Catheterization of the right jugular vein.

achieve the lead tip in the right ventricle. Exposure of the lead through an SVC tributary, such as the right IJV, can enhance the effectiveness of dilatation, by using the same technique and tools as in the presence of exposed leads. Once exposed through the IJV, free-floating leads can be managed in the same way as exposed leads.

The right IJV is percutaneously cannulated using an 11 Fr introducer. A Lasso is advanced via the jugular vein, the proximal end of the lead is grasped and then exposed. The lead exposure from the right IJV allows the insertion of a stylet and sheaths as described for a standard approach through the venous entry site. When the length of the lead does not allow the lead to be exposed, the Lasso (Osypka GmbH) is used as an extension of the lead and dilation is performed by a dilating sheath, previously inserted over the lasso. In our experience, this approach results in the removal of all the leads submitted to the procedure without complications.

Complex VEA Extraction

Fibrosis propagation occurs along the lead which becomes increasingly dense with time (Figure 12.1). Patient and lead-related factors account for the quantity

and quality of adherences [26–31]. Usually, the venous entry site, the curve into the SVC, and the region from the anode ring to the lead tip are sites most likely to develop severe fibrosis [31]. A comprehensive knowledge of adherence location is key to a safe and effective transvenous procedure. The aim is dissection of all lead-related adherences from the venous entry site to the tip. Complications are commonly observed as the result of vascular or cardiac damage during dilatation. In the past, adherence rate and location have been described for standard pacing leads, and some predictors have been identified [11,31].

The SVC is a critical region for the shot angle between this vein and the right or left innominate vein. Particularly in case of presence of tenacious adherences in this region, the advancement of dilating sheaths, specially if powered, must expose the patient to risk of vein tearing. According to the "Pisa approach" [32], we use the IJV in order to reduce the shot angle between the sheath and the SVC during the dilating maneuver. In the presence of a difficult lead, it can be turned into a free-floating one, thus slipping it through some binding sites from the femoral vein, and then exposed through the IJV. At this point there is a "straight line" course all the way to the tip of the lead. Conventional dilatation of distal binding sites and the tip can be carried out. Regardless of the energy used, the straight course of the lead from the jugular vein to the heart facilitates dilatation and allows the use of large sheaths.

The VEA can be troublesome and risky in presence of:

1) Tight space between clavicle and first rib (as in medial access to intrathoracic subclavian vein).
2) Tenacious adherences in some critical points like innominate vein–SVC junction, SVC–right atrium

spring, right atrium, tricuspid valve, right ventricle. When, despite the use of a larger sheath, advancement of the sheath was stopped at any site of adherence for 5 minutes, or when dilatation was judged too risky, a cross over to ITA is considered. The approach through the IJV presents some advantages in these conditions. The straight course of the lead from the jugular vein to the SVC, right atrium, right ventricle allows the dilatation of adherences along the longitudinal axis of the lead. Using this

(a) (b)

(c) (d)

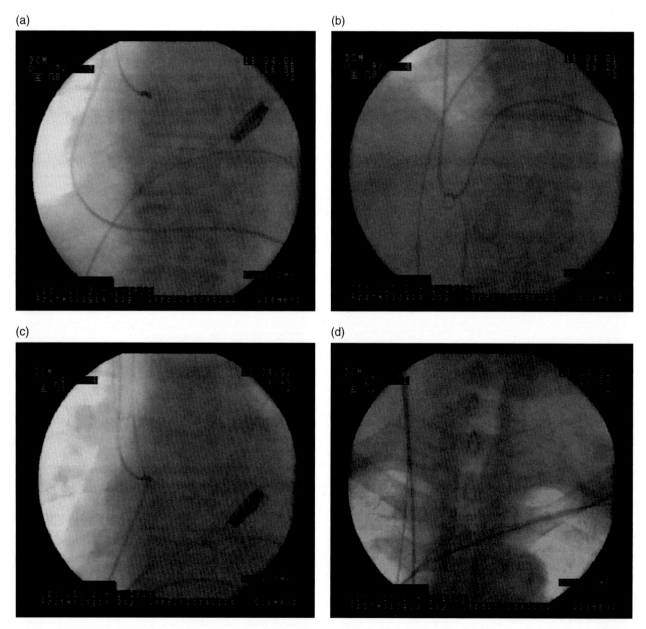

Figure 12.4 Fluoroscopic session of intra-procedural steps for internal transjugular approach (ITA) removal. (a) Dual chamber implantable cardioverter-defibrillator (ICD) with ineffective venous entry approach (VEA). (b) Using a transfemoral approach (TFA), the lead is grasped and pulled back in the venous system. (c) Using an ITA, the lead is grasped again and exteriorized. (d) A new mechanical dilatation is now performed from the right jugular vein.

technique, narrow bends (in leads inserted through the right site) and tight binding sites at the SVC are bypassed or safely dilated. In tight binding sites in the right chambers and tricuspid valve, the internal jugular approach allows better dilatation of adherences than through the vein of insertion because of the avoidance of long turns from venous entry access. The lead has to be made free from VEA up to the SVC. Then, through the right femoral vein, using a deflectable wire (Osypka) the lead is grasped and made intravascular. The next steps are exactly the same as described for intravascular leads (Figure 12.4).

Conclusions

Nowadays, transvenous approaches are the gold standard for cardiac lead extraction. In experienced hands, the overall success rate is about 90%, even if 10% of procedures continue to be challenging. The most common difficulties are related to the necessity of removal abandoned free floating leads or leads difficult to remove from the VEA. In all these cases, the ITA resulted in safe and effective complete lead removal. The incremental value of ITA is observed for both pacing and ICD leads, independently from procedural indication.

References

1 Bilgutay AM, Jensen NK, Schmidt WR, Garamella JJ, Lynch MF. Incarceration of transvenous pacemaker electrode: removal by traction. Am Heart J 1969;77:377–379.

2 Byrd CL, Schwartz SJ, Hedin N. Lead extraction: indications and techniques. Cardiol Clin 1992;10:735–748.

3 Imparato AM, Kim GE. Electrode complications in patients with permanent cardiac pacemakers: ten years' experience. Arch Surg 1972;105:705–710.

4 Myers MR, Parsonnet V, Bernstein AD. Extraction of implanted transvenous pacing leads: a review of a persistent clinical problem. Am Heart J 1991;121:881–888.

5 Wallace HW, Sherafat M, Blakemore WS. The stubborn pacemaker catheter. Surgery 1970;68:914–915.

6 del Rio A, Anguera I, Miro JM, Mont L, Fowler VG Jr, Azqueta M, et al. Surgical treatment of pacemaker and defibrillator lead endocarditis: the impact of electrode lead extraction on outcome. Chest 2003;124:1451–1459.

7 Frame R, Brodman RF, Furman S, Andrews CA, Gross JN. Surgical removal of infected transvenous pacemaker leads. Pacing Clin Electrophysiol 1993;16:2343–2348.

8 Love CJ, Wilkoff BL, Byrd CL, Belott PH, Brinker JA, Fearnot NE, et al. Recommendations for extraction of chronically implanted transvenous pacing and defibrillator leads: indications, facilities, training. North American Society of Pacing and Electrophysiology Lead Extraction Conference Faculty. Pacing Clin Electrophysiol 2000;23(4 Pt 1):544–551.

9 Wilkoff BL, Love CJ, Byrd CL, Bongiorni MG, Carrillo RG, Crossley GH 3rd, et al. Transvenous lead extraction: Heart Rhythm Society Expert consensus on facilities, training, indications, and patient management: this document was endorsed by the American Heart Association (AHA). Heart Rhythm 2009;6(7):1085–1104.

10 Robboy SJ, Harthorne JW, Leinbach RC, Sanders CA, Austen WG. Autopsy findings with permanent pervenous pacemakers. Circulation 1969;39(4):495–501.

11 Smith HJ, Fearnot NE, Byrd CL, Wilkoff BL, Love CJ, Sellers TD. Five years' experience with intravascular lead extraction: US lead extraction database. Pacing Clin Electrophysiol 1994;17(11 Pt 2):2016–2020.

12 Bongiorni MG, Zucchelli G, Soldati E, Arena G, Giannola G, Di Cori A, et al. Usefulness of mechanical transvenous dilation and location of areas of adherence in patients undergoing coronary sinus lead extraction. Europace 2007;9(1):69–73.

13 Segreti L, Di Cori A, Soldati E, Zucchelli G, Viani S, Paperini L, et al. Major predictors of fibrous adherences in transvenous implantable cardioverter-defibrillator lead extraction. Heart Rhythm 2014;11(12):2196–2201.

14 Verma A, Wilkoff BL. Intravascular pacemaker and defibrillator lead extraction: a state-of-the-art review. Heart Rhythm 2004;1(6):739–745.

15 Fearnot NE, Smith HJ, Goode LB, Byrd CL, Wilkoff BL, Sellers TD. Intravascular lead extraction using locking stylets, sheaths, and other techniques. Pacing Clin Electrophysiol 1990;13(12 Pt 2):1864–1870.

16 Yue A. System and lead extrations. In Timperley J, Leeson P, Mitchell ARJ, Betts T. (eds) Pacemaker and ICDs. O.M. Publications, 2008: 313–331.

17 Belott PH. Endocardial Lead Extraction. Futura, 1998: 142.

18 Byrd CL, Schwartz SJ, Hedin NB. Lead extraction: indications and techniques. Cardiol Clin 1992;10:735–748.

19 Bilgutay AM, Jensen NK, Schmidt WR, Garamella JJ, Lynch MF. Incarceration of transvenous pacemaker electrode: removal by traction. Am Heart J 1969;77(3):377–379.

20 Bongiorni, MG. Transvenous Lead Extraction: From Simple Traction to Internal Transjugular Approach. Springer Verlag, 2011.

21 Smith MC, Love CJ. Extraction of transvenous pacing and ICD leads. Pacing Clin Electrophysiol 2008;31(6):736–752.

22 Bongiorni MG, Soldati E, Zucchelli G, Di Cori A, Segreti L, De Lucia R, *et al.* Transvenous removal of pacing and implantable cardiac defibrillating leads using single sheath mechanical dilatation and multiple venous approaches: high success rate and safety in more than 2000 leads. Eur Heart J 2008;29(23):2886–2893.

23 Bongiorni MG, Giannola G, Arena G, Soldati E, Bartoli C, Lapira F, *et al.* Pacing and implantable cardioverter-defibrillator transvenous lead extraction. Ital Heart J 2005;6(3):261–266.

24 Sandring S. The anatomical basis of clinical practice. Gray's Anatomy, 40th edition. Churchill Livingstone, 2008.

25 Bongiorni MG. Techniques for transvenous leads extraction. Minerva Cardioangiol 2007;55(6): 771–781.

26 Bongiorni MG, Di Cori A, Segreti L, Zucchelli G, Viani S, Paperini L, *et al.* Transvenous extraction profile of Riata leads: procedural outcomes and technical complexity of mechanical removal. Heart Rhythm 2015;12(3):580–587.

27 Bongiorni MG, Segreti L, Di Cori A, Zucchelli G, Viani S, Paperini L, *et al.* Safety and efficacy of internal transjugular approach for transvenous extraction of implantable cardioverter defibrillator leads. Europace 2014;16(9):1356–1362.

28 Di Cori A, Bongiorni MG, Zucchelli G, Lilli A, Coluccia G, Fabiani I, *et al.* Short-term extraction profile of cardiac pacing leads with hybrid silicone-polyurethane insulator: a pilot study. Int J Cardiol 2013;9;168(4):4432–4433.

29 Maytin M, Carrillo RG, Baltodano P, Schaerf RH, Bongiorni MG, Di Cori A, *et al.* Multicenter experience with transvenous lead extraction of active fixation coronary sinus leads. Pacing Clin Electrophysiol 2012;35(6):641–647.

30 Di Cori A, Bongiorni MG, Zucchelli G, Segreti L, Viani S, de Lucia R, *et al.* Large, single-center experience in transvenous coronary sinus lead extraction: procedural outcomes and predictors for mechanical dilatation. Pacing Clin Electrophysiol 2012;35(2):215–222.

31 Di Cori A, Bongiorni MG, Zucchelli G, Segreti L, Viani S, Paperini L, *et al.* Transvenous extraction performance of expanded polytetrafluoroethylene covered ICD leads in comparison to traditional ICD leads in humans. Pacing Clin Electrophysiol 2010;33(11):1376–1381.

32 Kennergren C. European perspective on lead extraction: part II. Heart Rhythm 2008;5(2):320–323.

13

How to Perform Venoplasty for Access
Seth J. Worley

Medstar Heart & Vascular Institute Washington Hospital Center, Washington, DC, USA

Background

Fibrous occlusions develop in the subclavian/distal innominate vein and/or innominate/superior vena cava (SVC) in 13–35% of patients with existing leads. As indications for cardiovascular implantable electronic devices (CIEDs) expand and patients with existing CIED leads require additional or replacement leads, implanting physicians increasingly need to navigate these venous occlusions [1–8]. Subclavian obstruction is also a factor that prevents successful addition of an LV lead for cardiac resynchronization [9,10]. If crossing the occlusion followed by subclavian venoplasty is safe and does not damage the leads [11–18], it may be preferable to contralateral access, the supraclavicular approach [19,20], or powered sheath extraction, which pose additional risks [21–26].

Safety of Subclavian Venoplasty

We began performing subclavian venoplasty (SV) in 1999 and reported our results in 373 cases as of November 2010. Successful access was achieved in 371/373, with no adverse clinical outcome, no distal embolization (chronic occlusion no thrombus), no venous disruption (the veins are heavily encased in scar tissue), and no acute damage to the leads. To extend our safety data from 2010 [12], we identified 488 SV procedures performed by nine physicians at Lancaster General Hospital from January 27, 2004 to November 20, 2014 via an Electronic Health Record query. There were no acute clinical events in the cohort. It is unknown whether the pressure and mechanical stress to which existing leads are subjected during venoplasty affect long-term lead performance, so we looked for damage to existing leads becoming manifest over 12 months following venoplasty. Of the initial 488 patients, 20 were lost to follow-up. In the remaining 468 patients there were two atrial lead dislodgements and one insulation defect found in a pre-existing atrial lead. The atrial lead dislodgements were detected at 3 and 5 months post SV, respectively, while the insulation defect was detected at 9 months. When compared with a cohort who had lead replacement without venoplasty, there was no signal to suggest that venoplasty caused delayed lead damage.

In an attempt to acquire additional safety data, an email survey of 23 centers performing SV was conducted in 2015. All centers contacted responded. There was a mean of 19.4 ± 12.7 cases per center with no center reporting an adverse event. Based on the above it appears that SV is not only safe, but does not damage existing leads. Discussions of lead management should include venoplasty as a means to preserves venous access and assists in optimal lead placement. Because of the extensive fibrous tissue surrounding the leads (Figure 13.1), venoplasty is an intrinsically safe procedure: it is really fibroplasty not venoplasty. The safety experience described applies to patients with chronic leads (>2 years) where venoplasty was performed to add a lead(s). When SV is compared with progressively larger dilators, venoplasty is faster and there are problems with dilators; catheters remain difficult to manipulate throughout the procedure, central stenosis (SVC–right atrium junction) is not opened and dilators create a false sense of safety.

There are some situations where venoplasty may not be advisable such as along the SVC (Figure 13.2) and for a swollen arm developing within the first several months of implant. In the latter situation, fibrous tissue has not yet developed and larger balloons are required, increasing the likelihood of venous disruption: in this

How-to Manual for Pacemaker and ICD Devices: Procedures and Programming, First Edition. Edited by Amin Al-Ahmad, Andrea Natale, Paul J. Wang, James P. Daubert, and Luigi Padeletti.
© 2018 John Wiley & Sons, Inc. Published 2018 by John Wiley & Sons, Inc.
Companion website: www.wiley.com/go/al-ahmad/pacemakers_and_icds

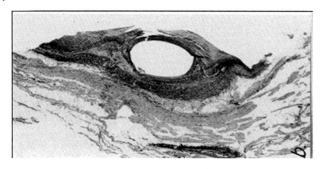

Figure 13.1 Example of the dense fibrous tissue that develops around the pacing lead.

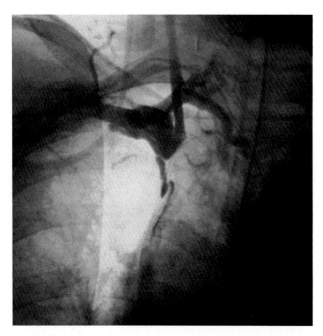

Figure 13.2 Right-sided venous obstruction that may not be safe to dilate. The predominant area off obstruction is along the lateral wall of superior vena cava (SVC) rather than within the subclavian innominate vein. Although a wire was easily advanced into the right atrium venoplasty was not performed because of the lack tissue surrounding the obstruction and the catastrophic nature of an SVC tear.

case venoplasty not fibroplasty. In addition, there is little evidence that venoplasty for a swollen arm produces lasting patency with clinical improvement resulting from collateral development.

Utility of Subclavian Venoplasty

Ji *et al.* [27] were able to evaluate the utility of SV at Montefiore Medical Center/Albert Einstein College of Medicine where some implanting physicians decided to adopt/learn venoplasty and others chose *not* to adopt/learn venoplasty. In 41 patients with subclavian vein occlusion who were sent for the addition of lead(s), 18 were performed by physicians who learned to perform SV, 23 by physicians who did not learn to perform SV. When the implanting physician was venoplasty competent, procedure times were shorter (2:31 hours venoplasty competent, 3:28 hours not venoplasty competent). When the implanting physician was venoplasty competent, implants were more successful: five implant failures in the 23 cases (21.5%) resulting from inability to gain venous access when the implanter was *not* venoplasty competent. There were no implant failures in the 18 cases when the implanter was venoplasty competent [27].

Step-by-Step Approach to Subclavian Venoplasty

1) In patients with previous leads, because of the possibility of subclavian obstruction, we now start venous access with a 15 cm stiffened dilator micro puncture kit (for details see Box 13.1) rather than using the 18 gauge needle and wire that comes with the sheath.

2) Perform an axillary vein venogram. While the contrast is flowing, enter the vein with the needle as far peripheral to the occlusion as possible (Figure 13.3; Videos 13.1, 13.3, and 13.4) without regard to the location of the rib. Unlike traditional axillary vein access, the needle should enter the body at a shallow angle (approximately 30 degrees).

3) To enter the vein peripheral to the occlusion it is often necessary to enter the vein through the skin rather than through the pocket. If the needle enters the vein at the site of occlusion, it will be difficult to advance the wire and any opening through which to advance the wire will be lost. Do not be concerned if it seems like there is a total occlusion, the peripheral venogram usually overestimates the severity of the obstruction.

4) Carefully advance the wire into the vein up to the site of obstruction. It is important not to disrupt the site of obstruction with the needle or the wire.

5) Carefully advance the 5 Fr dilator or stiffened dilator/5 Fr catheter over the wire (Videos 13.1, 13.3, and 13.5). The tip of the dilator should not be pushed beyond the tip of the wire. The goal is the get the tip of the dilator/catheter a few millimeters peripheral to the obstruction.

6) Attach a contrast injection system with hemostatic Y adapter to the hub of the dilator/catheter (Figure 13.4). An injection system similar to that shown in Figure 13.4(a) can be assembled from "spare parts" available in most labs or purchased more cost effectively as a kit (Box 13.1).

Box 13.1 Annotated list of equipment for crossing and dilating a subclavian obstruction/occlusion

Contrast injection system

Attached to the hub of the dilator from a 5 Fr sheath or the 5 Fr catheter of the micro-puncture system. Contrast injection through the system with the tip of the dilator/catheter at the site of occlusion will identify an opening through which to advance a wire. The Y adapter with rotating hemostatic valve allows the wire to be advanced through the dilator/catheter to cross the occlusion:

1) Contrast Injection System Worley Advanced Kit 1 CAK 1(comes w/contrast bowl and labels) (Order # K12-WORLEY1 Merit Medical); or
2) Worley Advanced Kit CAK 2 (without bowl and labels) (Order # K12-WORLEY2 Merit Medical).

Dilator from 5 Fr sheath

Prior to our recent conversion to a stiffened dilator micro-puncture kit, the dilator from a standard 5 Fr sheath would be advanced over the 0.035 inch J wire from a standard peel-away sheath. Conversion to stiffened micro-puncture kit was precipitated by:

1) Difficulty advancing a 0.035 inch wire into vein for initial venous access (easier using a 0.018 inch wire);
2) Difficulty advancing the dilator over the wire (not stiff enough);
3) Difficulty visualizing the tip of the dilator to be certain it was in the vein (not radiopaque).

5 Fr micro-puncture kit with radiopaque tip and stiffened dilator for initial venous access

The 21 gauge needle and angled tip 0.018 inch Nitinol wire can make initial venous access easier. The stiffened dilator (indicated by the S in the order number) provides support to advance over the wire through scar tissue and/or difficult anatomy when compared with a standard micro-puncture kit without a stiffened dilator. The stiffened dilator is also more radiopaque so you can be certain the tip is in the vein. Finally, the length of the catheter is 15 cm (usually 10 cm) to increase the likelihood that the tip of the 5 Fr catheter reaches beyond the stenosis (Order # S-MAK501N15BT) (Catheter = 5 Fr – 15 cm, wire = 0.018 inch × 60 cm Nitinol with platinum tip, needle = 21 G × 7 cm.

Wires for crossing subclavian obstructions

Angled polymer tip (PT) Nitinol wires with a hydrophilic coating (AKA glide wire or Terumo) are best for crossing subclavian obstructions These wires are available from multiple vendors with slightly different names. The polymer tip Nitinol construction, hydrophilic coating,

length, diameter, and tip configuration are all key issue. In general, 0.014 inch angioplasty wires have not been helpful in crossing subclavian occlusions. The majority of 0.014 inch angioplasty wires are made of stainless steel (not Nitinol). The tips of stainless steal wires are easily deformed by contact with the fibrous tissue where the Nitinol wire retail their shape.

1) 0.035 inch × 180 cm angled tip (not straight) wires are available from multiple vendors including Merit Medical Laureate wire (Order # LWSTDA35180 Merit Medical);
2) 0.018 inch × 180 cm angled tip (not straight) wire available from multiple vendors including Merit Medical Laureate wire (Order # LWSTDA18180 Merit Medical).

Torque device (AKA steering handle) for directing the angled tip wire

Because of the hydrophilic coating the wires are very slippery and the torque device is essential for the operator to direct the tip (caution: one size does not work for all size wires multiple vendors including Merit Medical).

1) Torque device for 0.014–0.018 inch wire;
2) Torque Device for 0.025–0.038 inch wires.

Catheters used to exchange from a polymer tip wire to an extra support wire and to cross a difficult subclavian obstruction/total occlusion

Catheters for wire exchange

The polymer tip wire used to cross the occlusion frequently does not provide sufficient support to advance the balloon across the occlusion. To provide adequate support the polymer tip wire needs to be exchanged for an extra support wire (Amplatz Extra Support). To exchange wires, a 4–5 Fr braided hydrophilic catheter works best. The metal braid and hydrophilic coating are essential. Similar catheters without metal braid (e.g., Terumo Glide Cath) do not have adequate stability to be advanced over the wire into the central circulation. On occasion a tight stenosis may require downsizing to a 4 Fr catheter. One of the angled tip catheters is used for both crossing a difficult occlusion and wire exchange. As an alternative to an angled tip catheter, the straight catheter can be used when the polymer tip wire advances to the central circulation without the need for an angled tip catheter.

Catheters for crossing difficult occlusions

To cross totally occluded subclavian, a properly shaped, angled tip, braided catheter with a hydrophilic coating is essential. To my surprise I also found that the length and

(Continued)

Box 13.1 (Continued)

angle of the tip are critical, slight variations in tip tangle and length are surprisingly important. The angled tip is used to direct the wire to more decisively, the braided catheter provides support to push the wire into the occlusion. Once the wire advances the catheter is worked up to the tip of the wire. I have the most experience with the 5 Fr version of the catheters listed. Similar catheters without metal braid (Terumo) do not have adequate torque control or support:

1) 5 Fr Impress KA 2 Hydrophilic Angiographic Catheter 5 Fr 65 cm (Order # 56538KA2-H Merit Medical);
2) 4 Fr Impress KA 2 Hydrophilic Angiographic Catheter 4 Fr 65 cm (Order # 46538KA2-H Merit Medical);
3) 4 Fr Impress STS Hydrophilic Straight Angiographic Catheter 4 Fr 65 cm (Order # 46538STS-H Merit Medical).

If both the 4 and 5 Fr KA 2 catheters (1 and 2 above) are available, the straight 4 Fr is optional (3 above).

J Tip Extra Stiff Support Wire to replace the polymer tip wire used to cross the obstruction

Note: Not all Amplatz Extra Stiff wires are created equal! For example, both the Boston Scientific and Cook are labeled "Amplatz Extra Stiff"; however, the support provided is very different. With "Extra Support" wires the total length, the coating, the tip (J tip not straight), the length of the floppy section after the J tip, and stiffness are the key issues. In my experience, the Cook Amplatz Extra Stiff Wire Guide provides the best option for providing stability in the coronary sinus (CS). The floppy section beyond the J tip of the Boston Scientific is too long to be useful in the CS. Cook wire details: 0.035 inch diameter, 180 cm total length, PTFE-Coated Stainless Steel, 3 mm curve J tip, 3 cm floppy tip length, and 7 cm taper length (THSCF-35-180-3-AES, Order # G03565). For providing support to advance a

balloon either wire is satisfactory; however, for providing support in the CS the correct wire (Cook) will make the difference between success and failure. Order the Cook for simplicity of inventory.

Balloons for subclavian venoplasty – Ultra-noncompliant and over the wire

Because a 0.035 inch polymer tip hydrophilic wire is usually used to cross the subclavian obstruction, you need a balloon with a 0.035 inch lumen to go over the wire.

1) To add one lead use a 6 mm diameter × 4 cm length × 75 cm. Example CONQUEST (Kevlar) Order # CQ-7564 Bard Peripheral Vascular Ultra-noncompliant: wire lumen 0.035 inch, over the wire, rated burst pressure 30 atm.
2) To add two leads or if there is elastic recoil use a 9 mm × 4 cm × 75 cm balloon Bard Peripheral Vascular Ultra-noncompliant: wire lumen 0.035 inch, over the wire, rated burst pressure 26 atm. Order # CQ-7594 Bard Peripheral Vascular.
3) When the 6–9 mm diameter balloon will not advance across the obstruction, use one of the 4 Fr braided hydrophilic catheter (above) to exchange the 0.035 inch wire for a 0.014 inch extra support wire and pre-dilate with a noncompliant rapid exchange coronary balloon (below). Once pre-dilated, replace the 0.014 inch wire for the 0.035 inch extra support wire and finish dilating with the 6–9 mm balloon.

Balloons for pre-dilation in the event the stenosis is too tight to allow the larger balloons to cross the obstruction (these are coronary balloons)

Noncompliant (RBP 18–20 atm) and rapid exchange available from multiple vendors (e.g., 3.0 × 15 mm, NC Sprinter from Medtronic).

---

7) Inject contrast to identify an opening in the occlusion (Figure 13.5). Do not be concerned if it seems as if there is a total occlusion. The majority of the time a wire can be passed, either alone with a torque device (Videos 13.1 and 13.5) or with the assistance of a braided angled tip catheter (Videos 13.3 and 13.4) even when no opening is immediately apparent (Figure 13.6).

8) Insert a 0.035–0.018 inch angled polymer tip Nitinol wire into the hemostatic valve. Nitinol angled polymer tip wires are available from several vendors (Box 13.1). In some cases, the 0.035 inch wire is too large to cross the obstruction. I find the 0.018 inch Nitinol polymer tip wire superior to a 0.014 inch

angioplasty wire because the angioplasty wire is stainless steel which is easily bent whereas the Nitinol of the 0.018 inch wire retains its shape.

9) Attach a torque device to the proximal end of the wire 5–10 cm from where it enters the hemostatic valve.
10) Close the hemostatic valve.
11) Use puffs of contrast and the torque device to direct the wire across the occlusion (Videos 13.1 and 13.5).
12) If the wire alone cannot be advanced across the obstruction, replace the 5 Fr dilator/5 Fr micro puncture catheter with and angled 4–5 Fr braided, hydrophilic catheter (Box 13.1). As detailed in Box 13.1, the angle and length of the tip as well as

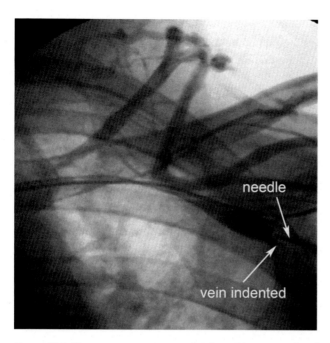

Figure 13.3 Venous access as contrast is injected into a peripheral vein. The occlusion with collaterals is apparent. The vein is entered peripheral to the occlusion. When the needle is inserted into the vein as contrast is flowing the vein can be seen to indent confirming where the needle enters the vein. When crossing an occlusion it is important to enter the vein as far peripheral to the occlusion as possible.

metal braid in the walls of the catheter are critical, substitution is not advised. The angled tip catheter is used to inject contrast and aim the wire toward an opening (Video 13.3). In addition, the catheter is stiff enough to be pushed into the occlusion followed by the wire (Video 13.4). I cannot say whether the 4 or 5 Fr angled catheter is superior. I have the most experience with the 5 Fr angled catheter and like the support provided.

13) Confirm that the wire has entered the heart.
   - Advance the wire until the tip enters either the pulmonary artery (PA) or the inferior vena cava (IVC). If the wire does not advance into the PA or IVC do not proceed.
   - Confirm in the right anterior oblique (RAO) and left anterior oblique (LAO) projections, that the wire follows the lead(s) to the SVC.

14) Replace the polymer tip wire with an Amplatz Extra Stiff wire using a braided 4–5 Fr catheter.
   - If the wire alone advanced, use either the 4 Fr straight or 4 Fr angled catheter.
   - If an angled tip catheter was required to advance the wire, use it for wire exchange.

15) Advance a 6–9 mm diameter by 4 cm ultra-noncompliant balloon over the Amplatz Extra Stiff wire (Box 13.1) to just beyond the SVC–innominate junction. Use a 9 mm balloon if the

plan is to add two leads or there is elastic recoil after 6 mm balloon inflation.

16) If the balloon will not track to the SVC–innominate junction, use the braided catheter to replace the 0.035 inch wire with two 180 cm 0.014 inch extra stiff angioplasty wires (any manufacturer will do). Pre-dilate the obstruction with a 4×15 mm non-compliant rapid exchange coronary balloon. Once dilated, use the braided catheter to replace the angioplasty wires with the Amplatz Extra Stiff wire and finish dilating with the 6–9 mm balloon.

17) Always perform the first inflation at or central to the SVC–innominate junction. Initially, we did not dilate at the SVC–innominate junction but when we tried to advance the sheath we found a stenosis requiring additional venoplasty in approximately 20% of cases. Because the profile of the balloon increases after the first inflation–deflation cycle (called "winging"), the balloon used for the more apparent proximal stenosis would not would advance through the central stenosis.

18) Inflate the balloon to the rated burst pressure (RBP) indicated on the balloon package (26–30 atm for the peripheral balloons listed in Box 13.1 and 18–20 atm for the coronary balloon).

19) Keep the balloon inflated until the pressure is stable at RBP and there is no residual waist. If the waist is not eliminated use "focused force venoplasty" (Figure 13.7).

20) Deflate the balloon by applying negative pressure to the inflation device.

21) Once the contrast is evacuated from the balloon, withdraw the balloon until the tip reaches the former tail position (head to tail overlap). Do not withdraw the balloon until the contrast is evacuated from the balloon (Figure 13.8).

22) Continue the head to tail overlap inflation until the tail of the balloon is visible in the pocket. The recommendation to continue until the tail visible in the pocket frequently produces concern but is essential and does no seem to cause excessive bleeding. If bleeding is a problem it is easily addressed with a hemostatic suture.

23) Advance a long (25 cm) sheath over the wire. Always use a long sheath after venoplasty. By definition, there is excessive elastic recoil if it is not very easy to advance the sheaths (similar to a virgin implant). If elastic recoil is present it is worth taking the time to upsize to a 9 mm diameter balloon. The other explanation for difficulty advancing the sheath is a residual peripheral stenosis from failure to inflate the balloon with the tail visible in the pocket as recommended.

24) If two leads are needed, advance two Amplatz Extra Stiff wires into the long sheath, and withdraw the sheath retaining the two wires.

(a)

(b)

(c)

(d)

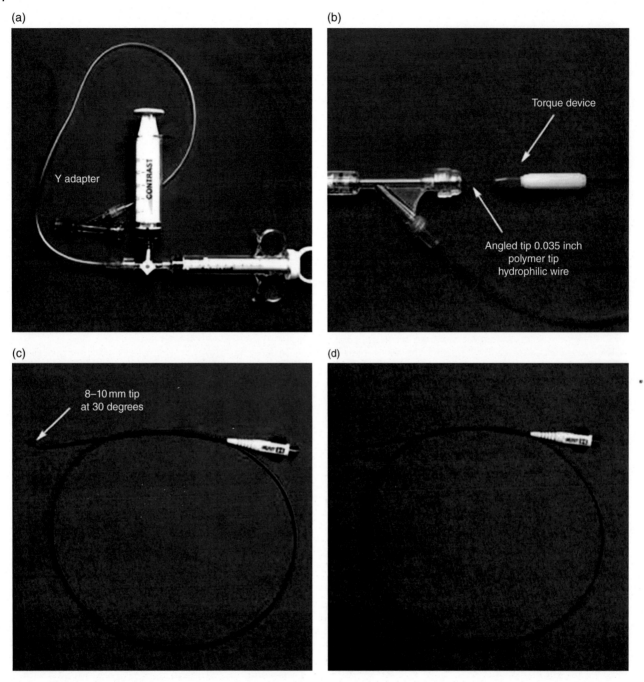

Figure 13.4 Equipment used to cross and dilate a subclavian obstruction. (a) The contrast injection system Contrast Injection System (Worley Advanced Kit 1 CAK 1 [includes contrast bowl and labels] order # K12-WORLEY1 Merit Medical or Worley Advanced Kit CAK 2 [without bowl and labels] Order # K12-WORLEY2 Merit Medical). (b) The 0.035 inch/150 cm angled polymer tip hydrophilic (Laureate wire Order # LWSTDA35150 Merit Medical) is advanced through the hemostatic valve of the Y adapter. A torque device is essential for directing the wire through the opening observed with local contrast injection. (c) The 5 Fr braided angled tip hydrophilic catheter (5 Fr 65 cm Impress KA-2 Hydrophilic Angiographic Catheter Order # 56538KA2-H Merit Medical) used to direct a wire through an occlusion (crossing catheter). The wire braid in the catheter provides torque control and "push-ability" that are important for crossing difficult obstructions. The length (6–8 mm) and angle (30 degrees) of the tip are also important. In my experience similar catheters with a longer tip or more acute angle are less effective. (d) The 4 Fr braided straight catheter (65 cm Impress Straight Hydrophilic Angiographic Catheter Order # 46538STS-H Merit Medical) used to exchange an existing wire for a more supportive wire over which to advance the balloon. I find that a braided hydrophilic catheter will advance through an obstruction when a non-braided catheter of the same French size will not advance.

(a)

(b)

(c)

(d)

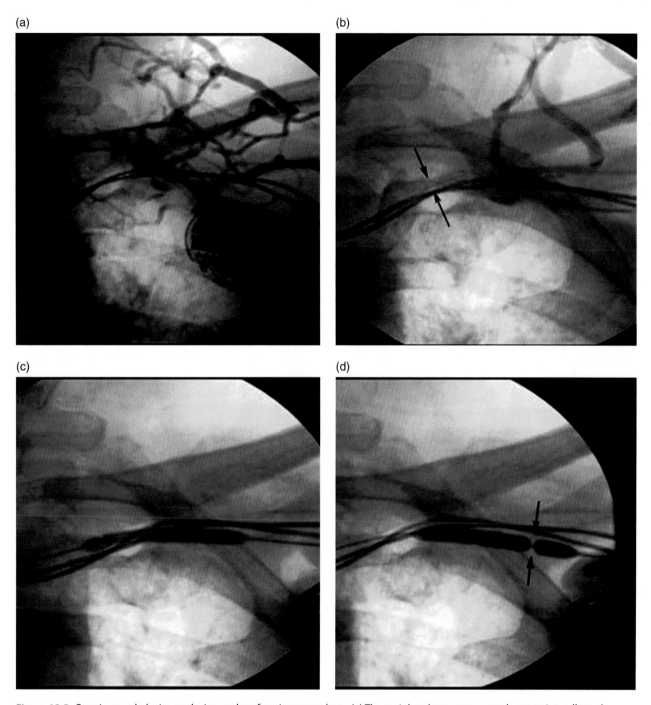

Figure 13.5 Crossing a subclavian occlusion and performing venoplasty. (a) The peripheral venogram reveals extensive collaterals suggesting total occlusion. (b) Injection at the site of occlusion through the dilator from a 5 Fr sheath (local venogram) reveals a stenosis not a total occlusion through which the wire is easily advanced. (c) A 6 mm × 4 cm non-compliant balloon is inflated at the site of occlusion seen on the venogram. (d) The balloon is inflated more peripherally, revealing a stenosis not appreciated on either the peripheral or local venogram.

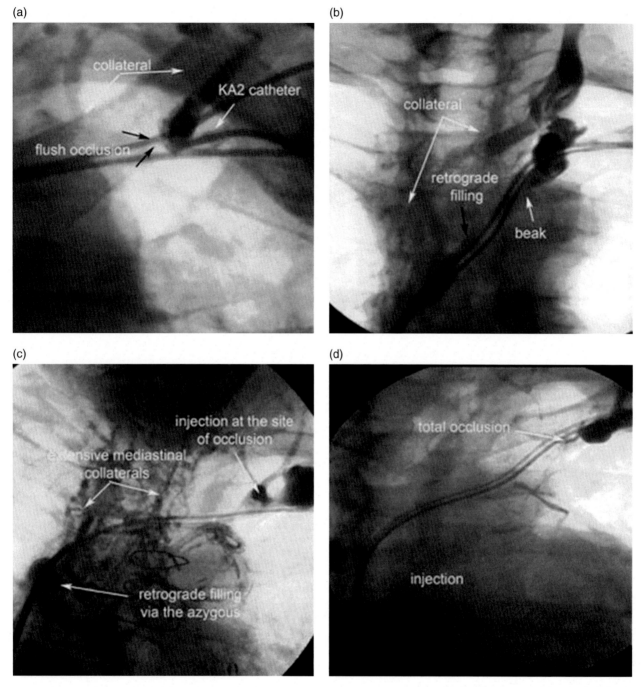

Figure 13.6 Subclavian occlusion despite injection at the site of occlusion (local venogram). (a) Injection with the angled tip hydrophilic braided crossing catheter (Figure 13.4c) at the site of obstruction reveals that the subclavian is flush occluded. Despite this the obstruction was crossed using the KA2 catheter and polymer tip hydrophilic wire. The KA2 was advanced into the right atrium, the hydrophilic wire exchanged for an extra support wire and venoplasty performed. (b) Injection at the site of occlusion reveals near total occlusion; however, contrast is seen to taper to a "beak." Directing the wire into the "beak" with the KA2 is associated with a good chance of successful crossing of the occlusion. Retrograde filling of contrast is also observed and is associated with successful crossing. The KA2 and glide wire were used to successfully cross the occlusion. (c) There is total occlusion at the site of injection though the dilator from a 5 Fr sheath. There is retrograde filling via collateral to the azygous vein. A beak at the site of occlusion suggests that crossing the occlusion is possible. Surprisingly, a 0.035 inch, angled polymer tip hydrophilic wire was easily passed through the occlusion without the need for the KA2. The glide wire was exchanged for a 0.035 inch super stiff wire using the 4 Fr braided hydrophilic exchange catheter (Figure 13.4d) but the 6 mm diameter balloon would not advance through the occlusion. The 0.035 inch wire was exchanged for a 0.018 inch wire and a 6 mm × 4 cm low profile balloon was advanced through the occlusion and venoplasty performed. (d) Total occlusion without a beak is seen with contrast injection at the site of occlusion. There is no retrograde filling of the innominate. Femoral access and injection at the site where the lead enters the SVC revealed flush occlusion. The obstruction could not be crossed.

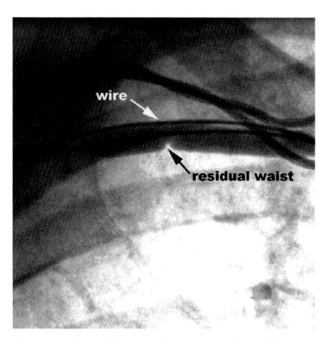

Figure 13.7 Focused force venoplasty (see text for details).

Balloon Options

Coronary balloons are too small (both length and diameter) for SV to add a lead. With a 0.035 inch wire across the obstruction it makes sense to start with a balloon designed to go over the wire (Box 13.1). When the stenosis is tight enough to require a 0.018 inch wire, the obstruction usually requires pre-dilation with a 4 mm coronary balloon before the 6–9 mm balloon will pass. As indicated in Box 13.1, the recommended balloon diameter is 6–9 mm and length 4–6 cm. The 9 mm balloon is useful if there is excess elastic recoil or if the intent is to add two leads. Alternatively, elastic recoil may be addressed with focused force venoplasty. If a 9 mm diameter balloon is not available for adding two leads, the stenosis can be re-dilated with the 6 mm balloon when the first long sheath (with dilator) is in place. The 6–9 mm balloons are 40–75 cm in length and can be over the wire without the need for exchange length wires. By comparison, coronary balloons are 120 cm in length, thus to avoid the need for 300 cm wires, rapid exchange models (not over the wire) are required.

Wire Exchange

The Nitinol angled polymer tip hydrophilic wire used to cross the occlusion often does not provide sufficient support to advance the balloon through the obstruction (Video 13.2). Accordingly, a 4–5 Fr braided hydrophilic catheter (Box 13.1) is advanced over the existing wire to

exchange for an Amplatz Extra Stiff wire. A variety of hydrophilic exchange catheters are available. We find that a braided catheter (wire braid incorporated into the wall) provides greater ability to advance through the obstruction.

Focused Force Venoplasty

Approximately 3% of cases require focused force venoplasty for a stenosis (Figure 13.8) refractory to an ultra-noncompliant balloon (RBP 30 atm). Focused force can also be attempted when there is excessive elastic recoil (i.e., when it remains difficult to manipulate the catheter after initial balloon dilation despite no visible waist). To apply focused force, remove the balloon, advance a long 5 Fr sheath over the wire (or a 6 Fr multipurpose guide not diagnostic catheter), advance two 0.035 inch J tip Amplatz Extra Stiff wires through the sheath/guide, remove the sheath/guide and advance the balloon over one of the wires. The balloon is then inflated to RBP against the wire beside the balloon. The stiff wire beside the balloon pressed against the fibrous tissue is more aggressive then the balloon alone. The procedure is also referred to as the poor man's cutting balloon.

How to Cross a Difficult Subclavian Occlusion

The key to success is to enter the vein peripheral to the occlusion at a shallow angle (30 degrees). To this end it is best to enter the vein while contrast is flowing to confirm where the needle enters the vein (Videos 13.1, 13.3, and 13.4). To achieve the proper angle (30 degrees off the skin), it is usually necessary to stick through the skin peripheral to the pocket then pull the wire into the pocket. In many cases the angled polymer tip Nitinol wire crosses the occlusion. If not, the 5 Fr dilator/5 Fr micro puncture catheter is replaced with a braided angled hydrophilic catheter (Box 13.1) to provide direction and support for the wire.

Combining Femoral Extraction and Venoplasty

In some cases, it may be impossible to cross a total subclavian obstruction which brings up the use of extraction for venous access. Pre-pectoral extraction with powered or mechanical sheaths requires termination of the procedure to arrange for OR back-up because of the risk of SVC laceration and perforation. However, in many cases,

(a)

(b)

(c)

(d)

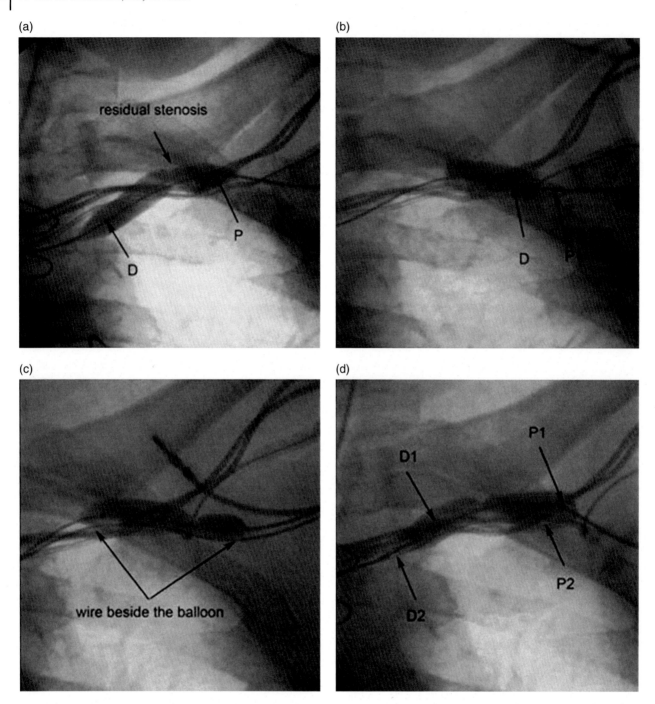

Figure 13.8 Difficult subclavian obstruction with extensive elastic recoil. (a) The balloon is inflated with a residual waist. The distal (D) and proximal (P) markers on the balloon catheter are separated by 4 cm. (b) The balloon is withdraw before the contrast is fully removed. The proximal (P) and distal (D) markers on the balloon are closer together indicating that the tip of the balloon is folded back on itself making it larger and more difficult to remove. (c) After the balloon is re-advanced, a wire is advanced beside the balloon and the balloon inflated against the wire (focused force venoplasty). (d) A second balloon is advanced beside the first and both balloons inflated simultaneously. D1, P1 are the distal and proximal markers on the first balloon. D2, P2 are the distal and proximal markers on the second balloon.

combining femoral extraction of an existing lead with venoplasty can avoid the need for OR back-up particularly in patients with prior sternotomy. For example, if there is an existing active fixation atrial lead in a patient with prior OHS the lead can be used for access as illustrated in Figure 13.9. Conversely, retained wire femoral extraction of an "old" passive fixation atrial lead in a patient without previous OHS could result in perforation at the site of attachment of the tip of the lead to the myocardium.

(a)

(b)

(c)

(d)

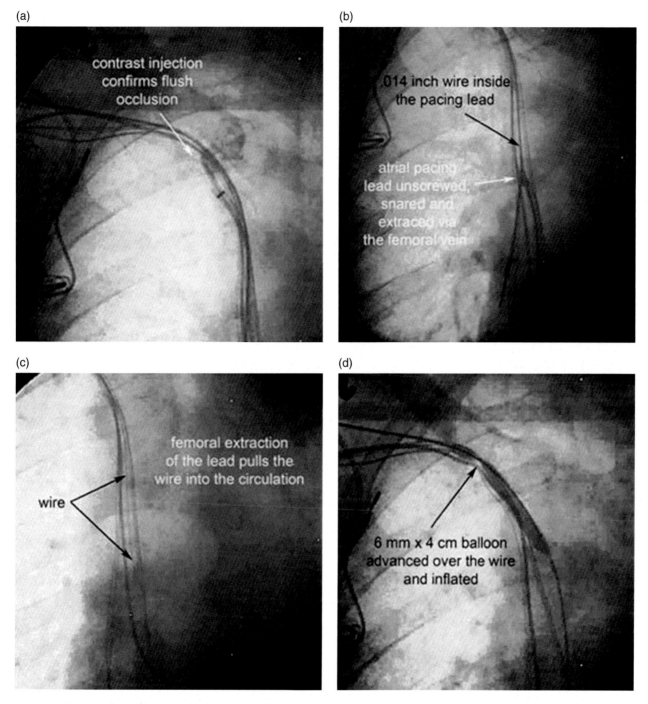

Figure 13.9 Retained wire femoral extraction followed by venoplasty in a case of total occlusion not able to be crossed. (a) Femoral access and contrast injection confirms that the right innominate is flush occluded at the SVC. It was not possible to advance a wire from either direction despite using the KA2. (b) The suture sleeve of the active fixation atrial lead was released and the screw retracted in an unsuccessful attempt to use the wire under the insulation technique to advance a wire into the circulation. Subsequently, the IS-1 connector was removed and a 300 cm 0.014 inch angioplasty wire advanced to the tip of the lead. A 25 mm loop snare (6 Fr × 100 cm snare catheter + a loop 25 mm diameter 120 cm in length "One Snare" order # ONE2500 Merit Medical) was advanced through a long sheath over the tip and closed on the body of the atrial lead containing the angioplasty wire. (c) The atrial lead is extracted via the femoral vein pulling the angioplasty wire into the circulation. The 0.014 inch angioplasty wire is exchanged for a 0.035 inch super stiff wire using the 4 Fr braided hydrophilic exchange catheter (Figure 13.4d). (d) A 6 mm × 4 cm noncompliant balloon was advanced over the Amplatz wire and inflated to it's rated burst pressure. The first inflation was at the subclavian SVC junction with subsequent overlapping inflations until the tail of the balloon was seen in the pocket.

How to Make a Subclavian Obstruction Difficult to Cross

An attempt at venous access in a patient with existing lead(s) before a venogram is often successful. However, if there is an obstruction the initial blind attempt(s) can disrupt the venous anatomy making it impossible to cross the occlusion. If the artery is entered inadvertently the subsequent hematoma will compress the vein making access even more difficult. If you start with a frozen venogram or ultrasound it will not be clear where the needle enters the vein relative to the obstruction. If the needle enters the vein at the site of occlusion the wire will not advance and/or an existing opening will be obscured.

References

1 Bracke F, Meijer A, Gelder B. Venous occlusion of the access vein in patients referred for lead extraction: influence of patient and lead characteristics. PacingClin Electrophysiol 2003;26:1649–1652.

2 Lickfett L, Bitzen A, Arepally A, Nasir K, Wolpert C, Jeong KM, *et al.* Incidence of venous obstruction following insertion of an implantable cardioverter defibrillator: a study of systematic contrast venography on patients presenting for their first elective ICD generator replacement. Europace 2004;6:25–31.

3 Spittell P, Vleietstra R, Hayes D, Higano S. Venous obstruction due to permanent transvenous pacemaker electrodes: treatment with percutaneous transluminal balloon venoplasty. Pacing Clin Electrophysiol 1990;13:271–274.

4 Spittell PC, Hayes DL. Venous complications after insertion of a transvenous pacemaker. Mayo Clin Proc 1992;67:258–265.

5 Oginosawa Y, Abe H, Nakashima Y. The incidence and risk factors for venous obstruction after implantation of transvenous pacing leads. Pacing Clin Electrophysiol 2002;25:1605–1611.

6 Haghjoo M, Nikoo MH, Fazelifar AF, Alizadeh A, Emkanjoo Z, Sadr-Ameli MA. Predictors of venous obstruction following pacemaker or implantable cardioverter defibrillator implantation: a contrast venographic study on 100 patients admitted for generator change, lead revision, or device upgrade. Europace 2007;9:328–332.

7 Bulur S, Vural A, Yazıcı M, Ertaş G, Özhan H, Ural D. Incidence and predictors of subclavian vein obstruction following biventricular device implantation. J Interv Card Electrophysiol 2010;29:199–202.

8 Sticherling C, Chough SP, Baker RL, Wasmer K, Oral H, Tada H, *et al.* Prevalence of central venous occlusion in patients with chronic defibrillator leads. Am Heart J 2001;141:813–816.

9 Poole JE, Gleva MJ, Mela T, Chung MK, Uslan DZ, Borge R, *et al.* REPLACE registry investigators. Circulation 2010;122:1553–1561.

10 Duray GZ, Israel CW, Pajitnev D, Hohnloser SH. Upgrading to biventricular pacing/defibrillation systems in right ventricular paced congestive heart failure patients: prospective assessment of procedural parameters and response rate. Europace 2008;10:48–52.

11 McCotter CJ, Angle JF, Prudente LA, Mounsey JP,Ferguson JD, *et al.* Placement of transvenous pacemaker and ICD leads across total chronic occlusions. Pacing Clin Electrophysiol 2005;28:921–925.

12 Worley S, Gohn DC, Pulliam RW, Raifsnider MA, Ebersole BI, Tuzi J. Subclavian venoplasty by the implanting physicians in 373 patients over 11 years. Heart Rhythm 2011;8:526–533.

13 Worley SJ. Implant venoplasty: dilatation of subclavian and coronary veins to facilitate device implantation: indications, frequency, methods, and complications. J Cardiovasc Electrophysiol 2008;19:1004–1007.

14 Worley SJ, Gohn DC, Pulliam RW. Over the wire lead extraction and focused force venoplasty to regain venous access in a totally occluded subclavian vein. J Interv Card Electrophysiol 2008;23:135–137.

15 Worley SJ, Gohn DC, Smith TL. Micro-dissection to open totally occluded subclavian veins. EP Lab Digest EP, September 2003.

16 Worley SJ, Gohn DC, Pulliam RW. Needle directed re-entry to cross a subclavian occlusion following failed microdissection. Pacing Clin Electrophysiol 2007;30:1562–1565.

17 Baerlocher MO, Asch MR, Myers A. Successful recanalization of a longstanding complete left subclavian vein occlusion by radiofrequency perforation with use of a radiofrequency guide wire. J Vasc Interv Radiol 2006;17:1703–1706.

18 Worley SJ, Gohn DC, Pulliam RW. Excimer laser to open refractory subclavian occlusion in 12 consecutive patients. Heart Rhythm 2010;7:634–638.

19 Antonelli D, Freedberg NA, Rosenfeld T. Lead insertion by supraclavicular approach of subclavian vein puncture. Pacing Clin Electrophysiol 2001;24:379–380.

20 Fox DJ, Petkar S, Davidson NC, Fitzpatrick AP. Upgrading patients with chronic defibrillator leads to a biventricular system and reducing patient risk: contralateral LV lead placement. Pacing Clin Electrophysiol 2006;29:1025–1027.

21 Jones S, Eckart R, Albert C, Epstein L. Large, single-center, single-operator experience with transvenous lead extraction: outcomes and changing indications. Heart Rhythm 2008;5:520–525.

22 Byrd CL, Wilkoff BL, Love CJ, Sellers TD, Reiser C. Clinical study of the laser sheath for lead extraction: the total experience in the United States. Pacing Clin Electrophysiol 2002;25:804–808.

23 Wilkoff BL, Byrd C, Love CJ, Hayes DL, Sellers TD, Schaerf R, *et al.* Pacemaker lead extraction with the laser sheath: results of the pacing lead extraction with the excimer sheath (PLEXES) trial. J Am Coll Cardiol 1999;33:1671–1676.

24 Bongiomi MG, Giannola G, Arena G, Zucchelli G, Paperini L, Viani S, *et al.* Pacing and implantable cardioverterdefibrillator transvenous lead extraction. Ital Heart J 2005;6:261–266.

25 Hauser RG, Katsiyiannis WT, Gornick CC, Almquist AK, Kallinen LM. Deaths and cardiovascular injuries due to device assisted implantable cardioverter-defibrillator and pacemaker lead extraction. Europace 2010;12:395–401.

26 Venkataraman G, Hayes D, Strickberger SA. Does the risk-benefit analysis favor the extraction of failed sterile pacemaker and defibrillator leads? J Cardiovasc Electrophysiol 2009;20:1413–1415.

27 Ji SY, Gunderwar S, Palma EC. Subclavian venoplasty may reduce implant times and implant failures in the era of increasing device upgrades. Pacing Clin Electrophysiol 2012;35:444–448.

 To watch the videos, please log in to the Companion Website: www.wiley.com/go/al-ahmad/pacemakers_and_icds

Video 13.1 Use of a 5 Fr 15 cm stiffened dilator micro-puncture kit for venous access. See video annotation for details.

Video 13.2 Exchanging the polymer tip wire used to cross the obstruction for an extra support wire using a 4 Fr hydrophilic catheter. The exchange was necessary because the polymer tip wire did not provide sufficient support to advance the balloon through the occlusion. See video annotation for details.

Video 13.3 Use of an angled tip hydrophilic catheter to provide wire direction for crossing a total subclavian obstruction. The despite the use of a torque device, the polymer tip wire could not be directed through the dilator of a 5 Fr sheath toward the center of the occlusion. The dilator was replaced with an angled tip hydrophilic braided angiographic catheter (for details see Box 13.1). The angle on the tip of the catheter made it possible to direct the wire across the occlusion.

Video 13.4 Use of an angled tip hydrophilic catheter to provide support to push through a total subclavian occlusion. The wire alone did not have sufficient support to advance into the total occlusion. The 5 Fr angled tip catheter was stiff enough to enter the occlusion. The wire was then advanced beyond the tip of the catheter and the catheter advanced over the wire to successfully cross the occlusion.

Video 13.5 Crossing an apparent total using the contrast injection system, the dilator from a 5 Fr sheath and a polymer tip wire. See video annotation for details.

14

How to Perform Defibrillation Threshold Testing

Chad Brodt and Marco V. Perez

Cardiac Electrophysiology & Arrhythmia Service, Stanford University Medical Center, Stanford, CA, USA

The implantable cardioverter-defibrillator (ICD) was developed as a life-saving device, initially for secondary prevention of ventricular arrhythmias and later for primary prevention. Clinical trials in multiple high-risk patient groups over the past several decades have shown, overwhelmingly, the ability of these devices to rescue individuals from sudden cardiac death (SCD). However, their success is dependent on the principle that these devices are capable of detecting a ventricular arrhythmia and delivering an effective intervention with a high probability of success. Notably, the clinical trials that have demonstrated efficacy of the ICD included defibrillation threshold (DFT) testing as part of the implantation protocol.

The DFT_{50}, often referred to as simply the DFT, is the shock energy required to successfully defibrillate 50% of the time. The term DFT, however, is often used, albeit somewhat inaccurately, to refer simply to the lowest amount of energy necessary to defibrillate successfully, or convert the myocardium from ventricular fibrillation (VF) to sinus rhythm, during testing. DFT testing has traditionally been performed during implantation to assure high probability of success.

A better understanding of shock delivery and improved technology has led to the development of high-output devices, pectoral devices that actively participate in energy delivery and biphasic waveforms that improve the probability of successful shock. Early devices utilized the truncated exponential monophasic waveform to depolarize the myocardium. The effect on the transmembrane potential peaks with a pulse width of approximately 5 ms. Modern devices use a biphasic waveform because the residual charge at the end of a monophasic impulse would leave the myocardium in a proarrhythmic state. The second phase of the shock functions to eliminate the transmembrane potential that would leave the tissue primed for propagation.

In light of these advances, the risks of failure to rescue a patient from ventricular fibrillation during DFT testing and the possible detrimental effects of shocks themselves have led to a debate about the need for routine DFT testing. Although there is a trend away from performing DFTs routinely, a 2010 review found the majority (71%) of ICD implants are still performed with DFT testing, based on the National Cardiovascular Data Registry [1]. The decision to perform DFTs must consider the balance of risks of mortality from a failure to identify a high DFT that would result in patient SCD versus the risk of failure to defibrillate a patient during DFT testing. Even among implanting physicians who have opted not to perform DFTs routinely, there are still important clinical scenarios when DFTs may be predictably high or when additional information is required for optimal device programming, thus maintaining an important role for DFT testing in all electrophysiology practices. There are many available protocols reviewed in this chapter to determine DFTs, including step-up and step-down protocols and the calculation of the upper limit of vulnerability (ULV), which correlates well with DFTs.

Reasons for DFT Testing

Although a test that guarantees successful defibrillation in all clinical scenarios is not possible, the goal of DFT testing is to estimate the energy at which the likelihood of defibrillation is high. Additional goals in DFT testing are to confirm adequate sensing of VF, to verify the electrical integrity of the device and lead system and to verify that all connections are intact. Much of this can be

How-to Manual for Pacemaker and ICD Devices: Procedures and Programming, First Edition. Edited by Amin Al-Ahmad, Andrea Natale, Paul J. Wang, James P. Daubert, and Luigi Padeletti.
© 2018 John Wiley & Sons, Inc. Published 2018 by John Wiley & Sons, Inc.
Companion website: www.wiley.com/go/al-ahmad/pacemakers_and_icds

estimated by checking pacing thresholds and impedances, as well as checking sensing thresholds during sinus rhythm. Rarely, however, an insulation failure can only be detected with high-voltage testing, or VF signal amplitude does not correlate with amplitudes during sinus rhythm [2]. In addition, testing during implantation can help identify patients with high DFTs who need system revision or modification that can be carried out immediately, at the time of implant.

Possibly one of the most important arguments in favor of DFT testing is that the major clinical trials that have demonstrated the efficacy of ICD therapy were carried out with DFT testing as part of the implantation protocol. The goal in the Multicenter Automatic Defibrillator Implantation Trial II was to achieve a safety margin of 10 J. However, the recently published SIMPLE trial looked at 2500 patients undergoing initial ICD implantation and were randomized to undergo DFT testing vs. no testing [3]. The patients were followed for a mean of 3.1 years and results show that there is no significant difference in shock efficacy or reduction of arrhythmic death between groups.

In theory, only patients who have predictably high DFTs could be selected for DFT testing. Factors that have been shown to be associated with high DFTs (Table 14.1) include obesity, enlarged left ventricular size or mass, a low ejection fraction, right-sided implantation, advanced heart failure, very wide QRS, and non-ischemic cardiomyopathy. However, these factors are not reliable and some studies have suggested that none of these clinical variables were sufficiently good predictors [4]. There are also many medications that are known to impact DFTs. Antiarrhythmic drugs from the Vaughan Williams Classifications Ib (mexiletine, lidocaine) and IV (verapamil, diltiazem) can increase DFTs,

while the class II (beta blockers) and class III (sotalol, dofetilide, ibutilide) decrease DFTs. The exception is amiodarone, a class III agent, whose long-term use is associated with increased DFTs.

The primary challenge in estimating the true DFT is the probabilistic nature of defibrillation. In pacing, the strength–duration curve to elicit myocardial capture is thought of as nearly an all-or-nothing phenomenon. This is attributed to the relatively stable conditions at which pacing occurs. The defibrillation strength–duration curve is more probabilistic (Figure 14.1), in part because the energy delivery affects the tissue in varying states of depolarization and repolarization. Other factors, such as electrolyte levels, medications, and left ventricular function, can also affect the likelihood of defibrillation at any given energy. Every patient has a different curve, which can change over time.

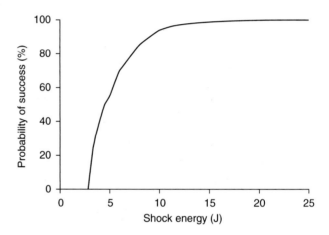

Figure 14.1 Theoretical defibrillation curve depicting the probability of successful defibrillation with increasing doses of energy.

Table 14.1 Factors that may influence decision to perform defibrillation threshold (DFT) testing.

Factors that may predict high DFTs	Contraindications to DFT testing	Factors that may increase risk of death from failure to defibrillate during DFT testing
Advanced heart failure	Atrial or ventricular thrombi	Advanced heart failure
Low ejection fraction	Atrial fibrillation without adequate anticoagulation	Severe COPD
Enlarged left ventricular size or mass	Hemodynamic instability or ongoing inotropic support	Obesity
Higher body surface area	Severe aortic stenosis	Three vessel or left main coronary artery disease
Right-sided implantation	Active coronary ischemia	
Wide QRS (>200 ms)	Recent stroke or TIA	
Non-ischemic cardiomyopathy	Recent percutaneous coronary intervention	
Use of medications that raise DFTs		

COPD, chronic obstrucive pulmonary disease; TIA, transient ischemic attack.

This uncertainty in predicting the effective energy to successfully defibrillate is one of the impetuses behind DFT testing.

An important argument that was originally made in favor of DFT testing was that a precise measurement of the DFT then allowed the clinician to program energy delivery at a relatively lower energy output. With modern devices, patients will typically have DFTs in the single digits. Even accounting for a 10 J window, the final energy programmed could remain relatively low, which would in turn result in quicker charge time and energy delivery to the patient during an episode of ventricular tachyarrhythmia. A quicker delivery time could mean the difference between syncope and no syncope. However, charge times in modern devices have become short enough that this concern has, for the most part, been mitigated. The use of lower shock energy, however, could lengthen the longevity of the device battery and, theoretically, result in less myocardial damage.

Arguments Against Routine DFT Testing

As previously noted, while 71% of implantations were performed with DFT testing in a recent registry survey [1], the remaining implantations did not include DFT testing which reflects the measurable trend away from routine DFT testing. This trend is likely a result of a combination of factors that include improvement in technologies, as described earlier, resulting in lower likelihood of unsuccessful DFTs. The likelihood of identifying high DFTs is approximately 2–12%. However, with high energy devices, the estimated percentage of ICDs that would need revision because of high DFTs is approximately 3% [5]. There are additional factors that are likely influencing the trend away from routine DFT testing.

One of the major concerns during DFT testing is the risk of death because of inability to rescue a patient from VF. The risk of prolonged resuscitation after multiple failed internal and external shocks in one study was 0.14% [6]. Beyond the mortality risk, there may also be other morbidities associated with induction of VF. Induction of VF and the subsequent shock to follow results in a period of myocardial depression that may not be well tolerated, particularly by those with left ventricular dysfunction and decompensated heart failure. Concerns have been raised that transient hypotension resulting from induction of VF could result in impaired cognitive function, myocardial ischemia, and strokes. The presence of underlying atrial fibrillation at the time of DFT could result in a thromboembolic event if the patient is not properly anticoagulated. It has been

difficult to determine which of these complications are caused by the DFT testing itself, versus the implant procedure or the underlying heart disease. Nevertheless, there are several contraindications to DFT testing which are meant to minimize the risk of major morbidities from VF induction (Table 14.1).

There have been prospective studies that have attempted to characterize the safety of foregoing DFT testing in the clinical setting. In one Italian study of 1284 patients who underwent ICD implant without DFT testing and followed for 2 years [7], there were a total of 144 patients who required shock therapy. Of these, six patients (0.5% of total implant population) had ineffective ventricular shocks during follow-up. This was not significantly different from the 836 patients who underwent DFT testing at the time of implant (0.8%). Although the patients in this study that did not undergo DFT testing may have been selected as low-risk patients, this study does support the growing sentiment that it may be safe to forego DFT testing in some groups of patients undergoing ICD implant. The SIMPLE trial was a randomized trial published in 2015 that found that foregoing DFT testing was non-inferior to routine DFT testing for arrhythmic death or failed appropriate shock [3]. Of note, this trial excluded patients with expected right-sided implants.

In addition to these arguments, there are other factors that may explain the trend away from routine DFT testing. The increase in the use of aggressive antitachycardia pacing (ATP) therapy, in combination with the implementation programming changes that delay ICD therapies, are resulting in a decrease in the number of ICD shocks needed. In the scenario where an ICD shock is needed and the first ICD shock fails, modern devices are typically programmed to deliver up to six additional shocks which increase the likelihood of successful defibrillation. Finally, there are costs associated with DFT testing, which include greater utilization of staff and other resources such as anesthesia. Some of these factors may even raise barriers that limit the appropriate use of ICD implantation.

Decision to Perform DFT Test

As with all clinical decisions, the decision to test depends on the risks and benefits involved. Ultimately, the risks of DFT testing, including the small increase in risk of death or morbidity, have to be balanced with the risks of not testing, which includes death from failure to deliver appropriate ICD shock therapy in the field. Contraindications, as well as other clinical factors that predict high DFTs or mortality from testing (Table 14.1), should be taken into account.

An additional factor that should be considered is the likelihood that a patient will have a clinical, life-threatening ventricular arrhythmia. In those with the highest likelihood of ventricular tachyarrhythmias, such as those being implanted for secondary prevention, a stronger argument for DFT testing could be made.

Despite all of the arguments against DFT testing, it is important to note that DFT testing has traditionally been considered standard of care. While these standards may be evolving with the publication of new trials and expert consensus statements [3,8], this argument may have medicolegal implications in cases where DFT testing is not performed in a patient without clear contraindications to testing.

DFT Testing Strategies

When planning an ICD implantation, it is important to know ahead of time whether DFT testing will be performed. The intention of DFT testing will require a team that can provide adequate anesthesia for this part of the procedure. The staff should be trained in the various protocols and aware of their responsibilities regarding stand-by external defibrillation if needed. Those in atrial fibrillation or atrial flutter who require DFT testing will also need to have a documented strategy for the minimization of stroke risk because DFT testing can result in conversion to sinus rhythm. For DFT testing that is performed at the time of initial ICD implant or generator change, an appropriate time for testing is after the leads have been tested, the generator connected and inserted into the pocket, and the incision is prepared for closure.

The first step of DFT testing is induction of VF, which may be carried out using one of three different strategies: delivery of alternating current (AC) voltage; using very high rate stimulation; or, most commonly, by delivering a shock on the T-wave. Classically, VF was induced by applying direct current (DC) voltage using an external battery connected to epicardial leads. This method has a very high success rate of VF induction, but internal delivery of DC voltage remains an option only in a small number of ICD systems. The T-wave shock method is currently the most popular and relies on the principle that the myocardium is vulnerable to VF when sufficient energy delivery is timed within a window surrounding the peak of the T-wave. This can be performed during sinus rhythm or, more commonly, after a pacing drive train of 8 beats at 400 ms. A 1 J shock on the peak of the T-wave, which is typically about 300 ms after the last paced impulse, will usually induce VF. If unsuccessful, analysis of the electrograms will allow optimization of T-wave shock timing, or a scan at 20 ms intervals, usually before the peak of the T-wave, can be performed. The final strategy, very high frequency stimulation, is generally not as efficacious as the shock on T-wave approach. However, it can be helpful when the peak of the T-wave is difficult to measure, or shock on T-wave is unsuccessful despite scanning. Very high frequency stimulation is performed by pacing between 10 and 50 Hz for several seconds until VF is induced.

The next step of DFT testing is evaluation for undersensing of VF. R-waves amplitudes during sinus rhythm generally correlate well with those during VF. Undersensing is rare if the R-wave amplitude during sinus rhythm is >5 mV. The VF amplitude varies, so it is typical that some beats during VF will be undersensed (Figure 14.2). These dropouts are acceptable as long as they are not long enough to prevent the device from delivering adequate therapy. A "worst-case" sensing threshold, ranging from 1.0 to 1.2 mV, depending on manufacturer, is usually adequate to assess proper detection during DFT testing. Testing can also be important in scenarios where interference occurs with other leads or devices. If the defibrillator lead does not demonstrate adequate sensing, either the existing lead must be repositioned to a location with larger R-wave amplitude, or a secondary bipolar pacing lead can be placed in the right ventricle for detection. The presence of existing hardware, such as abandoned leads or pulse generators,

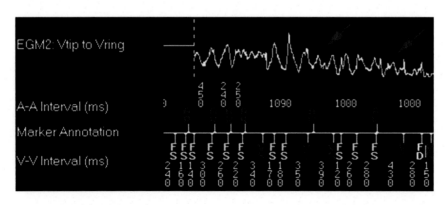

Figure 14.2 Sensing of ventricular fibrillation (VF) during defibrillation threshold (DFT) testing. Red arrows point to VF signals that were undersensed.

Figure 14.3 Interaction between new high-voltage lead and old lead noted only during VF induction. Red arrows point to examples of clipped signals that represent electrical noise caused by a new lead contacting the abandoned lead.

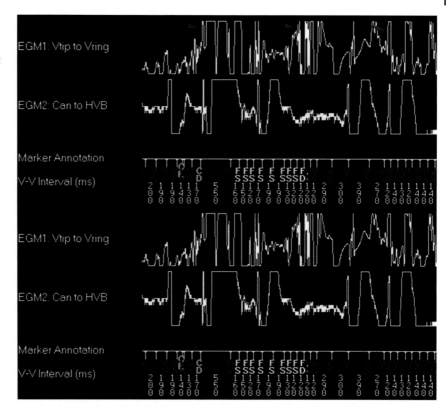

can lead to interaction only during VF induction (Figure 14.3) and may therefore prompt testing with a focus on adequate sensing.

Finally, there are many approaches that can be used to measure the DFT itself. These approaches vary in the total number of shocks delivered, precise estimate of the DFT, and amount of time the patient may remain in VF. The goal of testing is to determine the lowest energy required for successful defibrillation. A traditional method is the step-down (SD) approach, where defibrillation is attempted starting at an arbitrary value, typically 15 or 20 J. If successful, the testing is reattempted sequentially at steps of 5 J lower energy each time until failure to defibrillate. This approach has the advantage of measuring the DFT with relatively good precision without leaving the patient in VF for prolonged periods of time. Using this method, the lowest successful shock is termed the "DFT", and closely approximates the DFT_{70}, which is the energy able to successfully defibrillate 70% of the time. Programming the device to double the DFT_{70} would result in high confidence of successful defibrillation. However, if the DFT calculated is greater than half the maximum device output, then repeating the DFT test and demonstrating that the energy output is successful a second and third time increases the confidence and allows one to program smaller safety windows of 15–10 J, respectively.

The step-up (SU) approach begins with the first defibrillation attempt at 5 J with sequential increase in the energy dose by 5 J until successful defibrillation is achieved. This approach minimizes the total number of induction attempts, but may result in a prolonged episode of VF and if needed results in multiple shocks.

Another popular protocol for DFT testing, which is used at our institution, is the verification method, also called an efficacy protocol. This method does not measure the precise DFT, but ensures a high likelihood of defibrillation success at the maximum output of the defibrillator. After induction, energy is delivered at a desired safety margin below the maximum programmable output. For single shock testing, a 20 J safety margin results in a >90% probability of successful defibrillation at the first maximal output shock. We typically perform two tests at 25 J providing a safety margin of 10 J in devices with a maximal output of 35 J. This similarly results in a high probability of successful defibrillation at the device maximum programmable output. This method helps to minimize the total number of ICD shocks during testing.

An alternative strategy to predict successful defibrillation that also minimizes number of shocks delivered is to assess the upper limit of vulnerability (ULV). The vulnerable period is a time interval, within about 40 ms, near the peak of the T-wave during which a shock using an amount of energy within a certain range results in VF induction. The upper limit of this range is defined as the upper limit of vulnerability, and correlates strongly with the DFT. To identify the ULV, one can begin with a shock on the T-wave peak at approximately 20 J, then repeat the same shock energy delivery at 20 and 40 ms before the T-wave peak. Next, one can begin decreasing the amount of energy used by small increments, such as 5 J, and similarly scan at 0, 20, and 40 ms before the T-wave peak. The energy at which VF is first induced is then defined as the ULV. Using this method, VF is only induced (and converted) once. The final device programming should be made using at least a 10 J safety margin above the ULV.

When performing DFT tests, it is advisable to wait 5–10 minutes between VF inductions in order to allow for hemodynamic recovery. In the event that an initial shock fails to defibrillate, a back-up internal defibrillation at the maximum output of the device should follow promptly. While waiting for the device to charge for the rescue shock, an external defibrillator should be charged to provide back-up defibrillation if the maximum output internal shock does not work. The defibrillation pads are often placed in non-standard locations during ICD implantation, which can result in a failure to defibrillate, so the implanting physician should be prepared to deliver an external shock with paddles at maximum output in a more standard location. Because of the potential for worsening electromechanical dissociation with prolonged VF, the physician and staff should be prepared to perform adequate resuscitation efforts if necessary.

How to Manage High DFTs

In the event that the device does not allow the operator to program an adequate safety margin above the measured DFT, the implanting practitioner will need to either change the mode of energy delivery or change the hardware used for energy delivery. The first step is to review the device set up and patient to ensure that all the connections are adequate and that a pneumothorax has not developed. One should also ensure that the distal RV coil is programmed as the anode because this will typically result in the lowest DFT. With biphasic devices, switching polarity so that the RV coil is programmed as the cathode will improve the DFT in only 18% of patients. Another programmable option, found in only a few devices, is to change the biphasic waveform of the device, for example, from a fixed tilt waveform to a shorter tuned waveform.

Next, one should check that the RV coil position is as apical and septal as possible for best results; however, in some patients, a high septal position may prove more successful. One delivery strategy is to screw the tip of the RV lead into the high basal septum, near the outflow, and then prolapse the remaining lead so that the proximal end of the RV coil is situated near the apex of the RV. If still unsuccessful, and a single coil lead was used initially, the RV lead could be swapped out for a dual coil lead containing an SVC coil. On the contrary, if a dual coil system was used, and the impedances are less than 40, then one may try to remove the SVC coil from the shock vector.

(a)

(b)

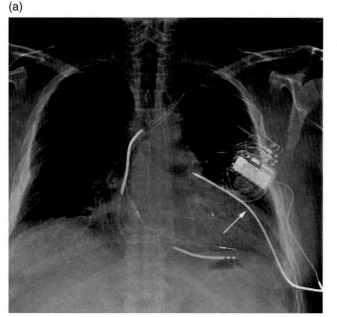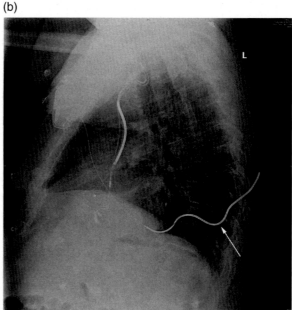

Figure 14.4 Anteroposterior (a) and lateral (b) chest X-rays in a patient with a subcutaneous electrode implanted. White arrow points to the subcutaneous lead.

If these basic changes fail, then most patients will need to move towards placement of additional hardware. For those in whom an endovascular device has failed, switching to a subcutaneous ICD system may be a good option. In patients who require pacing for other indications, one may consider concomitant use of an endovascular pacemaker and a subcutaneous ICD. If the patient is not a candidate for a subcutaneous ICD, or if adequate DFT are not found with the subcutaneous device, then placement of additional leads to an existing endovascular system can decrease impedance, improve the shock vector, and decrease the DFTs. A common next step is to add a long subcutaneous posterior electrode. This electrode can be inserted laterally and tracked subcutaneously along the back, towards the spine (Figure 14.4). The insertion can be at the lateral edge of the pocket, or at a separate, lower, and more lateral incision site. The tip of the lead is ideally placed near the base of the left ventricle as seen on an anteroposterior view.

Alternatively, additional coils could be placed in the azygos vein or the coronary sinus. The azygos vain can be found by exploring immediately superior to the right atrium–superior vena cava junction using a curved stylet. However, extraction of a lead placed in the azygos or coronary sinus is challenging in the case of an infection or malfunction. Other locations that can be explored with independent coiled leads include brachiocephalic and left subclavian veins.

If none of these additional coil locations result in adequate DFTs, then a trial of sotalol may be enough to lower the DFTs to an acceptable level. It is necessary to remember not to give with concomitant amiodarone, and that a period of amiodarone washout will be required prior to re-testing DFTs. A failure of all of these techniques may then result in surgical consultation for placement of an additional coil in the epicardial space. It also important to recognize that clinical judgment is crucial to safely addressing high DFTs. If a patient has failed multiple DFT tests, it may be advisable to reschedule for further testing at a later date to allow appropriate recovery.

References

1 Russo AM, Wang Y, Al-Khatib SM, Curtis JP, Lampert R. Patient, physician, and procedural factors influencing the use of defibrillation testing during initial implantable cardioverter defibrillator insertion: findings from the NCDR(R). Pacing Clin Electrophysiol 2013;36:1522–1531.

2 Ruetz LL, Koehler JL, Brown ML, Jackson TE, Belk P, Swerdlow CD. Sinus rhythm R-wave amplitude as a predictor of ventricular fibrillation undersensing in patients with implantable cardioverter-defibrillator. Heart Rhythm 2015;12(12):2411–2418.

3 Healy JS, Hohnloser SH, Glikson M, Neuzner J, Mabo P, Vinolas X, et al. Cardioverter defibrillator implantation without induction of ventricular fibrillation: a single-blind, non-inferiority, randomized controlled trial (SIMPLE). Lancet 2015;385:785–791.

4 Hohnloser SH, Dorian P, Roberts R, Gent M, Israel CW, Champagne J, et al. Effect of amiodarone and sotalol on ventricular defibrillation threshold: the optimal pharmacological therapy in cardioverter defibrillator patients (OPTIC) trial. Circulation 2006;114:104–109.

5 Russo AM, Sauer W, Gerstenfeld EP, Hsia HH, Lin D, Cooper JM, et al. Defibrillation threshold testing: is it really necessary at the time of implantable cardioverter-defibrillator insertion? Heart Rhythm 2005;2:456–461.

6 Birnie D, Tung S, Simpson C, Crystal E, Exner D, Ayala Paredes FA, et al. Complications associated with defibrillation threshold testing: the Canadian experience. Heart Rhythm 2008;5:387–390.

7 Brignole M, Occhetta E, Bongiorni MG, Proclemer A, Favale S, Iacopino S, et al. Clinical evaluation of defibrillation testing in an unselected population of 2,120 consecutive patients undergoing first implantable cardioverter-defibrillator implant. J Am Coll Cardiol 2012;60:981–987.

8 Wilkoff BL, Fauchier L, Stiles MK, Morillo CA, Al-Khatib SM, Almendral J, et al. 2015 HRS/EHRA/APHRS/SOLAECE expert consensus statement on optimal implantable cardioverter-defibrillator programming and testing. Heart Rhythm 2016;13(2):e50–86.

15

Use of Chest X-ray, Computed Tomography and 3-D Imaging to Evaluate Lead Location

Brett D. Atwater

Duke University Health System, Durham, NC, USA

Implantable cardiac leads provide effective treatment for bradyarrhythmia and heart failure and prevention of sudden cardiac death. Leads may be placed through the vasculature via an endocardial approach, or surgically via an epicardial approach. Chest radiography is useful for pre-operative planning, intraoperative assessment of anatomy for proper device positioning, and postoperative assessment of lead position and surgical complication including pneumothorax, pleural effusion, and pericardial effusion. This chapter describes methods for evaluating lead position using standard X-ray imaging, and indications for the incorporation of computed tomography and other three-dimensional (3-D) imaging for lead localization.

Chest X-ray Identification of Lead Insertion Site

Endovascular leads may be inserted in any central venous location, including cephalic, axillary, subclavian, innominate, internal jugular, femoral, iliac, or hepatic; however, in most labs, the preferred implantation sites include the cephalic, axillary, or subclavian veins. Identification of lead insertion sites prior to device generator change or insertion of additional leads is helpful for procedural planning. Clues as to the insertion site may be obtained on radiography; a more lateral insertion position suggests a cephalic site (Figure 15.1), while a more medial insertion site suggests a subclavian or axillary site (Figure 15.2). An extreme medial technique may be used for placement of leads in cases of occlusion of the axillary or subclavian vein. This may be identified on X-ray by an insertion point at or near the sterno-clavicular junction

(Figure 15.3). Tunneled leads may also me identified on X-ray as a lead that does not follow the course of any vascular bed (Figure 15.4).

X-Ray Right Ventricular Lead Tip Localization

The right ventricle (RV) is usually divided into three distinct anatomic regions when describing the position of the tip of a pacing or defibrillation lead: free wall, septum, and apex (Figure 15.5). Historically, the RV apex has been the preferred location for RV lead position, owing to the high degree of lead stability with tined or passive fixation leads, low pacing capture thresholds, and low defibrillation threshold values during high voltage therapies. More recent studies have suggested that pacing from the RV septum may provide more physiologic activation of the left and right ventricle, minimizing the negative hemodynamic effects of RV pacing. Enthusiasm for septal positioning of RV leads increased after data showed only a small increase in defibrillation threshold in this position relative to the apex. Unfortunately, inadvertent RV lead tip position on the free wall is associated with a higher risk of procedure-related complications including RV perforation, left anterior descending artery perforation, chest wall stimulation, and worsening RV and left ventricular (LV) dyssynchrony and function than placement on the interventricular septum or apex. In studies using 3-D echocardiography or 3-D CT imaging, the incidence of inadvertent RV free wall lead placement is as high as 50% when a RV septal location is targeted. Steep left anterior oblique (LAO) projections are used to assess septal versus free wall positions with

How-to Manual for Pacemaker and ICD Devices: Procedures and Programming, First Edition. Edited by Amin Al-Ahmad, Andrea Natale, Paul J. Wang, James P. Daubert, and Luigi Padeletti.
© 2018 John Wiley & Sons, Inc. Published 2018 by John Wiley & Sons, Inc.
Companion website: www.wiley.com/go/al-ahmad/pacemakers_and_icds

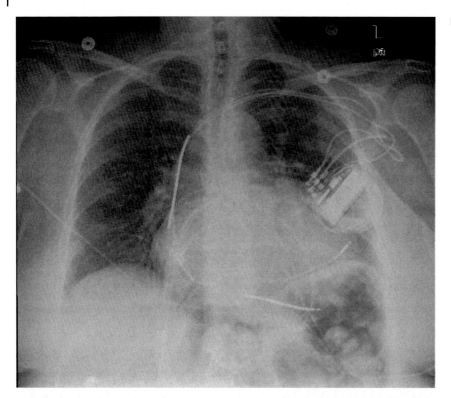

Figure 15.1 Cephalic vein insertion.

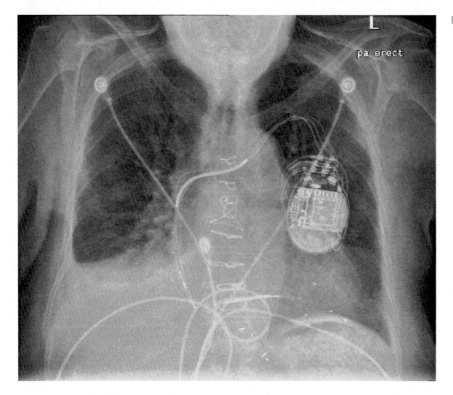

Figure 15.2 Axillary vein insertion.

anterior facing lead tips indicating free wall positions and posterior facing lead tips indicating septal positions. Prior work has compared the use of right anterior oblique (RAO) 30 degree and LAO 40 degree fluoroscopy to evaluate RV lead tip position using cardiac CT as the gold standard [1]. Implanting physicians attempted to place all RV lead tips in the mid-RV septum using LAO 40 degree and posterior-anterior (PA) fluoroscopy. Cardiac CT verified that 59% of the RV lead tips were inadvertently placed in the RV anterior-free wall while

Figure 15.3 Extreme medial technique posterior-anterior (PA) view.

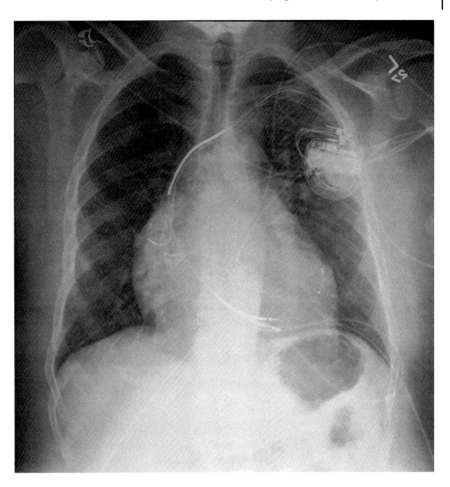

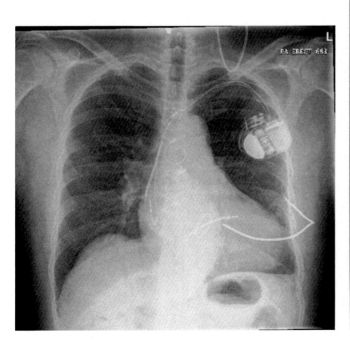

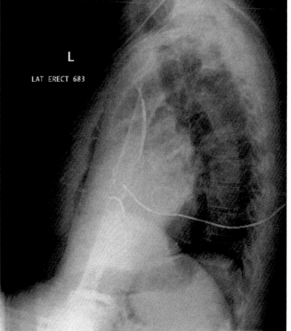

Figure 15.4 PA and lateral X-ray of tunneled high voltage lead.

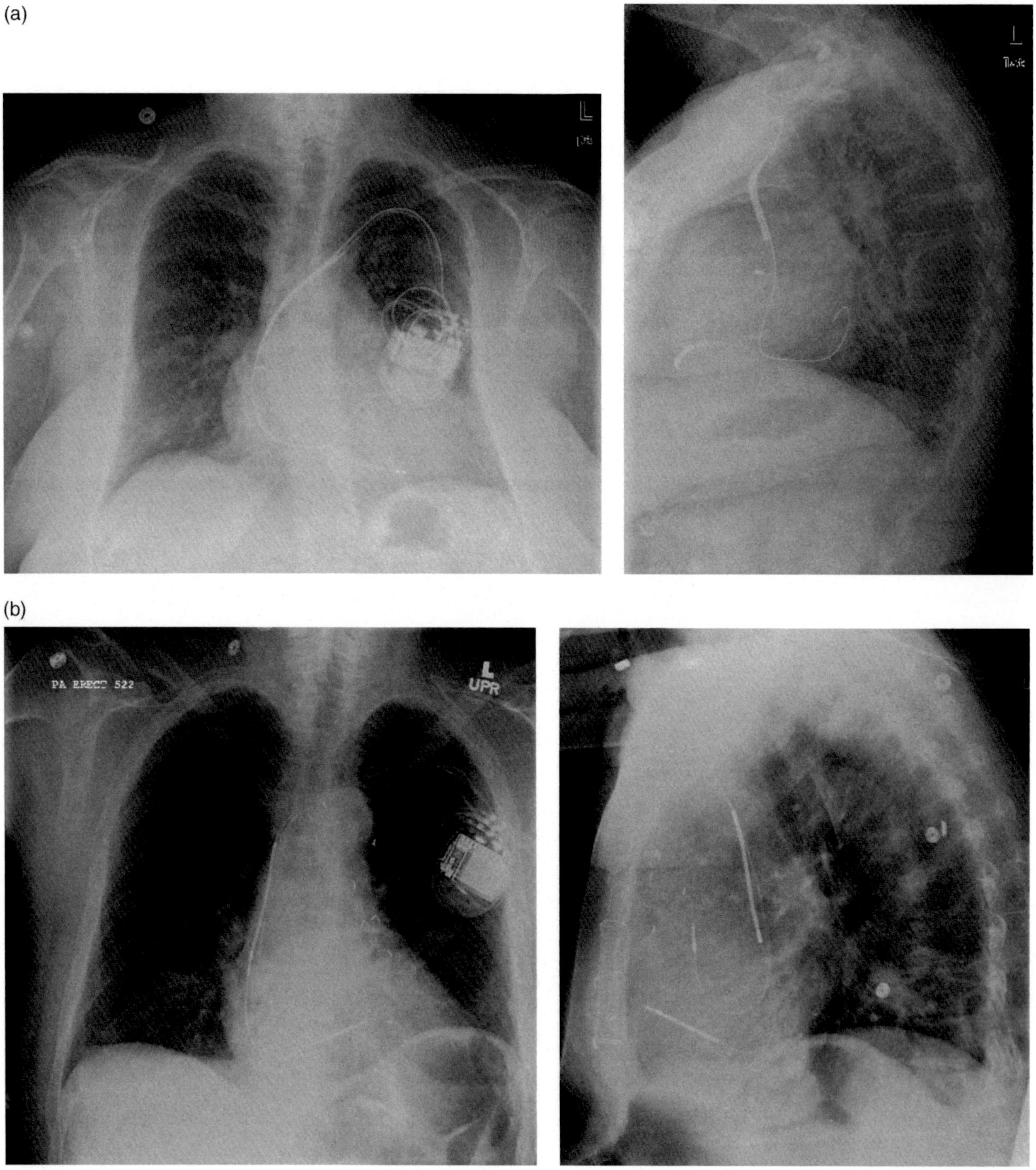

(a)

(b)

Figure 15.5 The right ventricule (RV) is usually divided into three anatomically distinct regions for identification of lead tip position. (a) An RV apical position is typically identified by a lead tip extending towards the leftward side of the cardiac silhouette in either an right anterior oblique (RAO) or PA angulation, usually associated with a downward direction to the lead tip. (b) An RV free wall location is identified by an anteriorly directed lead tip terminating near the sternum on a steep left anterior oblique (LAO) angulation and a position away from the cardiac border on an RAO or PA projection.

41% were correctly placed in the mid-septum. RAO 30 degree fluoroscopy provided better discrimination of septal lead tip position than LAO 40 degree (positive predictive value for septal placement 94.7% and negative predictive value of 90.6%). Numerous studies have evaluated the reproducibility and accuracy of X-ray imaging compared with CT imaging for RV lead tip localization. We recently showed limited ability to distinguish RV free wall locations from RV septal locations using X-ray.

(c)

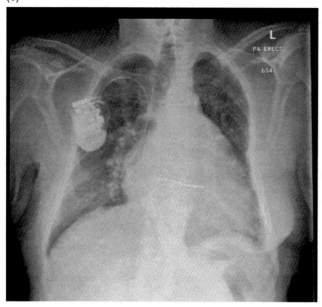
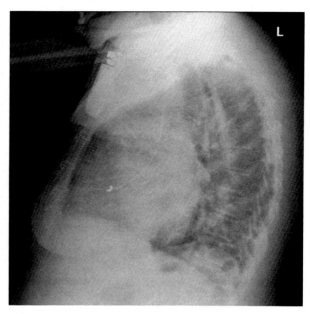

Figure 15.5 (Cont'd) (c) An RV septal lead position is identified by a posteriorly directed lead tip terminating away from the sternum on a steep LAO angulation and a position away from the cardiac border on an RAO or PA projection. (All lead tip locations in these figures were confirmed by 3-D reconstructed CT imaging.)

X-ray Left Ventricular Lead Tip Localization

Pacing leads are usually placed in a LV location along with a RV lead to deliver cardiac resynchronization therapy (CRT). Pacing is then provided from either both ventricular leads simultaneously or with a predefined offset, or from the LV lead alone with an attempt to provide fusion with conduction down the remaining ventricular conduction system. Numerous studies have shown that CRT provides improved ventricular hemodynamics, reverse remodeling of LV dilation, improvements in heart failure symptom severity, fewer heart failure related hospitalizations, and mortality reduction than placebo, especially among patients with a left bundle branch block on surface ECG. Unfortunately, not all patients respond to CRT and LV lead tip location is a key determinate of the likelihood of response.

The RAO, LAO, PA, and lateral X-ray views are used to identify LV lead tip position. Optimal RAO and LAO angulation are dependent on the degree of heart rotation within the thorax. The RAO view should maximally foreshorten the AV groove while the LAO view should minimally foreshorten the AV groove. One easy way to achieve this in a patient with prior LV lead placement is to angle the X-ray view to maximally and minimally foreshorten the portion of the LV lead body that rests within the coronary sinus and great cardiac vein.

Various LV segmentation strategies have been advocated to describe LV lead position. The 15-segment method divides the longitudinal LV axis into three segments (base, middle, and apex) using the RAO or PA X-ray projection. The short LV axis is divided into five segments (anterior, anterior-lateral, lateral, posterior-lateral, and posterior) using the LAO X-ray projection (Figure 15.6). Recent work has demonstrated that the 15-segment method lacks accuracy and reproducibility compared to simpler methods combining the base and middle LV segments (to create a "non-apical" segment) and the anterior-lateral, lateral, and posterior-lateral segments (to create a "lateral" segment) to produce a 6-segment method.

X-ray Identification of Alternative LV Lead Implantation Techniques

Left ventricular leads are usually implanted using an endovascular strategy, coursing through the coronary sinus into one of the ventricular branches to provide an LV epicardial position or by a surgical approach using a mini-thoracotomy approach to provide direct access to the epicardial heart surface. Recently, an endovascular endocardial approach has been described where the LV lead is advanced to the LV cavity through either a trans-aortic or trans-septal route. The trans-septal route can

(a) (b)

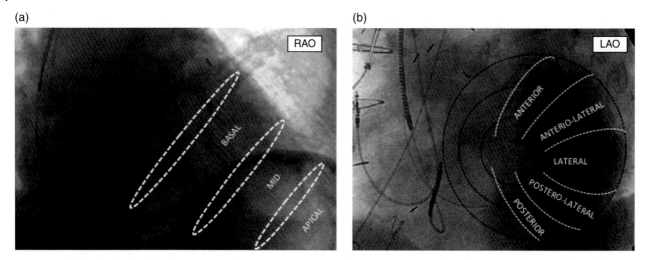

Figure 15.6 Classification of left ventricular lead location using standardized X-ray views. (a) Right anterior oblique (RAO) view is representative of the long axis of the heart. This view allows segmentation of the left ventricle into basal, mid-ventricular, and apical segments. (b) Left anterior oblique (LAO) view is representative of the short axis of the heart. This view allows segmentation of the left ventricle into anterior, anteriolateral, lateral, posteriolateral, and posterior segments.

(a) (b)

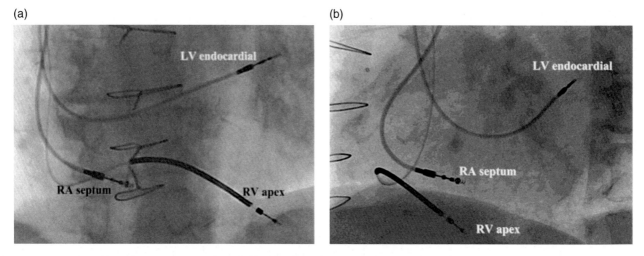

Figure 15.7 PA and lateral images an LV endocardial lead implanted by a trans-intra-atrial septal puncture. (a) is an RAO projection and (b) is an LAO projection. *Source*: van Gelder 2007 [3]. Reproduced with permission of Elsevier.

be achieved by puncture through either the inter-atrial septum followed by a course through the mitral valve to the LV cavity (Figure 15.7), or through a puncture through the inter-ventricular septum to the LV cavity (Figure 15.8). These approaches are used rarely, usually in cases of previous failed attempts at LV lead placement by the coronary sinus. An endovascular endocardial approach can be identified on X-ray by a posterior lead tip location within the cardiac silhouette without a course through the coronary sinus. An epicardial approach can be identified by a screw-in type active fixation and a lead tip that terminates outside of the cardiac silhouette (Figure 15.9).

X-Ray Identification of Alternative Defibrillator Lead Implantation Techniques

Defibrillator shocks are usually successful in restoring normal rhythm when delivered between a coil positioned within the RV, superior vena cava (SVC), and/or the defibrillator housing. Occasionally, the defibrillation threshold is higher than the maximum amount of energy deliverable from the defibrillator device and alternative defibrillator vectors are needed. Historically, these were

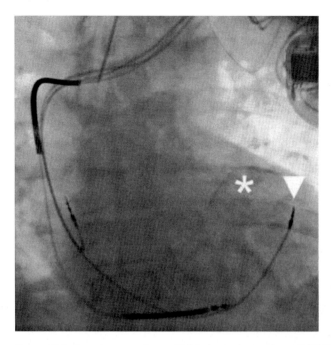
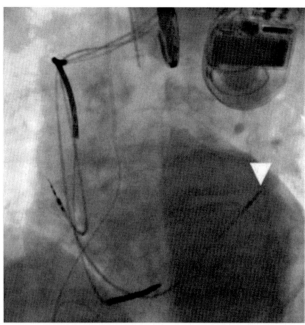

Figure 15.8 Anterior-posterior, and LAO views of an endocardial LV lead positioned by the trans-inter-ventricular septum technique. The left ventricular lead tip is marked by the arrowheads. The asterisk marks a left ventricular aneurysm. *Source*: Gamble 2013 [4]. Reproduced with permission of Elsevier.

Figure 15.9 Epicardial array, epicardial LV leads, epicardial RA lead, and endocardial RV lead.

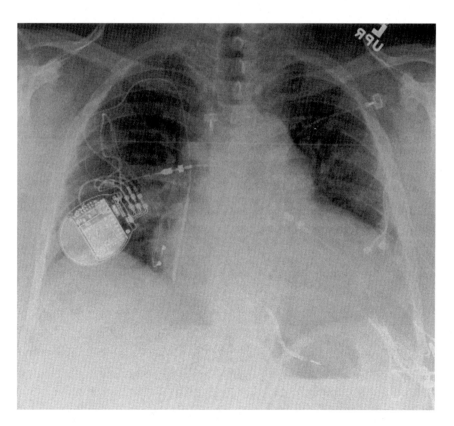

achieved through surgical positioning of epicardial defibrillator patches or subcutaneous coils (Figure 15.9). Newer methods involving alternative endovascular locations and subcutaneous tunneling to place shock coils have largely replaced the need for open surgical procedures. These positions can be identified easily on chest X-ray. The azygous coil location can be identified by a lead that transverses down the right side of the spine on the PA radiograph and that has an extremely posterior course near the spine on the lateral radiograph (Figure 15.10). A coronary sinus shock coil configuration can be identified by a lead coursing along the valve annulus in the PA view and coursing posteriorly in the lateral radiograph (Figure 15.11). Subcutaneously tunneled leads can be identified by their superficial course that does not follow a vascular pattern (Figure 15.4). Anatomic variations may also be identified easily after device implantation by following the course of leads placed through the

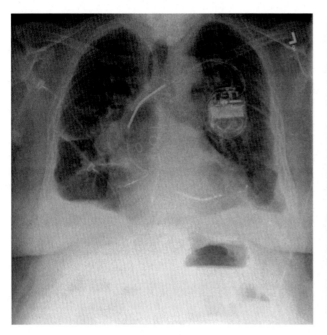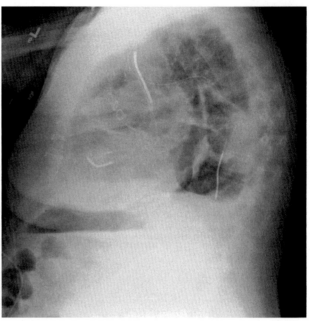

Figure 15.10 PA and lateral image of shock coil in azygous vein. The coil courses along the right side of the spine in the RAO projection and is very posterior in the lateral projection.

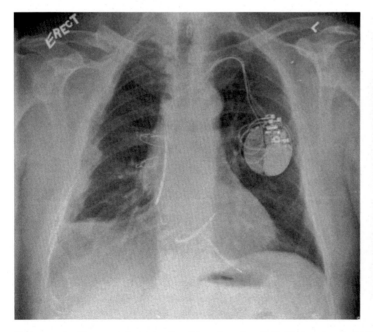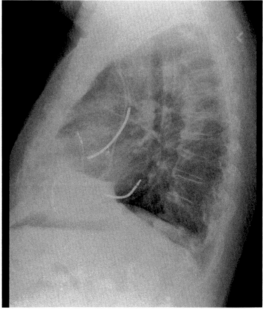

Figure 15.11 Coronary sinus shock coil location after defibrillation threshold (DFT) was found to be elevated with a shock coil in an azygous position. PA and lateral images. The coronary sinus position can be identified in X-ray by a lead coursing along the valve annulus in the PA view and coursing posteriorly in the lateral view.

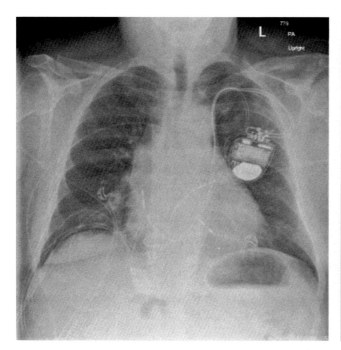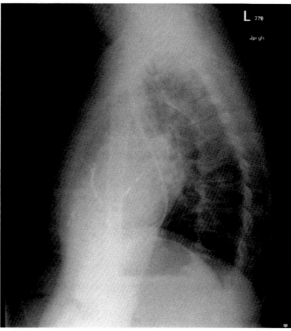

Figure 15.12 PA and lateral X-ray views obtained after a bi-ventricular ICD upgrade from prior pacemaker implantation. The pre-procedure X-ray demonstrated that the prior pacemaker was implanted through the left-sided superior vena cava, alerting implanting operators to expect a more difficult upgrade procedure.

anatomy. A common example is device implantation through a left-sided SVC approach (Figure 15.12).

X-ray Identification of Device Implant Complications

Complications occur in 1–3% of pacemaker implantation procedures and 3–6% of defibrillator implantation procedures. Some complications including pneumothorax, hemothorax, lead dislodgement, and cardiac perforation can be identified by X-ray, even in the absence of patient symptoms. While the utility of routine post-device implantation X-ray imaging has been debated in the literature, it is currently performed at most hospitals. Pneumothorax can be identified on X-ray by a linear opacity, usually located at the apex in an upright patient, but occasionally located in the sulcus or lateral lung field in dependent patients (Figure 15.13). The size of the pneumothorax is usually determined by measurement of the distance between the chest wall and the lung. An air rim of 2 cm at the level of the hilum or 3 cm at the apex differentiates a "small" and "large" pneumothorax. Small pneumothoraxes can usually be managed medically with high flow oxygen supplementation while large pneumothoraxes usually require placement of a chest tube. Less commonly, tension pneumothorax may be identified by absence of parenchymal findings in one lung field accompanied by mediastinal shift away from

the collapsed lung although this diagnosis is made clinically when hypotension and hypoxia accompany a radiographic diagnosis of pneumothorax. Tension pneumothorax should be treated urgently or emergently with either needle decompression or prompt chest tube insertion. Hemothorax may be identified by radiopaque density in the pleural space with accompanied collapse of the lung.

Lead dislodgement can be identified when a lead is not in its intended position. Typically, RV septal leads dislodge to either the RV apex or right atrium while RV apical leads dislodge to the right atrium or the inferior vena cava (IVC). RA leads usually dislodge to either the IVC or the SVC. More rarely, leads dislodge and advance forward, and can cause cardiac perforation. This may occur if excess slack is applied to the lead body at implantation. This can be identified when the lead tip exits the cardiac silhouette, and is occasionally accompanied by enlargement of the cardiac silhouette, indicative of hemoparicardium.

X-ray Identification of Lead Failure

Pacing and defibrillation leads undergo tremendous stress in the human body, with dramatic bending and twisting forces applied by the normal motion of the heart, chest, and arms and by the forces applied by sutures used to tie the leads in position. These forces

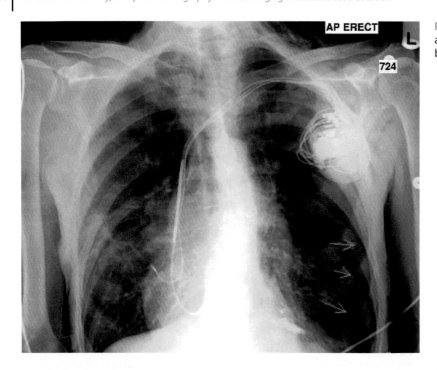

Figure 15.13 A large left-sided pneumothorax after device implantation. This was managed by chest tube placement.

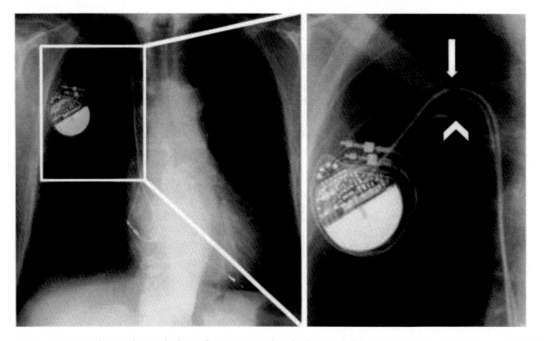

Figure 15.14 PA chest radiograph shows fracture (arrowhead) of ventricle lead and insulation breach (arrow) of atrial lead in subclavian vein adjacent to clavicle [5].

may cause lead insulation breach and lead fracture. Insulation breach can be identified as an interruption of the normal lead diameter on X-ray (Figure 15.14). Conductor fracture can be identified by interruption of the conductor cable. Image magnification may be helpful in some cases.

X-ray imaging is recommended for evaluation of all St. Jude Medical Riata defibrillation leads to evaluate for externalized electrical conductors. X-ray examination should be performed in two steps:

- Step 1: Examine the entire visible length of the lead focusing on areas where conductors appear to be separated from the rest of the lead. An externalized conductor exists if all of the lead conductors do not fit within the shock electrode shadow width.

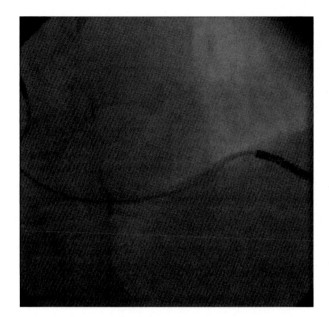

Figure 15.15 X-ray image of confirmed electrode cable externalization in St. Jude Medical Riata defibrillation lead. *Source*: Chan 2012 [6]. Reproduced with permission of John Wiley & Sons.

- Step 2: Examine the radius of curvature of each conductor. In most cases, externalized conductors have a different radius of curvature than the rest of the lead body. If the suspected externalized conductor occurs on the inside of a bend, the center of the conductor length has a radius of curvature that is larger than the rest of the lead body. If the externalized conductors occur on the outside of a bend, the externalized conductor will have a smaller radius of curvature than the rest of the lead body (Figure 15.15).

If a lead fulfills criteria in either step 1 or 2, conductor externalization is confirmed. At this point, little guidance has been put forward on the correct clinical course to take after identification of externalized conductor cables. Some advocate routine lead extraction followed by re-implantation of another lead. Others recommend capping the recalled Riata lead followed by placement of another lead. Still others recommend continuing to use leads with externalized conductors with intensified remote monitoring practices.

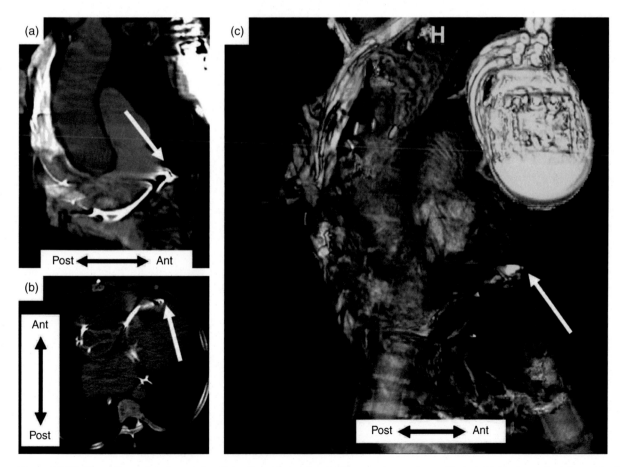

Figure 15.16 Three-dimensional reconstruction of two-dimensional CT images in a patient with device infection, prior left ventricular assist device prior to lead extraction. (a,b) Sagittal and coronal images demonstrate a high, anterior right ventricular lead position. (c) 3-D reconstruction demonstrates an anterior/free wall RV lead position with possible micro-perforation.

(a) (b) (c)

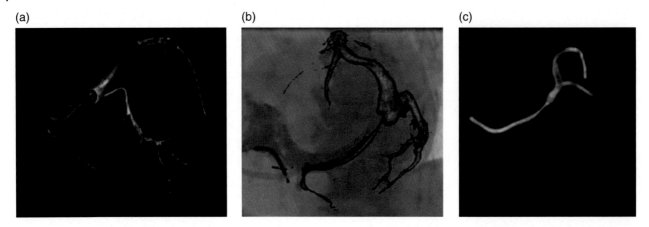

Figure 15.17 (a) 3-D reconstruction and segmentation of coronary sinus anatomy acquired by high-speed rotational angiography during CRT implantation (Dyna-CT, Seimens AG). (b) Integration of 3-D coronary sinus anatomy into real-time fluoroscopy to improve implanter understanding of 3-D left ventricular anatomy (Dyna-CT, Seimens AG). (c) 3-D reconstruction of coronary sinus anatomy acquired by high-speed rotational angiography during CRT implantation also incorporating LV activation timing to facilitate implantation of LV lead using both anatomical and electrical conduction information (Cardioguide, Medtronic Inc.)

CT and 3-D Imaging for Identifying Lead Location

X-ray imaging using multiple views is usually adequate for routine gross identification of pacing lead location. However, X-ray imaging is frequently inadequate when more detailed information about lead location is desired. These limitations result from an inability to control for cardiac rotation within the thorax and the inability to image cardiac soft tissues. When more detail is required, cardiac CT and 3-D imaging can be extremely helpful.

In our center, we employ cardiac CT with 3-D reconstruction routinely before lead extraction procedures (Figure 15.16). Using this technique, our operators have identified previously unknown cases of lead tip RV perforation, SVC lead perforation, and inadvertent lead placement in the splenic vein prior to extraction procedures. In these cases, elective open sternotomy extraction procedures were performed rather laser lead extraction and all leads were removed safely [2].

Three-dimensional imaging is also used commonly in many centers prior to and during cardiac resynchronization therapy implantation procedures to identify areas of LV scar, and branches of the coronary sinus venous system suitable for placement of LV leads. These images may then be imported into some fluoroscopy systems to be displayed in real time on the fluoroscopy screen to help ensure LV lead placement in a favored location. Alternatively, 3-D imaging may be acquired during the implantation procedure using either rotational angiography (Figure 15.17a,b) or electroanatomic mapping of the LV venous system (Figure 15.17c). The mapping procedures offer not only anatomic information about the venous system, but also the ability to identify the latest point of electrical activation. A building base of evidence suggests that placement of LV leads in areas of late electrical activation leads to superior outcomes in CRT.

Conlusions

X-ray imaging is extremely useful before, during, and after device implantation for identification of pacing and defibrillator lead location. More detailed information can be obtained using CT and other 3-D imaging techniques when needed.

References

1 Osmancik P, Stros P, Herman D, Curila K, Petr R. The insufficiency of left anterior oblique and the usefulness of right anterior oblique projection for correct localization of a computed tomography-verified right ventricular lead into the midseptum. Circ Arrhythm Electrophysiol 2013;6(4):719–725.

2 Lewis RK, Pokorney SD, Greenfield RA, Hranitzky PM, Hegland DD, Schroder JN, *et al.* Preprocedural ECG-gated computed tomography for prevention of complications during lead extraction. Pacing Clin Electrophysiol 2014;37(10):1297–1305.

3 van Gelder BM, Scheffer MG, Meijer A, Bracke FA. Transseptal endocardial left ventricular pacing: an alternative technique for coronary sinus lead placement in cardiac resynchronization therapy. Heart Rhythm 2007;4(4):454–460.

4 Gamble JH, Bashir Y, Rajappan K, Betts TR. Left ventricular endocardial pacing via the interventricular septum for cardiac resynchronization therapy: first report. Heart Rhythm 2013;10(12):1812–1814.

5 Lanzman RS, Winter J, Blondin D, Fürst G, Scherer A, Miese FR, *et al.* Where does it lead? Imaging features of cardiovascular implantable electronic devices on chest radiograph and CT. Korean J Radiol 2011;12(5):611–619.

6 Chan CW, Chiang CS. An ICD lead with failure of outer insulation goes undetected by regular measurements. Pacing Clin Electrophysiol 2012;35(9):e261–262.

16

How to Evaluate Postoperative Device Complications

Dan Sorajja and Win-Kuang Shen

Division of Cardiovascular Diseases, Mayo Clinic Arizona, Phoenix, AZ, USA

Annually, hundreds of thousands of pacemakers and internal cardioverter-defibrillator (ICD) implantations occur worldwide, usually without adverse events. However, the procedure is not without risk, as there are many potential complications related to the procedure itself that can occur immediately or in a delayed setting (Table 16.1). Of note, the incidence of these complications is inversely related to the procedural volume of the implanting physician and center [1,2]. This chapter discusses postoperative device complications including their risk factors, presentation, and management.

Lead Dislodgement

As fixation mechanisms have improved, lead dislodgement has become less frequent. However, this complication still occurs, being least common with generator changes (<1%), more common in new lead implantations (1.1–4.4%), with higher rates seen in pediatric populations as well as coronary sinus leads, which may dislodge in up to 3–10% of patients [1,3]. Coronary sinus lead dislodgement occurs at a higher rate, likely because of anatomic limitations for lead placement that must balance lead position stability with adequate thresholds while avoiding diaphragmatic stimulation. For non-epicardial leads, the ventricular lead dislodges at a lower rate than the atrial lead, which typically has to curve anteriorly and superiorly to gain adequate contact with myocardium [1]. Some lead dislodgments are attributable to Twiddler's syndrome (Figure 16.1), which may be conscious or unconscious patient manipulation of the pulse generator. To hinder repeat twiddling, an option is to place the device in a subpectoral position. Another option is to place the device inside an antibiotic sleeve, and then use sutures in multiple locations to anchor the sleeve (containing the pulse generator) to the pocket floor.

Dislodgement can be microdislodgement, in which the lead tip has moved but is unapparent visually, but enough to impair its function. In contrast, lead macrodislodgement is evident visually, such as on fluoroscopy or radiography.

With microdislodgement, usually the impedance remains normal while the threshold worsens. With macrodislodgement, common findings include loss of sensing, increased capture threshold, or inability to capture. This loss of capture can result in pacemaker syndrome, such as with atrial lead dislodgement leading to loss of AV synchrony. The lead may also dislodge to a position with inadvertent stimulation, such as the phrenic nerve or pocket stimulation of the brachial plexus. These leads require revision.

While lead revision is the likely course of action for a lead dislodgement, prevention should also be addressed. Signs that the lead is in adequate contact with myocardium include adequate sensing and a current of injury, as well as direct visualization of movement of the lead in coordination with the heart. Securing the lead to the suture sleeve, with proper anchoring to the pocket floor, should be standard procedure. Postoperative activity restrictions should be discussed with the patient and given as written instructions. A sling should be worn for 24 hours to remind the patient of the arm movement restriction, but afterward the sling should not be worn during daytime activities to avoid orthopedic complications such as frozen shoulder. For patients who sleep with their arm above their head, use of the sling only while sleeping is encouraged. Otherwise, patients should restrict their driving for at least 7 days post-procedure.

How-to Manual for Pacemaker and ICD Devices: Procedures and Programming, First Edition. Edited by Amin Al-Ahmad, Andrea Natale, Paul J. Wang, James P. Daubert, and Luigi Padeletti.
© 2018 John Wiley & Sons, Inc. Published 2018 by John Wiley & Sons, Inc.
Companion website: www.wiley.com/go/al-ahmad/pacemakers_and_icds

Table 16.1 Device complications, incidence, and timing [1–5].

Complications	Incidence (%)
Early complications (within 6 months post-implantation)	
Lead dislodgement, loss of capture	0.2–10
Lead or insulation damage	2.7–3.6
Bleeding, swelling, hematoma	0.1–2.3
Infection	0.7–1.9
Pneumothorax	0.5–1.6
Pain	0.2–1.4
Cardiac perforation, tamponade, pericarditis	0.09–1.4
Perioperative death	0.4–1.3
Erosion	NA
Inadvertent left ventricular lead placement	NA
Lead block connection problem	NA
Extracardiac stimulation	NA
Late complications (after 6 months post-implantation)	
Lead fracture	2.7–3.6
Thrombosis	0.03–3.5
Infection	0.7–1.9

Pneumothorax

Typical venous approaches to placement of new pacemaker and defibrillator leads include the axillary approach, subclavian approach, and cephalic vein cut-down. Pneumothorax is avoided with a cephalic cut-down approach, while an axillary (extrathoracic subclavian) approach has a lower risk than a subclavian approach. Other factors increasing the risk of pneumothorax include older patients, female gender, and a lower body mass index [2,3]. A micropuncture access kit may decrease the risk of pneumothorax, as will use of contrast injection because of the improved ability to target the venous system. Overall, the risk of pneumothorax is 1–2% [1–3].

Pneumothorax should be suspected when there is aspiration of air with the introducer needle, or there are systemic symptoms such as respiratory distress, hypotension, or chest discomfort. These findings manifest within 48 hours after new lead placement.

After a new lead implantation, post-procedure care should include an immediate chest X-ray to inspect for possible pneumothorax. This X-ray should be performed during inspiration with the patient upright. A small asymptomatic pneumothorax (Figure 16.2), comprising less than 15% of the lung field, can be managed with observation and supplement oxygenation, which can increase the reabsorption of the pneumothorax up to fourfold faster. The rate of reabsorption is estimated to be 1–2% daily with conservative measures, and may take several weeks to resolve. In the interim, these patients should be instructed to avoid air travel and deep sea diving until the pneumothorax is full resolved. However, larger pneumothoraces (those greater than 15% of the lung field) and those associated with hemodynamic compromise or significant bleeding into the thoracic cavity (hemopneumothorax) should be considered for chest tube placement. Management of pneumothorax should be primarily guided by the symptoms rather than the size of the pneumothorax. Small pneumothoraces can cause significant hemodynamic compromise, and chest tube placement may be warranted.

For hemopneumothorax, prevention is key. When access to the vein is obtained, the guide wire should be advance to below the diaphragm confirming placement in the inferior vena cava (IVC), not the arterial side, prior to dilatation with an introducer sheath. Use of an axillary approach is preferred as it allows for manual compression in this situation.

Bleeding, Swelling, and Hematoma

In patients on antiplatelets and/or anticoagulants, bleeding is more common throughout the procedure such as exposing the pectoral fascia and with creating the pacemaker pocket. Bleeding more commonly occurs during new device and lead implantations than during generator changes, when fibrosis typically limits the bleeding (Figure 16.3) [2,4].

Typical bleeding sites include subcutaneous vessels and exposed muscle fascia. Bleeding from the skin incision can be minimized with use of pulsed plasma radiofrequency energy (PEAK plasmablade) instead of a traditional scalpel, but this bleeding is likely inconsequential for most procedures. When bleeding occurs from multiple diffuse spots within the pocket (an "oozer"), electrocautery can be helpful in addition to gentle compression. Other options include using topical thrombin, thrombin-coated mesh, and Gelfoam. If the bleeding is limited to superficial bleeding, consider an ice pack or a pressure dressing. When the muscle fascia is split or torn, reapproximating the edges will reduce bleeding. For patients with high venous pressure or if a venous access site was double-wired to place multiple leads, bleeding around the lead suture sleeve can occur even if properly placed. Manual pressure or a purse string suture placed around the leads at their access site will facilitate hemostasis (Figure 16.3).

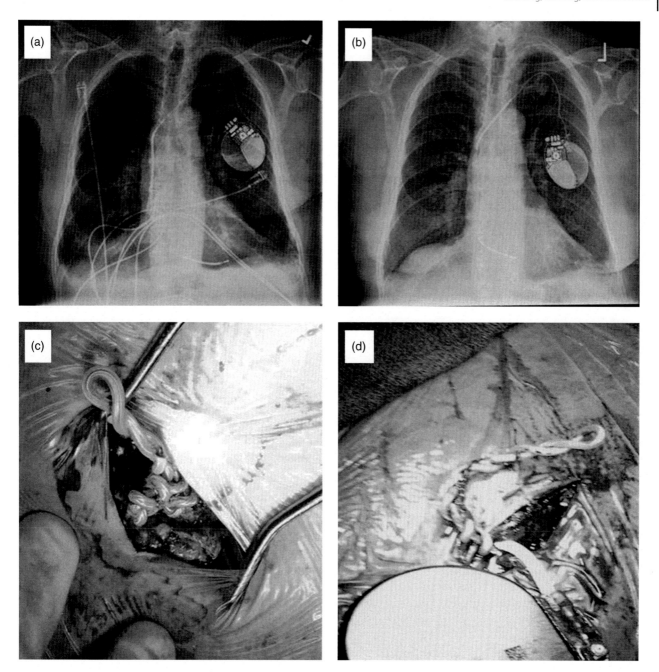

Figure 16.1 (a) Device at 1 day post implantation. (b) 1 month post implantation, and the coil is retracted to the innominate vein, while coiling of the lead is now apparent just superior to the pulse generator. (c) A lead from a Twiddler. (d) The same Twiddler lead as in panel (c) out of the pocket.

Prevention has a role in reducing the occurrence of postoperative bleeding. For patients on warfarin, bleeding complication is low when the international normaized ratio (INR) is less than 2.5 without disruption of warfarin therapy. Novel anticoagulants (dabigatran, rivaroxaban, apixaban) and clopidogrel should be held for at least 3 half-lives if possible. Heparin and low molecular weight heparin are especially associated with increased bleeding and hematoma formation. These

drugs should be discontinued prior to the procedure, and held at least 24–48 hours post device implantation.

At device follow-up, if ecchymosis is present, no further treatment than reassurance is required. Hematoma formation should be assessed for the rapidity of its formation, ability to control pain, and possible pocket erosion. Aspiration should not be attempted as it is unlikely to completely evacuate the hematoma while also increasing the risk of device infection. If the hematoma

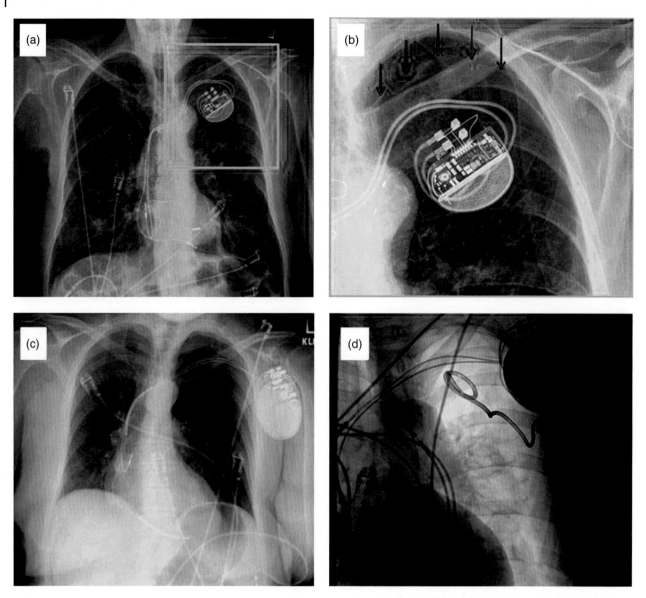

Figure 16.2 (a) Chest X-ray with minimal pneumothorax. (b) Panel (a) X-ray enlarged with arrows demarcating the margin of the pneumothorax, which was managed conservatively. (c) Large left-sided pneumothorax. (d) A pigtail catheter placed for the pneumothorax in panel (c).

continues to enlarge or the pain cannot be controlled, then the evacuation of the hematoma should be performed under sterile operating room conditions. Anticoagulation should be held if possible until bleeding has been controlled.

Pain

When patients present with pain immediately after a device implantation, the pain usually is caused by swelling, and typically responds to analgesics such as acetaminophen. Occasionally, this pain requires a narcotic in combination with the acetaminophen. Further from the time of device implantation, other possible contributors to pain should be considered, such as the device location being too superficial or lateral, nerve entrapment, or an allergy to a device component. However, the most worrisome complication that must be considered is infection.

If the device is placed too laterally or the device is not anchored properly, it can cause significant discomfort from irritation of the axillary nerve (or space). If the pain cannot be controlled, consideration should be given to affixing the device more medially. When the irritation is caused by the device swinging freely, non-absorbable suture or an encapsulating sleeve (e.g., AigisRx) can be

(a)

(b)

(c)

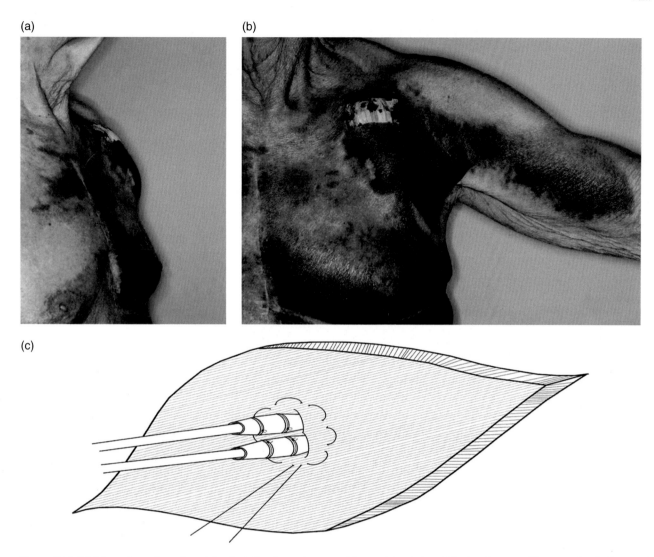

Figure 16.3 (a) A hematoma 1 week post implantation is most apparent from a lateral view with prominent swelling over the device pocket. (b) The same patient as in panel (a) with ecchymosis tracking down the chest and arm. He was on warfarin and clopidogrel during device implantation. (c) A device pocket floor is shown with two leads anchored to the floor with their suture sleeves. A pursestring suture encircling both leads can reduce bleeding, particularly in patients with high central venous pressure or when "double wiring" is required to access the vein.

used to anchor the device to the pocket floor. When the device is implanted too superficially within subcutaneous tissue rather than deep to the adipose tissue, the result can be very painful and difficult to control with medication. Usually, the pain is at the margin of the device, where pressure points exist. This complication frequently requires revision of the device to a deeper level, including submuscular implantation. For possible nerve entrapment, the device pocket can be "unroofed" but sometimes the device has to be relocated to the contralateral side to alleviate pressure on the nerve.

Several components that make up a pacing and defibrillating system have been shown to generate allergic reactions including: titanium, nickel, polychloroparaxylene, polyurethane, epoxy, mercury, cadmium,

chromate, silicone, and cobalt. On a similar note, combinations of these components make up several alloys used in devices, making an offending allergen not as apparent. Stainless steel (which contains nickel and chromium) can be found in many parts including the screws in a pacemaker or defibrillator, and the fixation portion of the pin and ring of the electrode lead. Many of these components are housed internally inside the pulse generator or inside the lead body, and therefore are not in direct contact with the patient. To determine if the patient has an allergy to a specific component, each of the manufacturers provides an allergy test kit to perform an epidermal skin test, but certain components such as titanium may elicit an allergic reaction despite negative testing. The risk of an allergic reaction should be weighed and considered fully with the patient, because the differential diagnosis includes infection, which requires removal of pulse generator and leads. Treatment for an allergic reaction includes topical steroids which is a temporizing measure. Other options include implantation of a gold-plated generator or a whole system coated with 0.2 mm PTFE surgical membrane.

Erosion

The development of erosion of the pulse generator is usually an indolent process occurring months to years after implantation. Superficial implantation of the pulse generator increases the risk or erosion. Another factor is the size of the device pocket being too small for the pulse generator, including new implantations but more so with device upgrades such as upgrading from a pacemaker to an ICD, or a biventricular device upgrade. Lateral placement of the pulse generator into the deltopectoral groove, where arm movement may create pressure on the device, also can lead to erosion. However, the most common cause of erosion is infection (Figure 16.4).

When erosion occurs, a revision of the pulse generator must be undertaken. The determination of whether there is infection should be made prior to performing a revision, as lack of visual purulent material during a revision is not satisfactory enough evidence to rule out infection. If the erosion occurs because of infection, then the leads must also be removed, and the new system should be implanted at a clean site (usually the contralateral side) after the infection has been cleared.

Infection

Superficial infection, which does not involve the device, is frequently caused by stitch abscess. This can typically be treated with oral antibiotics, usually for 7–10 days. Longer treatment up to 48 hours after resolution of erythema or signs of infection may be necessary.

The incidence of device infection after implantation is approximately 1% with slightly increased rates (up to 1.9%) seen with generator changes or device upgrade [1–5]. Other risk factors for infection include immunosuppression, diabetes, renal failure, pocket hematoma, longer case times, and additional operators [5]. Completed infusion of antibiotic within 60 minutes prior to implant can reduce the risk of infection by 80%, and good sterile technique should be employed. Counseling patients on postoperative care is also important, particularly avoidance of getting the implantation site wet for at least 48 hours post procedure.

Fever with systemic symptoms is more typical for early presentation (within 4 weeks post-procedure), infections with the causal agent predominantly being *Staphylococcus aureus*, which comprises almost 50% of all device infections [5]. These patients are more likely to be female and on anticoagulation. Of note, approximately 90% of cardiac device infection presents as a pocket infection. Frank erosion or purulent discharge is an obvious infection. However, device infection should be strongly considered when local erythema, serous drainage, skin adherence to the pulse generator, painful device pocket, or bacteremia are found. Of note, late presentations (after 4 weeks post procedure) of device infection

(a)

(b)

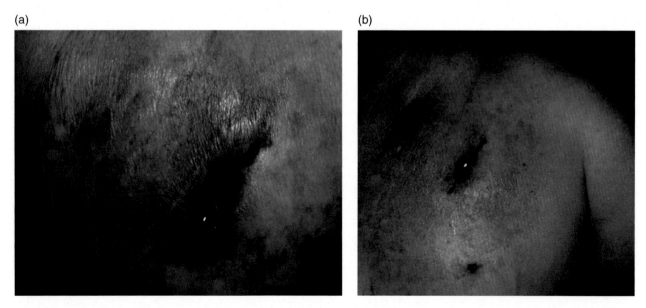

Figure 16.4 (a) Pus covering inapparent erosion with surrounding erythema. (b) Erosion is now apparent after the patient cleaned the wound himself.

typically lack fever, and the most frequent culprit is *Staphylococcus epidermidis*.

For possible device infection, the approach is to collect a suitable amount of evidence to determine if an infection is present, and whether there are sequelae from the infection such as cardiac valve vegetation or lead vegetation. Needle aspiration of a potentially infected pocket is not recommended; this test may potentially seed an uninfected pocket with infection. Blood cultures should be obtained prior to antibiotic administration. If blood cultures are obtained after antibiotics were given, and the cultures remain negative, the next step is a transesophageal echocardiogram. Positive blood cultures should result in a transesophageal echocardiogram to evaluate for possible vegetation involving the valve and lead. While transthoracic echocardiogram may have higher specificity, the sensitivity of the exam is insufficient for guiding therapy. Consultation with an expert in infectious diseases is recommended for all suspected device infections [5].

When there are sufficient data for a cardiac device infection, the whole system including the pulse generator and leads (including abandoned leads) should be removed, as approximately 50% of pocket infections have concomitant endovascular vegetations by transesophageal echocardiogram. Swab cultures from the pacemaker pocket and cultures of the lead tips should be obtained. After antibiotic treatment is started, serial blood cultures should be obtained, with the frequency depending on the suspected virulence of the causal organism and if definitive therapy (device system removal) has been performed [5].

Antibiotic duration will depend on the pathogen and its susceptibility. In general, pocket-site infection requires 14 days of antibiotics after device removal. If there are sequelae of infection (endocarditis, persistent bacteremia despite device removal), then antimicrobial therapy may be required for up to 6 weeks. Reimplantation of the device can occur after blood cultures (drawn after device removal) have been negative for at least 72 hours. If valvular infection is present, reimplantation of leads should occur at least 14 days after device removal. Reimplantation of the device should be not performed ipsilateral to the prior extraction site, and options include the contralateral side, epicardial, and iliac vein implantation [5].

Inadvertent Left Ventricular Lead Placement

Passing of the transvenous lead into the coronary sinus or middle cardiac vein and their branches sometimes occurs. The pacing configuration from the middle cardiac vein has a similar appearance to an apically paced right ventricular lead on the endocardium. In patients after tricuspid valve surgery, this placement may be

desirable, with adequate sensing typically seen but often with elevated capture threshold. Pericardial effusion or tamponade physiology may occur in the acute setting associated with vein perforation from the lead screw helix. As the lead matures over time if acute complications are not noted, worsening lead parameters are likely to be seen, thereby requiring revision.

Placement of a transvenous lead in the left ventricular cavity most commonly occurs when the lead passes inadvertently through a septal defect in the atrium or ventricle. The passage of a ventricular lead through an atrial septal defect can be recognized by the inability to lower the "takeoff" of the lead as it passes leftward because the takeoff will be limited by the inferior border of the atrial septal defect. In the left anterior oblique (LAO) view, the lead tip will be seen passing into the septum from the left. In the right anterior oblique (RAO) view, it should be possible to determine whether the lead crosses to the left side through the coronary sinus (inferior and posterior to tricuspid annulus fat stripe), atrial septal defect (closer to the vertebral column), or a ventricular septal defect (distal to tricuspid fat stripe and closer to sternum) (Figure 16.5).

Leads placed endocardially in the left ventricle require revision mainly because of the risk of thromboembolism, which also occurs with right-sided lead placement but is usually inconsequential. Anticoagulation should be initiated if the lead is to be left in the left ventricle, or there is a delay in therapy to revise the lead. Lead reposition or extraction should be considered when the left ventricular lead placement is detected.

Lead Block Connection Problems

If the lead pin is not adequately past the set screw or loosely connected, noise can be seen on monitoring but, more importantly, there can be failure of output, which may be intermittent or persistent. The noise is reproducible with manual manipulation of the device and lead. Other considerations for connection problems include air trapped in the header prior to lead insertion into the header, resulting in oversensing. Other causes include adaptors, such as with older leads to fit IS-1 headers, additional subcutaneous coils, or yokes for defibrillation.

Reconnection of the lead with the tip past the set screw is required. Visual inspection may show the lead pin not adequately passing through the connector block. With inadequately secured leads, gentle pulling of the lead at the header may completely disconnect the lead from the connector block without use of the wrench. Simple steps to ensure a connection without noise include "burping" of lead housing by placing the wrench in the connector block prior to connecting the lead, and wiping the lead

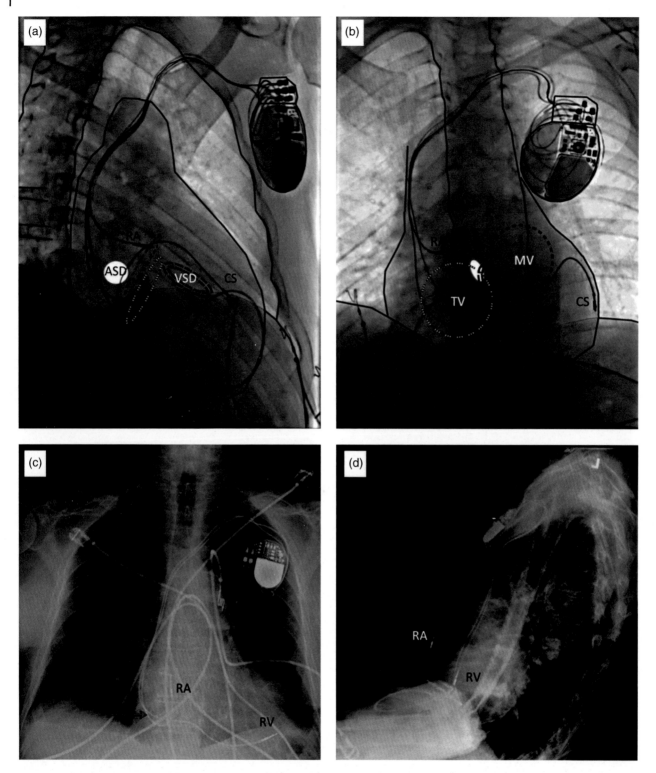

Figure 16.5 (a) A right anterior oblique (RAO) view is shown with the right atrial (RA), right ventricular (RV), and coronary sinus (CS) leads shown. Leads placed through an atrial septal defect (ASD, white circle) would be expected to have an inferior border or curve not lower than the ASD. Leads placed through a ventricular septal defect (VSD, double-dashed oval) would curve through this area. The profile of the tricuspid and mitral valves are seen and correspond to the visible fat-pad surrounding an annulus. (b) A left anterior oblique (LAO) view is shown of the same patients. (c) An RV lead is seen with a takeoff that is higher than the slack in the RA lead. The lead was inadvertently placed in the CS os, more specifically the middle cardiac vein. The lead has an unnatural curvature upward for an RV apical placement. (d) In the lateral film, the RV lead can be seen approaching the "septum" from the left side confirming the middle cardiac vein location.

tip and ring dry prior to connection. There are rare cases where the amount of lead insulation makes the lead diameter great enough to hinder advancement of the lead into the connector block. In these cases, placement of silicone oil on the lead body proximal to the lead electrode connectors should be considered. Use of forceps to advance the lead is discouraged, but non-teethed forceps (e.g., Debakey) are an option.

Lead or Insulation Damage

The median time to lead failure is 7 years, with the most common issue being insulation failure. More commonly, damage occurs with use of scalpels, scissors, or electrocautery such as during a generator change. Crush under the subclavian space (between the clavicle and first rib) is more likely to result in conductor problems rather than insulation failure.

While sensing abnormalities are more common, failure of the insulation can also result in abnormal pacing and, as a result, inappropriate shocks or no shock therapy may occur. Insulation damage is often unrecognized, but when significant enough can result in low impedance (less than 200 Ω). Chest X-rays typically do not reveal insulation issues. However, in some cases, fluoroscopy may detect insulation failure if there is externalization of the electrical conductors (e.g., St. Jude Riata leads).

Insulation damage, when apparent through other parameters of lead function, requires lead revision in most cases. The main aspect of managing insulation damage is prevention. For patients who are device-dependent or with occluded veins, consideration should be given to use of pulsed plasma radiofrequency energy (e.g., PEAK PlasmaBlade) which has a reduced thermal injury depth compared to standard electrocautery. In addition, avoidance of more lateral venous access can prevent subclavian crush and fatigue fractures from second or third rib stress from additional acute bends of the lead required to access the vein. For anchoring of leads to the pacemaker pocket, suture sleeves should be used to prevent damage to the lead or insulation, but overly tight suturing still can damage the insulation and conductor coils. Care should also be taken to avoid piercing the lead or insulation with the suturing needle.

Lead Fracture

Lead fracture is a complication that typically occurs late post procedure, at least 6 months after lead implantation in 2.7–3.6% of patients [1]. Sites of fractures are at stress points of the lead, such as coming out of the header block, at the costoclavicular space, and at suture sleeves.

Risk factors of lead fracture include younger age (<50 years old) and higher left ventricular ejection fraction (>45%), likely from increased activity and physical stress on the lead [1].

Without overt failure of sensing, impedance, or threshold of a device lead, impending lead fracture can sometimes be seen on a device check as non-physiologic noise, with a cycle length of less than 140 ms. The manifestations can vary, with sensing abnormalities or failure to capture or failure to output. If the fracture is complete, then the abnormalities are persistent and typically include failure to output. Occasionally, there may be intermittent capture with a complete fracture if the fracture intermittently has enough connection between the disjointed ends. In incomplete fractures, some of the device output is transmitted to the tissue but with failure to capture. For defibrillators, the noise that is sensed may result in inappropriate tachyarrhythmia therapy. Device programming algorithms have been designed to detect this non-physiologic noise, and with certain devices may be able to detect a fracture days before an inappropriate shock is delivered.

For management of lead fracture, the lead should be configured to sense and pace in a unipolar configuration, which may be able to "work around" the fracture. This situation is not ideal, and lead revision should be planned with timing based on the clinical scenario.

Rising Threshold and Exit Block

After achieving satisfactory pacing thresholds at the time of lead implantation, rising threshold and exit block manifests with progressively increasing threshold without any evident macrodislodgement or perforation. While microdislodgement is in the differential diagnosis initially, it typically does not have a continuing increase in the threshold. With steroid-eluting leads nowadays, exit block is less common, but rising threshold and exit block are still frequent with coronary sinus leads and epicardial leads. Although the etiology is unclear, one possible explanation is an increased reaction such as fibrosis at the lead–cardiac tissue interface.

Prevention may have a role in reducing the frequency of exit block; placement of the lead tip in a stable position that has limited movement (e.g., not acting as a hinge point) may help. Once exit block is present, the output of the lead will have to increase to maintain capture, and changing the pacing configuration or vector of the lead (e.g., unipolar, tip-to-coil) may facilitate this. Another option is a trial of steroids (dexamethasone 2 mg PO twice daily for 1 week), which may be able to lower the threshold sufficiently. However, the improvement may be temporary and limited to the time around steroid administration, so lead revision may ultimately be required. For patients undergoing lead revision for exit block, particularly with coronary sinus leads and epicardial leads without steroid elution, supplement steroid use for 1 month should be considered, as the steroid use will prevent chronic elevation in the lead threshold.

Extracardiac Stimulation

When leads dislodge, the extracardiac stimulation usually involves adjacent structures to the dislodgement, most commonly seen involving leads placed in the coronary sinus. A microdislodgement or macrodislodgement can have the same result.

The left phrenic nerve, which travels over the left lateral cardiac border, is not infrequently near the target site for a coronary sinus lead. To prevent this complication, the coronary sinus lead should be tested at high output (10 V) to assess for diaphragmatic stimulation, which if present should result in lead repositioning. When there are no other satisfactory coronary sinus lead positions (such as because of inappropriately high threshold or concern for lead position stability), the testing output should be titrated down to assess if there is an adequate safety margin between stimulating the phrenic nerve and left ventricular capture threshold. Different pacing vector configurations may be able to avoid phrenic nerve capture, which is facilitated by current coronary leads (particularly quadripolar leads) and pulse generators.

Less commonly, right phrenic nerve capture is seen with the right atrial lead. Repositioning of the lead is required if this phenomenon is observed. Although not extracardiac, the right atrial lead when placed in the appendage may be able to capture the right ventricular outflow tract. This finding also requires lead repositioning, usually to a position more lateral in the appendage or elsewhere in the right atrium.

The right ventricular lead, when placed away more inferiorly, may capture the diaphragm resulting in complaints of twitching or hiccups that may be positional. The right ventricular lead when placed anteriorly may result in intercostal muscle stimulation. Both of these situations frequently require lead revision if the pulse generator output cannot be reduced to capture cardiac myocardium without the extracardiac stimulation.

Cardiac Perforation, Tamponade, and Pericarditis

Lead perforation is a potential serious complication, with risk factors including elderly patients, low body mass index, and systemic steroid use [1]. Certain areas of the heart that are more prone to dissection include the right atrial free wall, right ventricular free wall, and distal coronary sinus. Lead perforation likely has an underrepresented frequency in studies as they are often asymptomatic and unrecognized. Symptomatic perforations are more common with ICD leads at a rate between 0.6–5% [1], while coronary sinus lead placement (1.3%) and pacemaker lead perforation (0.8–3%) are less common. In asymptomatic patients, diagnosis of perforation is detected by CT scan with rates of perforation being 15% with atrial leads and 6% with ventricular leads overall. While active fixation leads have lower rates of perforation in the right atrium (12% vs. 25% for passive fixation), passive fixation has lower rates of perforation with right ventricular pacemaker leads (5% vs. 7% for active fixation).

Diagnosis is frequently by CT scan for asymptomatic patients (Figure 16.6). Echocardiography may be helpful but usually the diagnosis is not apparent as a result of artifact on imaging from the lead. Impedance change is also typically not helpful. Of note, pericardial irritation may occur without any overt perforation. More typically, for leads placed in the right ventricle, perforation should be suspected when the paced rhythm is a right bundle pattern (suggesting pacing from the left ventricle), although apical right ventricular leads may also result in a right bundle pattern. Other signs of potential perforation include diaphragmatic stimulation, pericardial pain, and pericardial effusion with and without cardiac tamponade. These signs are apparent during lead implantation, but perforation may also result in slow hemodynamic worsening over 48 hours and reportedly even over 1 month from the time of implantation.

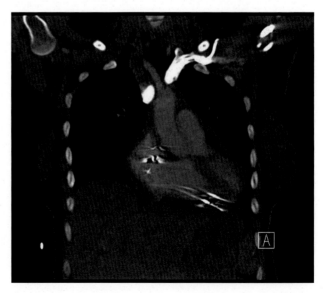

Figure 16.6 Coronal cuts through a computed tomography scan show the right ventricular lead perforating the myocardium anteriorly and inferiorly.

For management of patients with mild symptoms of pericardial irritation with and without perforation, observation with anti-inflammatory medications is reasonable and should resolve the symptoms during the course of treatment. High dose aspirin, colchicine, or even prednisone may be used depending on the severity of symptoms. For small pericardial effusions without tamponade, serial echocardiograms should be obtained to monitor for enlarging effusion size or tamponade physiology.

If there is a large effusion or one resulting in hemodynamic compromise, emergency treatment is required. For tamponade, pericardiocentesis should be performed using fluoroscopic or echocardiographic guidance, and a pigtail catheter should be left in the pericardial space. When the reaccumulation rate is less than 25 mL over 24 hours, then the pigtail catheter can be removed. Serial echocardiography should be performed to confirm a lack of reaccumulation, at which point lead revision is not required.

If there continues to be recurrent effusion, a pericardial window is not recommended, as it will not fix the underlying issue. A lead revision is required and this should be performed with either equipment ready for repeat pericardiocentesis if necessary or in an operating room with a cardiothoracic surgeon on standby.

Thrombosis

Post device implantation, thrombus attached to the right atrial and right ventricular leads can be detected with echocardiography in 9% of cases after 6 months of follow-up. Usually, patients are asymptomatic for these thrombi, with symptomatic thromboemboli seen in only 0.03–3.5% of cases [3]. When thrombus forms more proximally such as at the superior vena cava, there is concern for a higher likelihood of pulmonary embolism and development of superior vena cava syndrome (0.03–0.15%). With thrombosis involving the more proximal course of a transvenous lead, such as in the innominate or subclavian vein, the risk of pulmonary embolism decreases. The risk of vein stenosis or thrombosis increases with the numbers of leads, or increased diameter of leads, such as ICD leads.

These more proximal stenoses or occlusion can result in upper extremity swelling and pain if significant collateralization has not developed, with 1–3% of patients being symptomatic for this condition. In some cases, dilation of the superficial venous system is visible on physical examination (Figure 16.7).

Most thrombosis is asymptomatic, so no further management is usually required. If there are symptoms

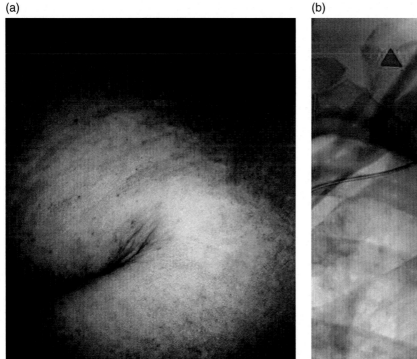
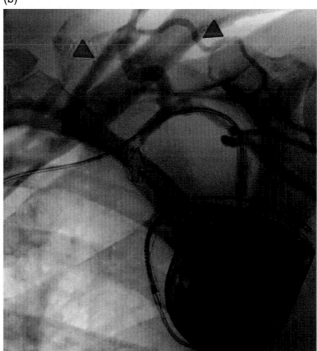

Figure 16.7 (a) Thrombosis apparent on physical examination resulting from extensive collateralization seen in superficial veins. (b) Same patient as in panel (a) with fluoroscopy and contrast injection confirming occlusion (arrow) of the subclavian vein with collateralization (arrowheads).

attributable to the thrombosis, or the potential for thromboembolism is great enough, then anticoagulation is recommended. Conservative measures such as arm elevation also help with symptom alleviation, which typically improve over weeks. Often, the venous stenosis or thrombosis is discovered during a lead revision or device upgrade. In these cases, venoplasty should be considered if there is expertise in opening the vein. With complete occlusions, this usually requires the use of alternative venous access.

Conclusions

With increasing indications for implantation of pacemakers and ICDs with an aging population, the number of devices will continue to grow every year. While most procedures occur smoothly, the risk of an adverse event is small but present. For physicians who perform device implantations or manage these patients, knowledge of the potential postoperative complications and their corresponding management is essential.

References

1 Armaganijan LV, Toff WD, Nielsen JC, Andersen HR, Connolly SJ, Ellenbogen KA, *et al.* Are elderly patients at increased risk of complications following pacemaker implantation? A meta-analysis of randomized trials. PACE. 2012;35:131–134.

2 Kirkfeldt RE, Johansen JB, Nohr EA, Jørgensen OD, Nielsen JC. Complications after cardiac implantable electronic device implantations: an analysis of a complete, nationwide cohort in Denmark. Euro Heart J 2014;35:1186–1194.

3 Peterson PN, Daugherty SL, Wang Y, Vidaillet HJ, Heidenreich PA, Curtis JP, *et al.* Gender differences in procedure-related adverse events in patients receiving implantable cardioverter-defibrillator therapy. Circulation 2009;119:1078–1084.

4 Poole JE, Gleva MJ, Mela T, Chung MK, Gottipaty V, Borge R, *et al.* Complication rates associated with pacemaker or implantable cardioverter-defibrillator generator replacements and upgrade procedures: results from the REPLACE registry. Circulation 2010;122:1553–1561.

5 Baddour LM, Epstein AE, Erickson CC, Knight BP, Levison ME, Lockhart PB, *et al.* Update on cardiovascular implantable electronic device infections and their management: a scientific statement from the American Heart Association. Circulation 2010;121:458–477.

Part Two

17

How to Program Pacemakers for Patients With Sinus Node Disease

Carsten W. Israel and Lucy Ekosso-Ejangue

J.W. Goethe University, Frankfurt, Germany
Department of Medicine – Cardiology, Evangelical Hospital Bielefeld, Bielefeld, Germany

Pacemaker therapy in sinus node disease (SND) alleviates symptoms rather than modifying prognosis. Causing symptoms by suboptimal programming therefore has a particularly important role.

Forms of SND are: permanent sinus bradycardia, intermittent sinoatrial (SA) block/arrest, sinus bradycardia alternating with atrial fibrillation (AF) and tachyarrhythmic ventricular response (brady-tachy syndrome), and chronotropic sinus node incompetence. SND associated with an AV block represents binodal disease.

Pacemaker programming in SND aims to maintain intrinsic conduction if the atrioventricular (AV) node function is normal. Single-chamber ventricular pacing in SND should be avoided because it can lead to pacemaker syndrome, cause AF, reduce exercise capacity and quality of life, and increase the risk of stroke [1].

Several decisions have to be made when programming a pacemaker in patients with SND: pacing mode, lower and upper pacing rate, sensor programming, AV delay programming, activation of specific algorithms, and memory functions.

Pacing Mode Programming in Different Forms of SND

The ideal pacing mode in SND is atrial pacing (AAI with or without sensor) which entirely avoids ventricular pacing and problems associated with blocked atrial premature beats (APBs), single non-conducted P waves, intermittent first degree AV block, retrograde conduction, and so on. Atrial pacing mode can be chosen in patients with normal AV conduction and sinus bradycardia, SA block/sinus arrest, or chronotropic incompetence (Table 17.1).

Patients with brady-tachy syndrome usually require drugs that slow AV conduction during AF and can cause iatrogenic AV block. Patients with bundle branch block and primary AV block may require ventricular pacing. The optimal pacing mode in these patients is DDI(R) or DDD(R) with mode switching to avoid rapid tracking of atrial tachyarrhythmias.

The risk of developing AV block in patients with SND is not clear. Upgrade from an AAI(R) to a DDD(R) pacemaker because of AV block occurred in the DANPACE trial in 9.3% of patients over the course of 5.4 years (1.7% per year) [2]. Pacemaker memory shows intermittent AV block in approximately 20% of patients with SND.

Implanting a dual-chamber pacemaker and programming it to AAI(R) avoids the need for reoperation if AV block develops. Unnecessary ventricular pacing can only occur in dual-chamber modes. The Wenckebach block heart rate should be assessed at each follow-up (even if the predictive value is unclear) and the device reprogrammed to DDD/DDI if atrial pacing at 120 bpm is not conducted 1 : 1 to the ventricle.

In individual patients with rare SA block or sinus arrest, VVI pacing might be considered. The pacing mode should be VVI, not VVIR, to avoid frequent ventricular asynchronous pacing and pacemaker syndrome. A hysteresis should be activated allowing pacing only if the rate falls below 40 bpm. Unfortunately, the frequency of "rare" SA block or sinus arrest is not clearly defined (one pause per day, per week, or every 3 months?). Patients with seemingly rare SA block or sinus arrest may develop more frequent episodes or persistent sinus bradycardia that causes frequent asynchronous VVI pacing. As 80% of patients with SND have retrograde ventriculo-atrial (VA) conduction, many (30%) develop pacemaker syndrome and would have better results with dual-chamber pacing.

How-to Manual for Pacemaker and ICD Devices: Procedures and Programming, First Edition. Edited by Amin Al-Ahmad, Andrea Natale, Paul J. Wang, James P. Daubert, and Luigi Padeletti.
© 2018 John Wiley & Sons, Inc. Published 2018 by John Wiley & Sons, Inc.
Companion website: www.wiley.com/go/al-ahmad/pacemakers_and_icds

Table 17.1 Programming pacing mode in patients with different forms of SND.

Permanent sinus bradycardia

1st choice: DDDR, DDIR, AAIR
2nd choice: DDD, DDI, AAI
   Contraindicated: VDD, VVI, VVIR

Intermittent SA block/sinusarrest (without permanent sinus bradycardia or chronotropic sinus node incompetence)

1st choice: DDD, DDI, AAI
2nd choice: DDDR, DDIR, AAIR, (in individual cases VVI with hysteresis 40 bpm)
   Contraindicated: VDD, VVIR

Brady-tachy syndrome (without chronotropic incompetence)

1st choice: DDD with mode switching, DDI
2nd choice: DDDR with mode switching, DDIR, AAIR
   Contraindicated: VDD, VVI, VVIR, DDD without mode switching

Chronotropic sinus node incompetence

1st choice: DDDR, DDIR, AAIR
2nd choice: DDD, DDI, AAI
   Contraindicated: VDD, VVI, VVIR

SND with PQ >300 ms, AV block 2nd/3rd degree, BBB (without chronotropic incompetencen)

1st choice: DDD
2nd choice: DDDR, DDI, DDIR
   Contraindicated: AAI, AAIR, VDD, VVI, VVIR

Mode Switching

Many patients with SND have paroxysmal AF causing rapid ventricular rates if the AV node functions normal. In tracking modes (DDD, DDDR), AF is tracked at the upper tracking limit leading to rapid ventricular pacing. Patients with SND can therefore be programmed to a non-tracking mode [AAI(R) or DDI(R)] as long as there is no AV block. In patients with AV block, the DDD(R) should be programmed together with automatic mode switching to DDI(R) mode to prevent rapid tracking of AF and to switch back to tracking as soon as AF has ceased. Switching should aim at DDI(R), not to VVI(R) or VDI(R), because pacing until device criteria for AF termination are fulfilled should be DDI(R), not VVI(R).

Mode switching algorithms detect AF differently (e.g., mean atrial rate, consecutive atrial beats, x out of y) with fast or slow reaction [3]. In general, fast reacting algorithms and settings that facilitate AF detection are to be preferred. Inappropriate mode switching because of farfield oversensing of ventricular signals in the atrium can be avoided by programming long postventricular atrial blanking (PVAB) periods (e.g., 150 ms), or according to farfield oversensing tests.

Table 17.2 Programming of parameters pertinent to mode switching.

Mode switching: activation in all patients programmed to DDD(R) mode

Activation of algorithms to discover blanked atrial flutter (without delay)

Atrial tachyarrhythmia detection rate: 170–180 bpm

Non-tracking mode during mode switching: DDI(R), not VVI(R)/VDI(R)

Postventricular atrial blanking (PVAB) period: long (e.g., 150 ms) to prevent oversensing of ventricular farfield signals in the atrium

High atrial sensitivity (0.2–0.3 mV) to avoid intermittent AF undersensing with switching back and forth (mode switching oscillations)

AV block during AF: lower rate different from sinus rhythm (e.g., 70 bpm during AF and 60 bpm during sinus rhythm)

Activation of stored bipolar atrial electrograms for mode switching or atrial tachyarrhythmia detection

The atrial tachyarrhythmia detection rate should be programmed to 170–180 bpm because blanking periods (AV delay, PVAB) and intermittent undersensing can cause sensed AF rates <200 bpm.

Atrial flutter at 220–250 bpm may pose a problem for mode switching if every second flutter potential occurs after a QRS in the PVAB (2 : 1 lock-in, blanked flutter). Some mode switching algorithms allow activation of a separate Atrial Flutter Reaction® (Boston-Scientific) or Blanked Flutter Search® (Medtronic Inc.). These algorithms should be activated (Table 17.2).

Lower Rate Programming

Programming the lower rate limit depends on the type of SND, patient symptoms, and atrial lead position (Table 17.3). Competition between intrinsic sinus rhythm and atrial pacing should be avoided because alternating excitation from different atrial sites can be proarrhythmic. The lower rate limit should be programmed either slower than the intrinsic sinus rate or faster if sinus bradycardia is symptomatic.

Symptoms such as exercise intolerance, fatigue, and so on, typically result from permanent sinus bradycardia and chronotropic incompetence [1]. To relieve these symptoms, a lower rate of 60 bpm may be required. In contrast, syncope results from asystolic pause. In patients with normal resting sinus rate but intermittent sinus arrest, it may be preferable to maintain intrinsic sinus rhythm and program a lower rate at 50 bpm or a hysteresis (pacing at 60 bpm, hysteresis 50 bpm).

Table 17.3 Arguments for different settings of lower rate programming.

Situation	Lower rate limit programming
Fatigue, dizziness at rest, resting heart rate <55 bpm	60 bpm
Syncope, usually no symptoms at rest, resting heart rate >55 bpm	50 bpm (or 60 bpm with sinus hysteresis)
Exercise intolerance, resting rate <55 bpm, sinus rate at maximum exercise <100 bpm	60 bpm, rate response on
Paroxysmal AF, sinus rate <55 bpm	60–70 bpm
Permanent sinus bradycardia <50 bpm	60 bpm, rate response on
Intermittent SA block/sinus arrest	50 bpm (or hysteresis)
Brady-tachy type with sinus bradycardia <55 bpm	60–70 bpm
Chronotropic incompetence, resting heart rate >55 bpm	50 bpm, rate response on
Chronotropic incompetence, resting heart rate <55 bpm	60 bpm, rate response on
Atrial pacing causing PQ prolongation to >250 ms	50 bpm
Atrial pacing not causing PQ prolongation	60 bpm
(Symptomatic) AV junctional rhythm at 50–60 bpm	Overdrive (70 bpm, atrial overdrive algorithms)

In some patients with SND of the brady-tachy type, AF may be associated with bradycardia or rate decrease (vagally induced AF). In these patients, a lower rate limit of ≥70 bpm may prevent AF recurrences.

Programming the lower rate should consider if atrial pacing prolongs PQ and increases the percentage of unnecessary right ventricular pacing. The lower pacing limit should be programmed rather low (50–60 bpm) if the patient tolerates this well and if atrial pacing causes PQ prolongation >270 ms or right ventricular pacing. If atrial pacing does not prolong PQ, side effects of atrial pacing (AV desynchronization, forced unnecessary right ventricular pacing leading to ventricular desynchronization) are unlikely and a lower rate limit of 60–70 bpm can be programmed more liberally.

Upper Sensor Rate and Sensor Programming

Data from randomized clinical trials did not show a benefit of rate-adaptive pacing. Thus, rate-adaptive pacing should be restricted to patients with severe chronotropic incompetence.

Table 17.4 Programming of parameters pertinent to rate-adaptive pacing.

Activation of rate-adaptive pacing: heart rate at anaerobic threshold ≤90–100 bpm or during maximal exercise (exercise test, 24 h Holter) ≤100 bpm

Maximal sensor rate: 110 bpm in less active patients, patients with coronary artery disease, and patients with heart failure

Sensor activation threshold: depending on sensor and algorithm; usually low, low-to-moderate, moderate (high in some sensors and e.g., thin patients)

Speed of sensor activation: fast

Sensor rate increase: fast in physically less fit patients, slow in physically fit patients

Sensor rate decay: slow

Activity of daily living: 85 (–95) bpm, cross-check short

Blended sensors: individually after 2 min defined physical activity test

Patients with SND should receive an exercise test or, if treadmill and bicycle exercise cannot be performed, a 24 h ECG Holter or telemetrc monitoring during normal daily activity. Patients with a heart rate <100 bpm when stopping exercise due to dyspnea or exertion, at the anaerobic threshold, or as maximum value during 24 h despite normal physical exercise most likely have severe chronotropic sinus node incompetence that can be improved by pacing.

In most patients aged >65 years, the maximum sensor rate should be limited to 110 bpm for three reasons:

1) Most patients perceive "overpacing" (i.e., pacing at a heart rate faster than necessary) as more uncomfortable than "underpacing" (i.e., pacing at a rate slower than optimal for metabolic demands);
2) Pacing at a rate >110–120 bpm may cause angina pectoris in patients with concomitant coronary artery disease;
3) Pacing at a rate >110–120 bpm can deteriorate hemodynamics in heart failure.

Programming of parameters pertinent to sensor function has to be individualized in the absence of study data (Table 17.4). The activity threshold triggering the sensor to increase the pacing rate should be programmed individually. The need for a rapid activity detection and rate increase is considered to be higher in less physically active patients. Most physical activities in daily life are short, so the sensor should react fast. The rate decay to the lower rate limit should be programmed slow to avoid rapid rate changes and to support the heart rate after anaerobic exercise.

Some devices offer a physical activity cross-check program. If this option is present, they increase the heart rate only moderately during "activity of daily living"

(ADL; e.g., to 85–95 bpm). Upon the threshold of activity being reached the device allows a further rate increase to the maximum sensor rate only if activity is confirmed. These algorithms should be activated to avoid inappropriately fast pacing rates. However, a slow cross-check can reduce the benefit of rate-adaptive pacing because the patient may be exhausted by the time the algorithm allows a further rate increase above the ADL rate.

Some dual-sensor devices offer sensor blending (e.g., Boston-Scientific). Rate-adaptive pacing can be optimized in these devices by an exercise test in which the patient performs a defined 2 minute activity protocol (e.g., walking slowly through a corridor for 30 s, climbing a stair for 30 s, walking down a stair for 30 s, walking fast through a corridor back to the device check-up room for 30 s). The heart rate during this 2 minute period can be stored, interrogated, and virtually modified by different sensor settings until a the sensor response is optimal.

Upper Tracking Rate

In SND patients with normal AV conduction, the upper tracking limit is meaningless. If a tracking mode [DDD, DDD(R)] is programmed, however, tracking should be limited to 110 bpm in most patients:

1) Paroxysmal AF can be tracked at the upper tracking limit before device criteria for arrhythmia detection are met and mode switching occurs. If mode switching fails (algorithm deactivated, significant AF undersensing), ongoing rapid tracking may occur.
2) Atrial flutter may not be detected due to 2 : 1 lock-in of every alternate flutter potential. Typical atrial flutter with an atrial rate of 240–250 bpm can only be tracked 2 : 1 if the upper tracking rate is ≥120 bpm. With an upper tracking rate of 110 bpm, Wenckebach block occurs, atrial flutter is no longer associated 2 : 1 with blanking times, and can be detected.
3) In patients with coronary artery disease and heart failure, tracking atrial rates >110 bpm may cause angina pectoris, ischemia, and deterioration of heart failure.

AV Delay: Sensed and Paced

Programming the AV delay after an intrinsic P wave (sensed AV delay) or atrial pacing (paced AV delay) depends on intrinsic AV conduction and atrial lead position, the latter determining paced AV conduction. Unnecessary right ventricular pacing should be avoided in patients with SND and narrow QRS. However, long first-degree AV block shortens diastolic

Table 17.5 Different steps in AV delay programming.

1) Measurement of spontaneous AV conduction after atrial sensing (device marker for atrial sensing to device marker for ventricular sensing)
2) Measurement of spontaneous AV conduction after atrial pacing (device marker for atrial pace to device marker for ventricular sensing)
3) Both <250 (−300) ms: program AV delay (sensed and paced) to 300 ms
4) AV conduction after atrial sensing <250 (−300) ms but after atrial pacing >250 (−300) ms: consider reprogramming to a low lower rate limit (e.g., 50 bpm), or program sensed and paced AV delay to shorter, optimized values (echocardiography, ECG)
5) AV conduction after atrial pacing <250 (−300) ms but after atrial sensing >250 (-300) ms (found in atrial septal pacing): consider reprogramming to a higher lower rate limit (e.g., 70 bpm), rate-adaptive mode, or activate atrial overdrive algorithms. Consider reprogramming to DDIR (no sensed AV delay)
6) AV conduction after atrial sensing and pacing >250 (−300) ms: program sensed and paced AV delay to shorter, optimized values (echocardiography, ECG)
7) Varying AV conduction with PQ >250 ms alternating with PQ <250 ms: activate AV hysteresis function (e.g., 100 ms) together with shorter settings (e.g., paced AV delay 200 ms, sensed AV delay 150 ms)
8) If long values for sensed and paced AV delay are programmed: check memory functions: (i) ventricular pacing <1%, (ii) endless loop tachycardia (inaccurately termed "PMT" in counters), (iii) occurrence of repetitive non-re-entrant VA synchrony (usually inappropriately stored as atrial high rate episode)

filling time and can cause mitral regurgitation and heart failure. Therefore, the decision whether to facilitate intrinsic AV conduction or normalize AV timing can be difficult. Intrinsic conduction with PQ >270 ms seems to be worse than right ventricular pacing at an optimized AV delay in most patients [4].

The sensed (spontaneous P wave, spontaneous QRS complex) and atrial paced (slightly above the sinus rate) intrinsic AV conduction should be checked. If both are below 250 (−300) ms, sensed and paced AV delays can be programmed to 300 ms (Table 17.5). This avoids unnecessary right ventricular pacing (with full capture, fusion, or pseudo-fusion) even if there is intermittent prolongation of the PQ time.

If only sensed AV conduction exceeds 250–300 ms but paced AV conduction does not (e.g., in atrial septal pacing; Figure 17.1), the atrial pacing rate can be programmed to provide predominantly atrial pacing (70 bpm, rate response, atrial overdrive). Otherwise, ventricular pacing can usually not be avoided without hemodynamic compromise and sensed and paced AV delays should be programmed to shorter, optimized values.

(a)

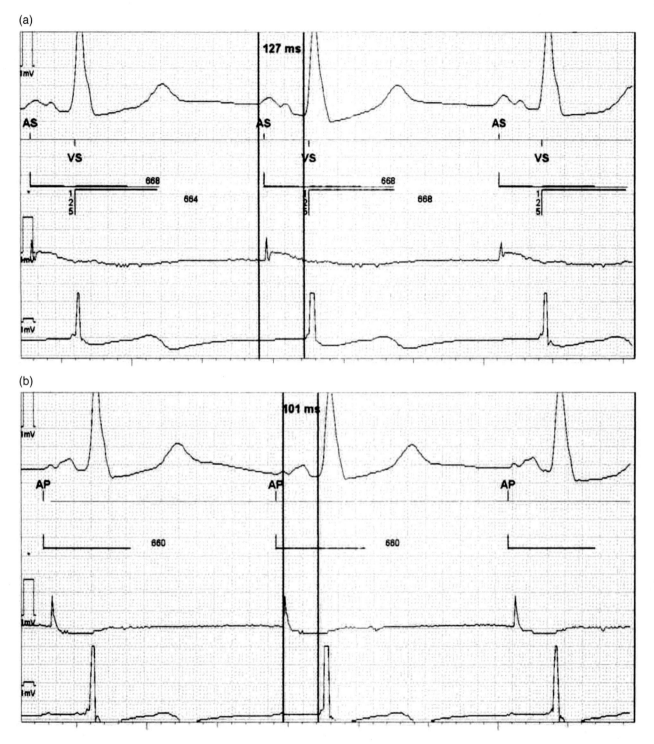

(b)

Figure 17.1 AV conduction during pacing from the atrium septum shorter than during atrial sensing. (a) During intrinsic sinus rhythm, PQ time is 127 ms, the double-peaked P wave indicates atrial conduction delay. Paper speed 100 mm/s. (b) During atrial pacing, PQ time decreases to 101 ms, the P wave is no longer double-peaked but narrower. Paper speed 100 mm/s.

If only paced AV conduction exceeds 250–300 ms (atrial lead positioned at the lateral atrial wall or right atrial appendage; Figure 17.2), the paced AV delay should be programmed to a value <270 ms, lower rate to 50 bpm, and the pacing mode to DDI(R).

If both atrial-sensed and paced AV conduction exceed 250–300 ms, the AV delay should be programmed to shorter values hemodynamically optimized for atrial sensing and atrial pacing. An easy method for AV delay optimization is to look at the interval between the end of

(a)

(b)

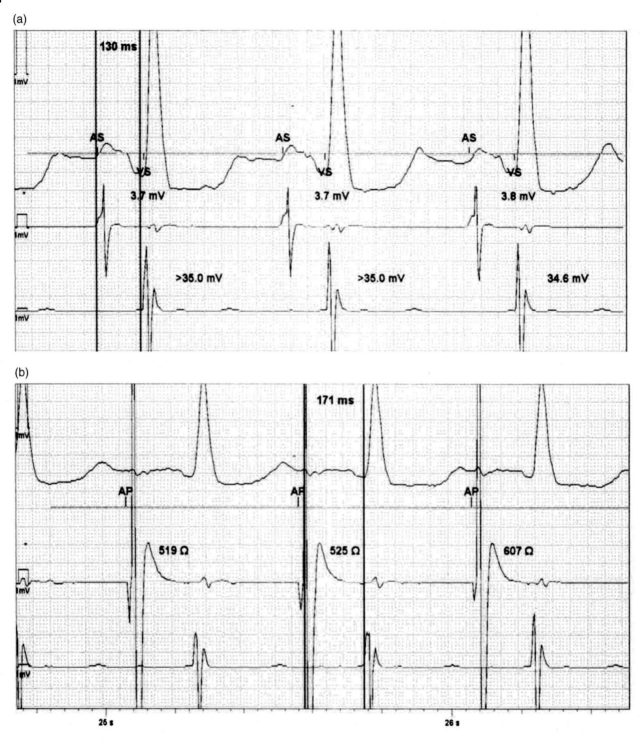

Figure 17.2 AV conduction during atrial pacing from the right atrial appendage longer than during atrial sensing. (a) During intrinsic sinus rhythm, PQ time is 130 ms, the P wave is double-peaked. Paper speed 100 mm/s. (b) During atrial pacing, PQ time increases to 171 ms, the P wave is now broad and flat. Paper speed 100 mm/s.

the P wave and the tip of the R wave. The ideal interval is 100 ms [5]. If this interval is, for example, 220 ms in a sequentially paced AV interval of 300 ms, it is 220−100 = 120 ms too long. The paced AV delay should be shortened to 300−120 = 180 ms (Figure 17.3) [5].

The paced AV delay starts with the atrial spike which occurs before the beginning of the P wave, while the sensed AV delay starts at the time when the atrial lead detects activity which (depending on the implantation site) can be late within the P wave. Therefore,

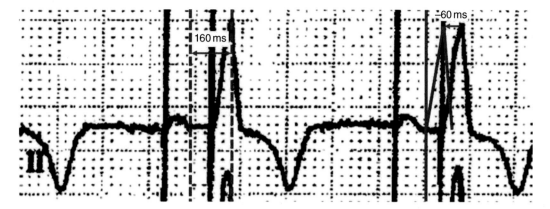

Figure 17.3 Optimizing the AV delay via the surface ECG. In this example, the paced P wave is very narrow, after the P wave there is a rather long PQ segment followed by ventricular pacing at a paced AV delay programmed to 200 ms. The interval between the end of the P wave and the peak of the R wave is 160 ms (left) but should be 100 ms (60 ms shorter). The paced AV delay should therefore be reduced by 60 ms to 140 ms (right).

hemodynamically optimal timing of ventricular pacing requires longer paced than sensed AV delays. Particularly implanting the atrial lead at the lateral free wall or in the right atrial appendage can cause flat, long P waves with significant prolongation of the intrinsic PQ time. Pacing from the atrial septum (high near Bachmann's bundle or low near the fossa ovalis or coronary sinus ostium) in contrast creates P waves and intrinsic AV conduction times shorter during atrial pacing than sensing. In these cases, the paced AV delay can be programmed to the same value as the sensed AV delay (the paced AV delay cannot be programmed shorter than the sensed AV delay in most devices). Septal placement of the atrial lead is therefore useful in patients with SND to prevent unnecessary right ventricular pacing and a paced AV block first degree at the same time.

Programming long AV delays (≥250 ms) is associated with several problems. First, the AV delay can be completely blanked. This deteriorates AF detection and can synchronize every second atrial flutter wave to the R wave causing 2 : 1 lock-in. Secondly, if AV conduction fails (vagally blocked sinus beats, blocked atrial premature beats), ventricular pacing can occur at long, non-physiologic AV intervals triggering endless loop tachycardia (ELT) with retrograde conduction through the AV node. Thirdly, retrograde ventriculo-atrial (VA) conduction of a premature ventricular beat can be followed by atrial pacing that is ineffective because it occurs in the myocardial atrial refractory period after a retrograde P wave. If this ineffective atrial paced beat is followed by ventricular pacing after a long AV delay, retrograde VA conduction can occur again and cause repetitive non-reentrant VA synchrony (RNRVAS).

Ventricular pacing at long AV delay can cause symptoms (e.g., palpitations, dyspnea, and thoracic discomfort) and deteriorate hemodynamic function. Therefore, programming more physiologic AV delays (e.g., paced AV delay 200 ms, sensed AV delay 150 ms) together with an automatic algorithm to search for intrinsic AV conduction by intermittently prolonging the AV delay (e.g., by 100 ms for one cycle) or with algorithms that provide AAI(R) pacing and switch to DDD(R) if significant AV block occurs are preferable in many SND patients.

If long AV delays are programmed, the device memory should be checked at each follow-up to verify that this setting allows AAI(R) pacing without ventricular stimulation. Ventricular pacing after atrial sensing (markers "AS-VP") and atrial pacing (markers "AP-VP") should not exceed 1%. Otherwise, the atrial paced or sensed AV delay can be increased if programmed to <250 ms or decreased to more physiologic values with an AV hysteresis or automatic AAI(R) ↔ DDD(R) switch. The occurrence of ELT and RNRVAS should be checked by looking through specific device memory functions including electrograms stored in response to detection of atrial high rates (Table 17.5).

Rate Adaptive AV Delay

Algorithms such as "dynamic" or "rate-adaptive" AV delay shorten the AV delay, can cause unnecessary right ventricular pacing in SND and should therefore be avoided. They are nominally "on" in some devices and have to be switched off.

In patients with binodal disease, rate-adaptive shortening of the AV delay may be activated, shortening of the AV time between lower and upper rate limit should be limited to 30–50 ms. Rate adaptive delays are used in

AV block patients to facilitate 1 : 1 conduction of high atrial rates. However, in SND, high atrial rates typically result from atrial tachyarrhythmias, which should not be tracked by the pacemaker.

AV Hysteresis Algorithms

Most patients with SND should be programmed to allow intrinsic AV conduction up to 250–300 ms while at the same time shorter, more physiological AV delays should be applied when AV conduction is impaired (spontaneous or drug-induced). Therefore, the use of AV hysteresis functions is recommended (Table 17.6). These prolong the AV delay as long as intrinsic AV conduction is detected but automatically shorten it if intrinsic conduction is lost. After programmable intervals (e.g., every 32 cycles, every minute), the algorithm automatically prolongs the AV delay again in search for recovery of intrinsic AV conduction. Empirically, patients with normal AV conduction and only intermittent PQ prolongation or AV block can be programmed to a sensed AV delay of 150 ms, a paced AV delay of 200 ms, and an extension of 100 ms during an automatic search for intrinsic AV conduction (i.e., 300 ms AV delay after atrial pacing, 250 ms AV delay after atrial sensing).

Some algorithms allow progressive AV delay prolongation as long as no intrinsic conduction is observed or search for intrinsic conduction prolonging the AV delay for more than one cycle. This is useful if the right

ventricular lead detects ventricular sensing late (descending limb of the QRS complex) or if AV conduction recovers slowly after more than one cycle.

Automatic AAI(R)↔ DDD(R) Switching Algorithms

Programming the pacemaker to AAI(R) represents the safest way to avoid ventricular pacing, ELT, and so on. However, results of AAI(R) pacing in SND are disappointing, as demonstrated in a large, randomized trial [2]. AAI(R) pacing with ventricular monitoring and switching to DDD(R) if criteria for AV block are fulfilled seems to be the best way to prevent unnecessary ventricular pacing and pacing at long AV delays at the same time. These algorithms, depicted as AAI(R)↔DDD(R), do not track single blocked P waves.

The Managed Ventricular Pacing (MVP®) algorithm by Medtronic switches from AAI(R) to DDD(R) if two out of four atrial events (sensed or paced) are not spontaneously conducted. This algorithm should not be used in patients with long first-degree AV block because it does not switch to DDD as long as there is a QRS after each P, even if the PQ period exceeds 400 ms.

Reply® DR devices by Sorin (Milan, Italy) offer a SafeR® mode to provide AAI(R)↔DDD(R) pacing. It can be activated together with normal sensed and paced AV delays (e.g., 155 and 210 ms; Table 17.7). The devices switches back to DDD(R) if the intrinsic AV interval exceeds a programmed value (nominally 300 ms at rest and 200 ms during exercise) for six consecutive cycles (primary AV block criterion), if 3 out of 12 atrial events are not conducted spontaneously (secondary AV block criterion), if two consecutive atrial events (paced or sensed) are not conducted (tertiary AV block criterion) and if no ventricular beat occurs within a programmed interval (nominally 3 s). The device switches back to AAI(R) mode after sensing 12 consecutive spontaneous ventricular events, every 100 paced ventricular cycles, or at least once daily.

Table 17.6 Examples for programming AV delays and AV hysteresis functions in some contemporary pacemakers.

Biotronik Effecta DR	Paced AV delay: 200 ms Sensed AV delay: 150 ms Dynamic AV delay: off AV delay hysteresis: medium AV repetitive hysteresis: 3 cycles
Boston-Scientific Insignia DR 1290/1291	AV delay (paced): 200 ms Sensed AV offset: −50 ms Dynamic AV delay: off AV delay increase: 50% AV search interval: 32 beats
Medtronic Sensia SEDR01	Paced AV delay: 200 ms Sensed AV delay: 150 ms Rate adaptive AV delay: off Search AV +: on Maximum increase to AV: 100 ms
St. Jude Medical Endurity DR	Paced AV delay: 200 ms Sensed AV delay: 150 ms Rate-adaptive AV delay: off Ventricular intrinsic preference (VIP): on, 100 ms Number of cycles for conduction search: 3

Table 17.7 Examples for programming devices incorporating MVP® or SafeR® algorithms for AAI(R)⇔DDD(R) switching.

Medtronic Adapta ADDR01	Paced AV delay: 200 ms Sensed AV delay: 150 ms Rate adaptive AV delay: off MVP: on
Sorin Reply DR	Pacing Mode: SafeR (AAI↔DDD) or SafeR-R (AAIR↔DDDR) Sensed AV delay: 155 ms Sense/Pace AV delay offset: 65 ms Exercise AV delay: (125–) 155 ms

Atrial Sensitivity and AF Detection

Patients with SND have known AF, are at high risk of developing new AF, or develop undetected AF. Therefore, atrial sensing should be programmed sensitive to optimize AF detection. Independently of the sensed P wave amplitude, bipolar atrial sensitivity set to 0.2–0.3 mV is favoured to reliably detect AF even if signals are intermittently very small. To avoid farfield oversensing of ventricular signals in the atrium, a PVAB of at least 100–150 ms should be programmed. Attempts to reduce the atrial sensitivity to 0.5–0.75 mV should be avoided because at these settings AF can no longer be reliably detected. Parts of the cardiac cycle are blanked in pacemakers (PVAB, most of the AV delay) and cannot be used for AF detection. Therefore, the AF detection rate should be programmed to 170–180 bpm.

PMT Intervention, PVC Reaction

Most patients with SND have normal retrograde VA conduction. This poses a risk for ELT and RNRVAS, particularly if long AV delays are programmed. Algorithms that react to premature ventricular complexes (PVC reaction) should be activated and set to "atrial pacing": After a PVC, the postventricular atrial refractory period (PVARP) is prolonged, after which AV sequential pacing occurs to prevent ELT. Similarly, a "PMT intervention" should be activated that stops tracking of high sinus rates suspicious of ELT.

Non-competitive Atrial Pacing (NCAP®)

Some devices offer specific algorithms that prevent atrial pacing within a short time after atrial refractory events (e.g., NCAP® in devices by Medtronic Inc.). These should be activated to prevent RNRVAS, particularly if long AV delays are programmed.

Atrial Preventive Pacing

Pacing can prevent AF in some patients with SND by preventing a rate decrease <60 bpm. In vagally induced paroxysmal AF, programming the lower rate limit to 70 bpm together with rate-adaptive pacing and a slow rate decay after exercise may reduce AF recurrences. Some devices offer atrial overdrive algorithms that adjust the atrial pacing rate just above the sinus rate to maintain continuous atrial pacing (e.g., Atrial Pacing Preference® in Medtronic devices, AF Suppression® in

Table 17.8 Pacemaker memory functions that should be checked in patients with SND.

Parameter	Memory data	Checked events
Atrial rate	Counters, histograms	1) High average rate? 2) Atrial sensed rates >170 bpm (AF?) 3) High atrial paced rates (sensor, preventive pacing algorithms?)
Ventricular rate	Counters, histograms	1) High average rate? 2) VP at upper tracking limit? 3) VS above upper tracking limit (AF with intrinsic AV conduction?)?
Sensor-indicated rate	Histograms	1) Appropriate rate increase?
Atrial pacing (%)	Counter	1) Progression of SND?
Ventricular pacing (%)	Counter	1) <1%?
AV conduction	Counters, histograms	1) AS-VS%, AP-VS% 2) Success of AV hysteresis/AV management algorithm?
Atrial tachyarrhythmia	Counters, histograms, stored EGMs	1) Cumulative time in AF (AF burden)? 2) No. of AF episodes 3) Duration of (longest) AF episode 4) Appropriate detection?
PMT	Counters, episodes, stored EGMs	1) Sinus tachycardia or true ELT?

AF, atrial fibrillation; AP, atrial pacing; AS, atrial sensing; AV, atrioventricular; EGM, electrogram; ELT, endless loop tachycardia; VP, ventricular pacing; VS, ventricular sensing.

St. Jude Medical devices) or increase the pacing rate after arrhythmias (Post Mode Switching Overdrive Pacing, PMOP®, Medtronic, Acceleration on PAC®, Sorin). The maximum rate during atrial preventive pacing should be limited to 100–110 bpm. Atrial pacing offers more antiarrhythmic properties if it starts from the septum (better right and left atrial synchronization, no prolongation of AV conduction, no forced right ventricular pacing). Pacing from the right atrial appendage or lateral free wall may be proarrhythmic by increasing the dispersion of atrial refractoriness, prolonging AV conduction and inducing unnecessary right ventricular pacing.

Proarrhythmia can be detected by pacemaker memory functions. The percentage of ventricular pacing, average atrial rate, and AF burden should be assessed at each follow-up.

Memory Functions

Activation and analysis of pacemaker memory functions is essential in optimizing programming of dual-chamber devices. The following parameters should be checked (Table 17.8): atrial and ventricular rates (particularly ventricular pacing at the maximum tracking rate), sensor-indicated rates, percentage of atrial and ventricular pacing, AV delay histogram, time in AF (AF burden), number of AF episodes, longest AF episode, atrial electrograms stored upon AF detection.

Atrial rate should be checked as appropriate in rate histograms. If rate-adaptive pacing is not activated or under-responsive, atrial rates may be close to 60 bpm. Rate-adaptive or preventive pacing may be over-reactive, producing a high proportion of atrial pacing at high rates. Atrial rates >170 bpm indicate frequent atrial premature beats or AF.

Table 17.9 Reaction to issues detected by checking pacemaker memory functions.

Finding	Solution
Max. atrial rate <90 bpm, most pacing close to lower rate limit	Activate sensor or program more responsive
High atrial pacing rates	Reduce sensor reactivity, reduce max. sensor/preventive pacing rate, deactivate preventive pacing
>1% ventricular pacing after atrial sensing	1) Prolong sensed AV delay (up to 270–300 ms)/activate AAI(R)↔DDD(R) algorithm, or 2) Set sensed AV delay to optimal values together with an AV rate hysteresis
>1% ventricular pacing after atrial pacing	1) Prolong paced AV delay (up to 300 ms)/activate AAI(R)↔DDD(R) algorithm, or 2) Set paced AV delay to optimal values together with an AV rate hysteresis
Increase in AF burden	1) Consider antiarrhythmic drugs 2) Increase atrial pacing rate or preventive pacing (particularly if from septum) 3) Consider reduction in atrial pacing rate/deactivation of preventive pacing (particularly if from RAA/lateral lead position)
AF episode >48 h duration	1) Consider oral anticoagulation
Inappropriate AF detection due to ventricular farfield oversensing in the atrium	1) Prolong PVAB (e.g., to 150 ms, do not decrease atrial sensitivity!)
Inappropriate AF detection due to RNRVAS	1) Change to AAI(R)↔DDD(R) mode if possible 2) Activate NCAP® or similar algorithm (300 ms) if available 3) Reduce sensor reactivity and max. sensor rate (e.g., to 90 bpm) 4) Shorten paced AV delay if other options fail
Stored PMTs (optimal: confirmed by EGM analysis)	1) Change to AAI(R)↔DDD(R) mode if available 2) Prolong PVARP 3) Activate PVC reaction and PMT intervention 4) Shorten paced AV delay if other options fail
Atrial flutter not detected	1) Activate specific atrial flutter detection algorithms 2) Reduce upper tracking limit to ≤100 bpm 3) Shorten PVAB and sensed AV delay if other options fail
AF (intermittently) not detected	1) Increase atrial sensitivity (e.g., to 0.1–0.2 mV) 2) Reduce atrial tachyarrhythmia detection rate (e.g., to 160 bpm) 3) Shorten PVAB and sensed AV delay if other options fail

AV delay programming should be checked and eventually optimized looking at AV histograms and percentages of ventricular pacing after atrial sensing (AS-VP) and pacing (AP-VP). Electrograms stored upon detection of atrial high rates should be checked for inappropriate detection of ventricular farfield oversensing or RNRVAS. If atrial high rate episodes of long duration (>48 hours) are appropriate, oral anticoagulation may be indicated. Electrograms stored upon detection of ELT should be checked for sinus tachycardia (Table 17.9).

References

1 Brignole M, Auricchio A, Baron-Esquivias G, Bordachar P, Boriani G, Breithardt OA, *et al.* 2013 ESC Guidelines on cardiac pacing and cardiac resynchronization therapy. Eur Heart J 2013;34:2281–2329.

2 Nielsen JC, Thomsen PE, Højberg S, Møller M, Vesterlund T, Dalsgaard D, *et al.* A comparison of single-lead atrial pacing with dual-chamber pacing in sick sinus syndrome. Eur Heart J 2011;32:686–696.

3 Israel CW. Analysis of mode switching algorithms in dual chamber pacemakers. Pacing Clin Electrophysiol 2002;25:380–393.

4 Iliev II, Yamachika S, Muta K, Hayano M, Ishimatsu T, Nakao K, *et al.* Preserving normal ventricular activation versus atrioventricular delay optimization during pacing: the role of intrinsic atrioventricular conduction and pacing rate. Pacing Clin Electrophysiol 2000;23:74–83.

5 Koglek W, Kranig W, Kowalski M, Stammwitz E, Brandl J, Oberbichler A, *et al.* A simple method for determining the AV interval in dual chamber stimulation. Herzschr Elektrophys 2004;15(Suppl 1):23–32.

18

How to Interpret Pacemaker Electrocardiograms

Giuseppe Bagliani[1], Stefania Sacchi[2,3], and Luigi Padeletti[4]

[1] *Department of Cardiology and Arrhythmology, Foligno General Hospital, Perugia, Italy*
[2] *Institute of Internal Medicine and Cardiology, University of Florence, Florence, Italy*
[3] *International Centre for Circulatory Health, National Heart and Lung Institute, Imperial College, London, UK*
[4] *IRCCS, MultiMedica, Sesto San Giovanni, Milan, Italy*

The artificial stimulation of the heart is based on its ability to respond to an electrical impulse with a depolarization of the cardiac chamber where the pacemaker (PM) lead is placed. In PM recipients, the myocardium is activated in parallel by both the natural excitation-conduction system and the implantable device. This latter detects the presence of spontaneous rhythm and in condition of reduced spontaneous activation, below a programmed heart rate, stimulates the heart, delivering artificial impulses [1].

Over the years, cardiac implantable electric devices evolved considerably from simple life-saving PMs to highly sophisticated pacing systems able to stimulate the atrial and ventricular chambers in a sequential manner, allowing physiologic stimulation. Several technologic algorithms have been progressed:

1) *Rate-responsive* function to increase the heart rate during physical activity under the regulation of special sensors;
2) *Rate-smoothing* function to gradually reduce the pacing rate when there is an abrupt decrease in the frequency of spontaneous rhythm;
3) *Automatic atrioventricular (AV) delay* function to physiologically modulate AV delay.

The knowledge of these complex properties is crucial to recognize PM functioning and avoid a mistaken diagnosis of malfunction. In the last few years, cardiac devices aimed to the resynchronization of the left ventricular mechanical activity in heart failure have also been developed. The electrocardiogram (ECG) is an essential tool to identify patients eligible for the procedure and verify the correct functioning of the system, according to the Guidelines [2].

Normal ECG, in PM Patients: Basic Principles of Interpretation

The ECG is an important tool to investigate the functioning of PM. The two main PM functions are sensing and pacing (Figure 18.1).

1) *Sensing function* is the ability of the PM to detect the spontaneous activity of a cardiac chamber. The level of sensing is broadly programmable to allow the exclusion of external noise signals, sources of dangerous malfunctions.
2) *Pacing function* is the ability of the PM to deliver electrical pulses activating a cardiac chamber. On ECG, artificial stimulation (spike) has a needle-like appearance and is usually recognizable from the spontaneous electrical activity for its very short duration and high slope.

Unipolar and Bipolar Configuring Pacing

The spike's morphology primarily depends on the stimulation's configuration (Figure 18.2). In the presence of unipolar configuration, the stimulus is provided between the electric pole at the apex of the lead and the metal generator can. On ECG recording, it results in a high deflection. Conversely, in the presence of bipolar configuration, the stimulus is provided between the two electric poles both placed at the tip of the lead, resulting in a substantially smaller deflection on ECG. Sometimes, the amplitude of the bipolar spike on the ECG surface is so low as to require a change of configuration to unipolar for better visualization.

How-to Manual for Pacemaker and ICD Devices: Procedures and Programming, First Edition. Edited by Amin Al-Ahmad, Andrea Natale, Paul J. Wang, James P. Daubert, and Luigi Padeletti.
© 2018 John Wiley & Sons, Inc. Published 2018 by John Wiley & Sons, Inc.
Companion website: www.wiley.com/go/al-ahmad/pacemakers_and_icds

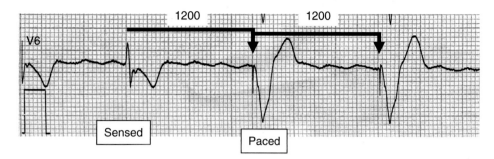

Figure 18.1 The functions of sensing and pacing of a single chamber pacemaker (VVI). A spontaneous ventricular event is sensed by the pacemaker that emits a stimulus after a programmed period of time (1.2 s in this case).

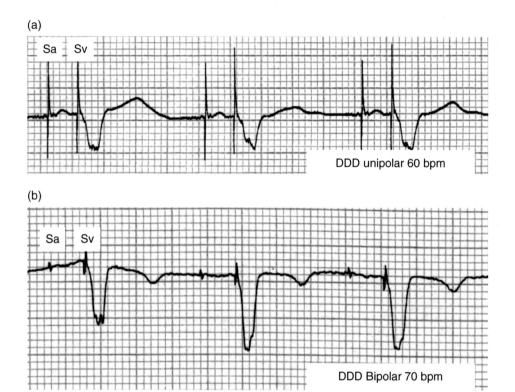

(a)

(b)

Figure 18.2 Unipolar and bipolar stimulation in a double pacemaker (DDD). (a) Unipolar pacing configuration: both atrial and ventricular stimulation are well evident. (b) Bipolar pacing configuration: atrial and ventricular stimulati are extremely low compared to the unipolar configuration.

Atrial and Ventricular Pacing

The lead for atrial pacing is commonly placed in the right appendage. In this case, the atrial depolarization following the atrial pacing is hardly visible on the surface ECG. Alternative sites for the atrial pacing lead are possible (in particular, inter-atrial septum) but they are less often used. The ventricular depolarization induced by ventricular pacing is usually evident on ECG and its morphology depends on the site of stimulation. Commonly, the right ventricular lead is placed in the apex of the right ventricle. In this case, the ventriculogram is characterized by a left intraventricular conduction delay morphology with an axis directed from the bottom to the top and towards the left (marked left axis deviation; Figure 18.3).

Concepts of Fusion and Pseudo-fusion

Fusion phenomenon results from the competition between the spontaneous and PM-induced activation of the ventricles, giving rise to an intermediate QRS morphology on the ECG surface (Figure 18.4). In the presence of a very delayed electric impulse, unable to depolarize the peri-lead portion of myocardium and

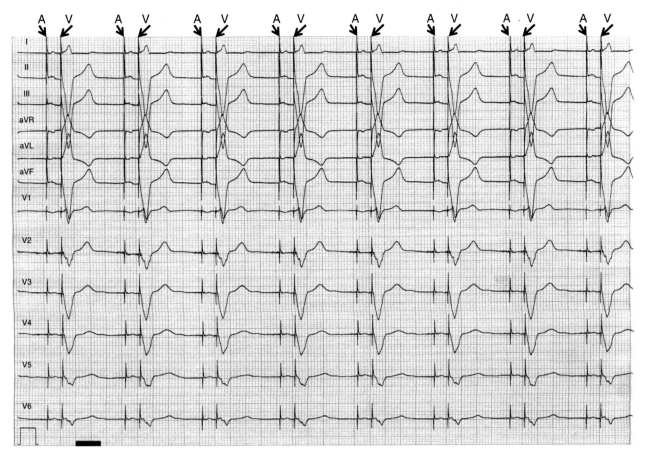

Figure 18.3 Right ventricular apex stimulation: QRS morphology. A pacemaker DDD is present as evident by the regular succession of stimuli in atrium and ventricle. The QRS originates from the apex of the right ventricle and spreads to the ventricular myocardium with a left ventricular conduction delay: therefore the QRS morphology type is left bundle branch block. The axis in the frontal plane is markedly deviated to the left.

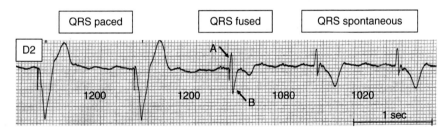

Figure 18.4 Paced, fused, and spontaneous QRS. The basic rhythm is atrial fibrillation with a single-chamber pacemaker (VVI) set to a frequency of 50 bpm (cycle of 1200 ms). The first two ventricular complexes are paced (P QRS) as evident by the presence of the spikes, a width of 180 ms and a monophasic and negative morphology in the inferior lead. The last two narrow QRS are spontaneous as evident by the lack of the spike. The third QRS has a morphology of fusion between the paced and spontaneous; its duration is only slightly increased (100 ms). The fusion is also evident at the level of the ventricular repolarization: the T wave is positive when the QRS is stimulated, negative when the QRS is spontaneous, and much less negative when the QRS is fused.

consequentially any portions of the cardiac chamber, a pseudo-fusion phenomenon is observed. In this case, despite the ventricular pacing, QRS morphology is like spontaneous QRS on the ECG surface (Figure 18.5).

Fusion and pseudo-fusion electrocardiographic findings should be always recognized to prevent an erroneous interpretation of abnormal PM function.

Hysteresis

In the presence of competition between spontaneous and paced rhythm, the first one can be favored, activating the hysteresis function. A pacing rate inferior to the programmed low pacing rate is set up (Figure 18.6). Hysteresis is the difference between the programmed

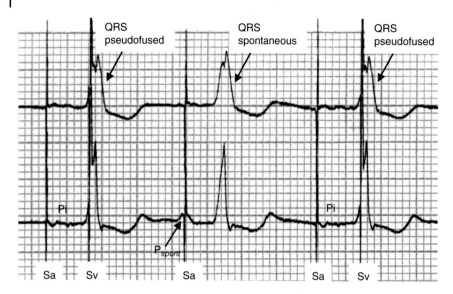

Figure 18.5 Atrial and ventricular pseudo-fusion. There are three cardiac cycles in the presence of dual-chamber pacemaker (DDD). Atrial pacing: the pacemaker delivers atrial stimuli (Ap) in all three cardiac cycles, but only in the first and third atrial depolarizations are induced (Pi); in the second cardiac cycle a spontaneous atrial activity (Pspont) and a spike realizing an atrial pseudo-fusion. Ventricular pacing: the pacemaker sends stimuli to the ventricles (Vp) only during the first and third cardiac cycle without any change of the QRS (ventricular pseudo-fusion).

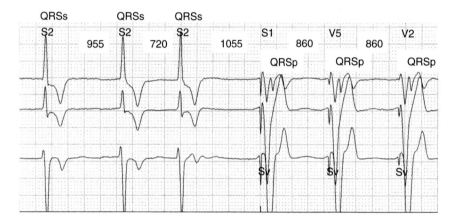

Figure 18.6 Hysteresis function in a VVI pacemaker. Atrial fibrillation is the basic rhythm. The first three are spontaneous ventricular complexes (QRSs) while the last three are induced by the pacemaker (QRSp) at ventricular cycle of 860 ms. The pacemaker intervenes after an interval (1055 ms) that is higher than that of stimulation (860 ms) for the presence of the hysteresis function by means of which we try to prefer the spontaneous rhythm.

low pacing rate and the effective heart rate leading to PM activation. It generally amounts to 10, 20, or 30 beats per minute (10 bpm in most of cases). This function can be applied to both single and dual chambers PMs.

Response to the Application of a Magnet

The simple analysis of the ECG changes induced by a magnet placed on the PM can allows immediate diagnosis of the PM mode of operation. Under the effect of magnet, the PM system loses sensing function and commutes to the asynchronous pacing mode (A00, V00, D00) at the maximum amplitude of the stimulus. Analysis of the ECG allows the identification of single or dual chamber stimulation (Figure 18.7). The pacing heart rate induced by the application of the magnet is termed magnetic frequency and is a marker of the battery charge level. A decreased magnetic frequency can be suggestive for an elective replacement. The asynchronous mode of pacing mediated by an external magnet can also be used to avoid an inappropriate stimulation of the PM during surgery requiring electrical devices. The asynchronous stimulation induced by the magnet can generate dangerous ventricular arrhythmias; for this reason its use requires appropriate precautions.

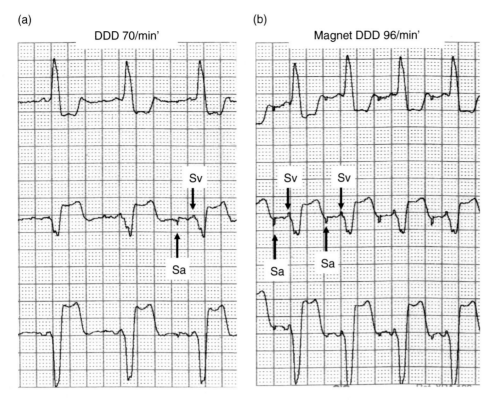

(a) DDD 70/min' (b) Magnet DDD 96/min'

Figure 18.7 The magnetic frequency of a pacemaker. (a) There is an artificial atrial and ventricular stimulation at a frequency of 70/min'. (b) The application of a magnet above the pulse generator provides a stimulation at a frequency of 96 bpm which therefore corresponds to the magnetic frequency.

Classifications of PM Functions by NBG Code (NASPE and BPEG Generic)

A simple code classification allows quick identification of both PM type and mode of operation. The code includes five positions [3]. The first three code positions (I, II, III) are related to the anti-bradycardia functions, the fourth position (IV) concerns the programming mode, and the fifth code position (V) identifies multisite pacing parameters:

I) *Paced chamber:* atrium (A), ventricle (V), both atrium and ventricle (D), none (0).
II) *Sensed chamber:* atrium (A), ventricle (V), both atrium and ventricle (D), none (0).
III) *Modality of response to a sensed event:* after a sensed event PM can be inhibited (I) or, in case of a sensed atrial event, the ventricle can be paced with a triggering mechanism (T); the letter D (dual) indicates that the device will respond to the sensed signal by either inhibiting the pacemaker response, tracking the sensed event, or inhibiting the output on the sensed channel and triggering an output to maintain AV synchrony.

IV) *Programming mode:* the fourth position identifies the characteristics of programmability. (0) indicates that PM has no programmable parameters; (P) indicates that it is limited to three or fewer parameters; (M) means that it can be programmed in more than three parameters; (R) classifies it as capable of a rate-responsive function, to vary the pacing rate depending on the physical activity of the patient.
V) The fifth position is used to indicate whether multisite pacing is present in none of the cardiac chambers (0), in one or both of the atria (A), in one or both of the ventricles (V), or a combination of A and V as just described (D).

Mode of PM Programming

Single Chamber Pacing: AAI(R), VVI(R)

In these modes of stimulation, only one cardiac chamber is paced, the right atrium or the right ventricle in the AAI and VVI mode, respectively. As a result of the detection of spontaneous activity, the PM is inhibited. The stimulus is delivered after a predetermined interval from a previous either spontaneous or induced event. The AAI mode is rarely used and the VVI mode is limited to cases with atrial fibrillation associated with low ventricular response.

Dual Chamber Pacemakers: DDD(R)

The DDD pacing mode is able to reproduce the physiologic events of normal heart. The DDD cardiac device detects spontaneous rhythm both in the atrium and in the ventricle. In the absence of spontaneous activity, when the heart rate falls below a predetermined frequency, DDD-PM sequentially paces atria and ventricles according to a programmed rate interval (LRI, lower rate interval). The AV delay, the interval between atrial and ventricular activation, is a programmable value. ECG in DDD(R)-PM recipients shows four patterns (Figure 18.8):

1) When atrial activity and conduction to the ventricles are normal, both atrial and ventricular PM channels are inhibited;
2) If there is an insufficient sinus activity and an impaired AV conduction, both atria and ventricles are stimulated;

3) If the atrial rate is low with a preserved AV conduction, the right atrium is stimulated at the programmed rate while the ventricular rhythm is spontaneous (this electrocardiographic pattern is no different from that of an AAI-PM);
4) When sinus atrial activation is preserved but the AV conduction is altered, after a spontaneous P wave, a ventricular spike appears.

Particular Aspects of the Dual-Chamber Pacing (DDD) Identifiable on the Surface ECG

Rate Responsive and Automatic AV Interval

The rate responsive (RR) is a function through which the stimulation systems increase their frequency of stimulation with physical activity. The PM is provided with a system of detection of physical activity (movement, muscle tremors, oxygen saturation, pH, respiratory rate, QT interval duration) that is able to increase the

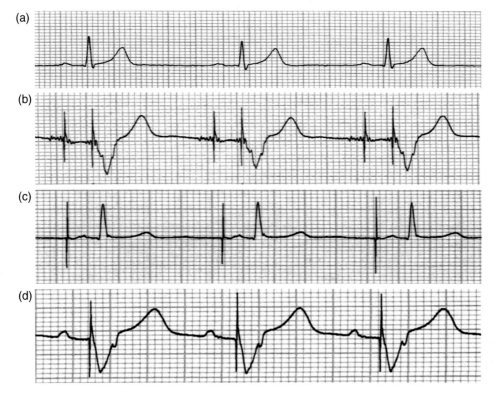

Figure 18.8 Possible ECG findings of a two-chamber pacemaker (DDD). (a) In the presence of normal atrial activity and normal atrioventricular (AV) conduction, both the atrial and ventricular channel are inhibited and therefore any stimulus of the pacemaker is evident. (b) In the presence of insufficient sinus activity and delayed atrioventricular conduction, both the atria and the ventricles will be stimulated. The classic electrocardiogram consisting of two stimuli (atrial and ventricular, respectively) separated by the programmed AV interval will therefore be evident. (c) The atrial rate is compromised while the AV conduction is preserved: the pacemaker stimulates the atria but not the ventricles. The electrocardiographic waveform is similar to that of a AAI pacemaker. (d) The atrial rate is preserved but the AV is so compromised that the pacemaker triggers to the ventricles of the spontaneous atrial depolarization.

frequency of depolarization of the PM until a maximum programmed value. There is also the possibility to program the slop of increasing heart rate. Most generators can also automatically shorten the AV interval as the frequency of stimulation increases.

Blanking Period and the Ventricular Safety Pacing (Committed)

The dual chamber pacing systems, albeit superior to standard single chamber pacing systems, present a number of problems that must be avoided with the introduction of specific functions.

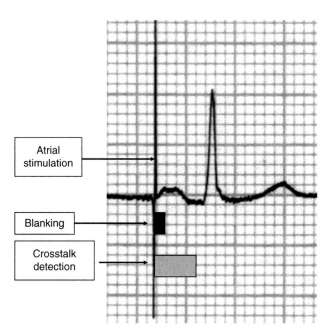

Figure 18.9 The blanking period and the period of ventricular safety. After an atrial stimulus, in the ventricular channel is generated a blanking interval that prevents the channel to be inhibited by the atrial depolarization. A subsequent interval is the window of detection of crosstalk in which each sensed event is followed by a ventricular safety pacing or "Committed."

One of the main problems with a dual chamber pacemaker is the possibility that the ventricular channel can be inhibited by atrial depolarization. This is the phenomenon of crosstalk, a dangerous situation causing asystole in patients without spontaneous heart rhythm. The probability of the crosstalk is also dependent on the amplitude of atrial depolarization and is therefore more likely with unipolar atrial stimulation. To avoid crosstalk, a blanking period is present in the ventricular channel which starts with atrial depolarization and generally lasts 15–50 ms. During the blanking period, sensing of the ventricular channel is abolished (Figure 18.9). After the blanking period, to avoid further ventricular electrical activity being inappropriately inhibited, was introduced a further period during which the PM responds to any sensed event by ventricular safety pacing. This mode of pacing is usually defined "committed" and is characterized by a particularly short AV interval (usually 110 ms; Figure 18.10).

Mechanisms of Control of High Ventricular Pacing Rates

AV trigger, typical of DDD pacing, is a mechanism by which the PM stimulates the ventricular chambers after a spontaneous atrial depolarization. In rapid atrial tachyarrhythmia, specific functions have been introduced in the pacemaker to avoid high ventricular rates. The primary mechanism performing such protection is the maximum tracking rate (MTR), the achievement of which is followed by a Wenckebach AV sequence. The delivery of ventricular stimulus is progressively delayed until an atrial activity that is not followed by the delivery of a stimulus in the ventricle (Figure 18.11). This function is made possible by the introduction of the post ventricular atrial refractory period (PVARP), which is a period of refractoriness of the atrial channel following a ventricular depolarization. During the PVARP, the PM cannot sense atrial activities. When in the course of an atrial tachycardia an atrial wave is inside the PVARP, it is

Figure 18.10 Ventricular safety pacing (Committed) in a DDD pacemaker. In the first two cardiac cycles there are both atrial and ventricular stimulation (AV interval 220 ms). In the following three cardiac cycles, ventricular safety pacing (committed) occurs, characterized by an AV interval of 110 ms. In the last cardiac cycle, the AV interval returned to baseline (220 ms).

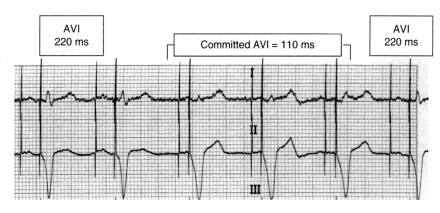

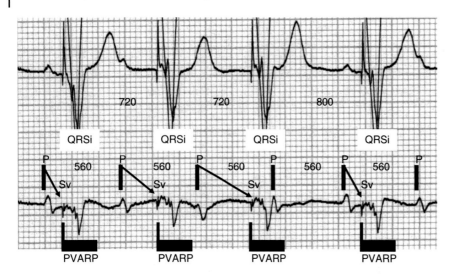

Figure 18.11 Mechanism of decremental AV conduction (Wenckebach-like) of the DDD pacemakers. An atrial tachycardia (cycle PP = 560 ms) is conducted to the ventricles at the maximum tracking rate (RR = 720 ms). There is an irregularity of RR intervals (720–720–800 ms) and the longest RR cycle is due to the fourth P-wave non-conducted to the ventricles because it falls within the post ventricular atrial refractory reriod (PVARP).The next P wave is regularly sensed and therefore it is triggered to the ventricles with the programmed AV interval. The AV interval exhibits a Wenckebach-like trend, with a progressive prolongation before the blocked P and a shortening after that.

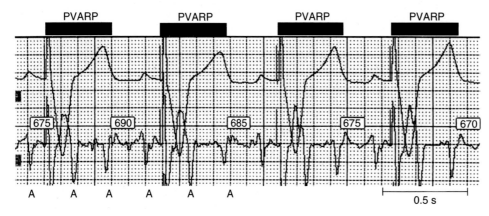

Figure 18.12 Atrial flutter with AV conduction 3 : 1 by a DDD pacemaker. Protective mechanism from high ventricular rates. Atrial recording (esophageal lead) shows an atrial flutter (cycle 230 ms) conducted to the ventricles by the pacemaker with an AV ratio of 3 : 1. This degree of block occurs because two F waves every three fall within the PVARP.

not perceived and therefore it becomes impossible to trigger and maintain the endless loop tachycardia (ELT).

When atrial tachycardia stabilizes at high frequencies, the point of 2 : 1 AV block is reached; this is made possible by the regular alternation of atrial depolarizations into the PVARP.

The values of both MTR and of the point of AV 2 : 1 block can be adjusted separately.

Pacemaker-Dependent Arrhythmias

The arrhythmias mediated by PMs are those in which the pacing system participates in the trigger and/or maintenance of the arrhythmia. We can divide

pacemaker-dependent arrhythmias into two subgroups depending on the role played by the stimulation system:

1) *Atrial tachyarrhythmias sensed by the atrial channel of the pacemaker and conducted passively to the ventricles* In this case, an atrial arrhythmia (atrial flutter, atrial tachycardia, or atrial fibrillation) may be sensed by the atrial lead of the PM and consequently transferred to the ventricle at the programmed MTR (Figure 18.12). In this case the pacemaker is not part of the electrogenetic mechanism of the arrhythmia but only contributes to the development of high ventricular rates.

2) *Re-entrant arrhythmias that have the PM as an integral part of a circuit* In such cases, also called

endless loop tachycardia (ELT) or pacemaker-mediated tachycardia (PMT), the stimulation system is an essential part of the electrogenetic circuit. These arrhythmias usually develop by an ectopic atrial beat (or a ventricular ectopic beat retroconducted to the atria). If such a premature atrial depolarization is

Endless loop tachycardia

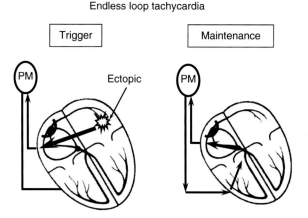

Figure 18.13 Endless loop tachycardia: trigger and maintenance. The diagram shows the trigger mechanism and the subsequent maintenance of a re-entrant pacemaker-mediated tachycardia. The trigger is usually an atrial ectopic beat that is sensed and triggered to the ventricles by the pacemaker. The impulse come back to the atria through retrograde conduction of the nodo-Hisian system. The maintenance is carried out by a mechanism in which the pacemaker is fundamental.

sensed by the atrial channel of the pacemaker, it will thus be triggered to the ventricles by the PM, returning to the atria by retrograde conduction in the nodo-Hisian system (Figure 18.13). In this circus mechanism of the ELT the PM, the atria, and the ventricles are an essential part of the re-entry circuit, and the AV ratio is 1 : 1. Figure 18.14 shows an example of ELT in which atrial activity has been recorded by a double atrial esophageal lead. The pacemakers have automatic systems for the interruption of such arrhythmias after a fixed number of beats. For preventing the ELT, many PMs have the ability to extend the PVARP after each premature beat.

Electrocardiographic Signs of Biventricular Pacing

The main purpose of the biventricular pacing is to re-synchronize the areas of myocardium that spontaneously depolarize late, recovering the contractile function. To better understand the ECG pattern of biventricular pacing, it should be remembered that the pattern of right ventricular pacing is characterized by a left intraventricular conduction delay morphology with marked left axis deviation (Figure 18.3). Regarding the left ventricular pacing ECG pattern, the stimulation of the left ventricle generates an activation front directed from

Figure 18.14 Endless loop tachycardia: pacemaker-mediated re-entrant tachycardia. Use of the esophageal lead in the identification of the electrogenetic mechanism. The ventricular depolarization induced by the pacemaker (Vp) is retroconducted to the atria through the AV conduction system (dark arrow). The atrial depolarization (A) is sensed in the atrial channel of the pacemaker with consequent depolarization of the ventricles (double arrow).

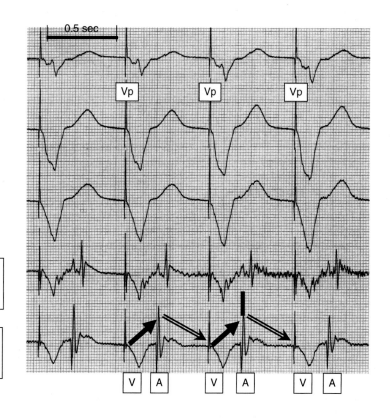

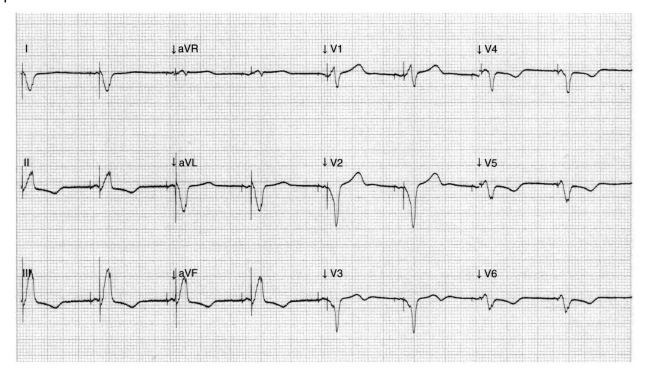

Figure 18.15 ECG in isolated left ventricular stimulation. The figure refers to an ECG in which ventricular pacing is performed from the lateral wall of the left ventricle. This mode of stimulation generates an activation front directed from left to the right with a QRS essentially negative in the derivations exploring the left ventricle (D1, aVL, V5, V6) and positive in lead V1. The Q wave in D1 and the R wave in V1 are characteristics of the stimulation from the lateral wall of the left ventricle.

the left to the right leading to an essentially negative QRS in D1. This right axis deviation in the frontal plane is associated with a typical morphology in V1 with a positive QRS initial component (Figure 18.15). In biventricular pacing, owing to the fusion of two fronts of activation (left and right), QRS duration is smaller than in a single left or right stimulation (Figure 18.16). Biventricular ECG pattern is characterized by an initial QRS negativity (Q-wave) in D1 and positivity (R waves) in V1, both generated by contribution of left ventricular pacing. The QRS axis in the frontal plane is intermediate between the left pacing axis directed from the bottom to the right and the right pacing one directed upward to the left. The timing programmability of both right and left ventricular channels is completely independent and a wide range of fusion morphologies between left and right ventricular activity can be realized (Figure 18.17). Figure 18.17(b) shows that early activation of the left ventricular chamber (Vs −30 ms) makes more evident the Q wave in D1 and R wave in V1, peculiar signs of the left ventricular activation. Conversely, when the left ventricular activation is delayed (Figure 18.17d; Vs 30 ms) both the Q wave in D1 and the R wave in V1 gradually reduce until they

disappear (Figure 18.17e, Vs 60 ms) and QRS morphology becomes similar to that from isolated right ventricular pacing. QRS axis in the frontal plane is directed:

1) **1** To the top and right side when the ventricular stimulation is simultaneous (Vs 0 ms);
2) Down and to the right side when the left ventricular stimulation is anticipated (Vs −30 ms);
3) Up and towards the left side when the right ventricular stimulation prevails (Vs 30 ms).

PM Malfunctions

A PM malfunction occurs when there is an alteration of both sensing and pacing functions, either alone or in combination [4].

Impairment of the Pacing Function

A defect in the pacing function is usually characterized by the inability of the PM electrical pulse to depolarize the cardiac chamber in which the lead is positioned.

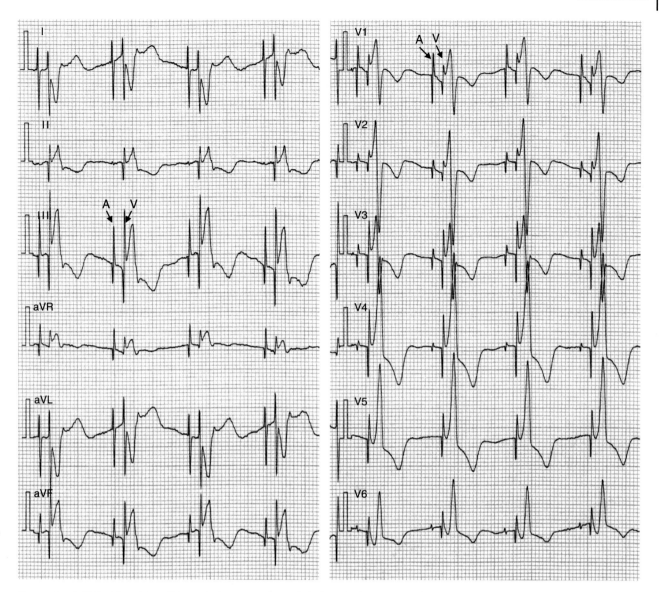

Figure 18.16 ECG with atrial and biventricular pacing (unipolar). The ECG shows a unipolar pacing in which an atrial stimulus (Ap) is followed by a ventricular stimulus (Vp) provided by a system of simultaneous biventricular pacing (first generation). The induced QRS is the result of a fusion between the left and right ventricular depolarization. The Q wave extension D1 and an R wave in lead V1 are typically generated by left ventricular depolarization. The QRS axis in the frontal plane is intermediate between the left ventricular pacing axis directed from the bottom to the right and the right ventricular pacing directed upward to the left.

ECG shows the presence of spikes not followed by depolarization waves. Pacing malfunctions can occur both at the atrial (Figure 18.18) and ventricular level (Figure 18.19). Lead dislodgment, fibrosis at the site of insertion, and battery discharge are the main causes of loss of pacing.

Impairment of the Sensing Function

Alterations in the sensing function can occur either from the PM's inability to detect the intrinsic depolarization of the chamber in which the PM lead is placed (under-sensing) or from an excess of sensing (over-sensing), resulting in a PM pacing inhibition.

Under-sensing on ECG is characterized by an emission of spikes despite the presence of spontaneous rhythm. This alteration can appear at both an atrial (Figure 18.20) and ventricular level (Figure 18.21).

Over-sensing occurs when electrical signals extraneous to the cardiac chamber's lead (muscle tremors or other) are recorded by the PM (Figure 18.22). It is an extremely dangerous phenomenon because the consequent cessation of pacing can lead to a prolonged asystole in PM-dependent patients.

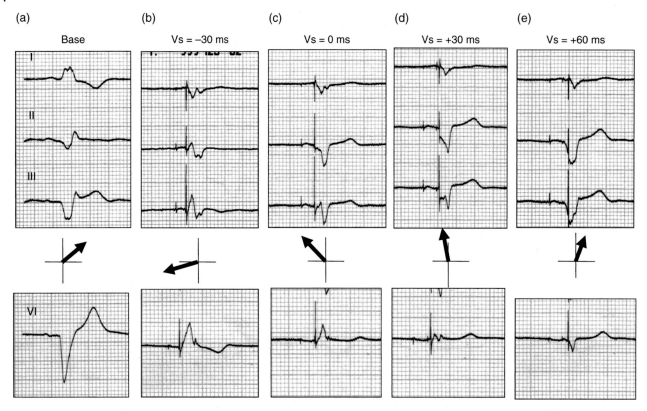

Figure 18.17 ECG changes of the QRS by biventricular pacing. The morphology of the QRS varies with the time sequence of the stimulation of the two ventricles. This figure shows morphologic variations of the QRS in leads D1, D2, D3, and V1 and the direction of the vector in the frontal plane with a second-generation biventricular pacing. (a) In basic conditions, a typical left bundle branch block is present. The QRS duration is 180 ms. (b) The stimulator is programmed so that left ventricular pacing advances of 30 ms right ventricular pacing and therefore the typical signs of left ventricular stimulation (Q wave in lead D1 and R wave in lead V1) appear well evident. D3 shows a positive QRS typically associated with right axis deviation. (c) Left and right ventricular pacing are delivered simultaneously. The morphology of the QRS is identical to that of a first-generation biventricular pacing. Compared with (b), reducing the component of left ventricular pacing reduces the R wave amplitude in V1 and Q wave in D1. For the same reason the axis of the QRS in the frontal plane moves upward as evident by the morphology of the QRS in D3. (d) Left ventricular pacing is delay of 30 ms compared to right ventricular one; there is a further reduction of the R wave amplitude in V1 and Q wave in D1. The axis of the QRS in the frontal plane shift to the left becoming negative in D3. (e) Left ventricular pacing is markedly delayed (60 ms) and the global ventricular depolarization is almost completely determined by right ventricular pacing. The QRS morphology is similar to that of the isolated right ventricular pacing.

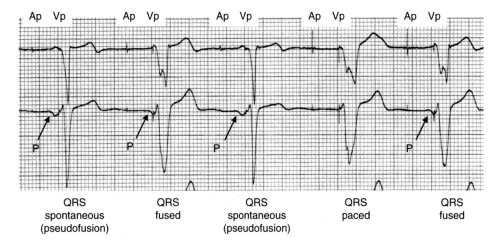

Figure 18.18 Impairment of atrial pacing in a DDD pacemaker. A DDD pacemaker delivers both atrial (Ap) and ventricular (Vp) spikes. An impaired pacing function at atrial level is observed because atrial stimuli (Ap) are not followed by corresponding atrial depolarization; occasionally, spontaneous P wave appears. The pacemaker constantly paces the ventricles but in the first and in the third complexes the spontaneous atrial activity (P) appears able to reach the ventricles generating QRS of normal morphology (pseudo-fusion).

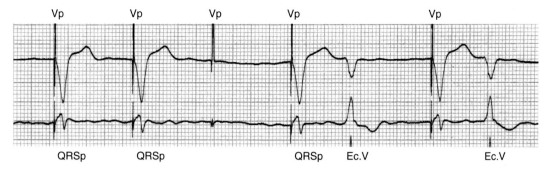

Figure 18.19 Occasional impairment of ventricular pacing in a VVI pacemaker. The basic rhythm in an atrial fibrillation with the presence of ventricular pacemaker (Vp). The third ventricular stimulus (Vp) is not followed by an appropriate ventricular depolarization. The fourth ventricular stimulus appears normally transmitted to the ventricles and the next ventricular ectopic ventricular beat is normally sensed by the pacemaker which waits before releasing a new ventricular stimulus.

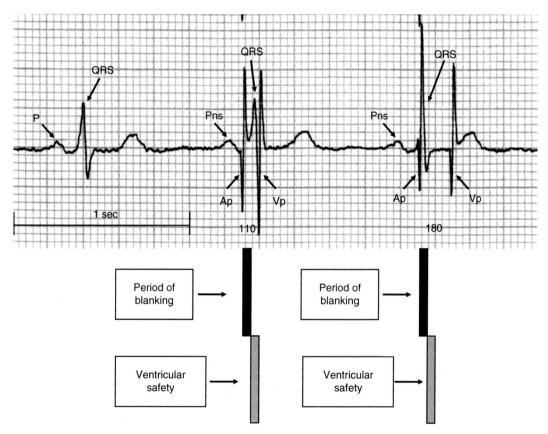

Figure 18.20 Impairment of atrial sensing in a DDD pacemaker, the blanking and ventricular safety periods. A sequence of three cardiac cycles in a patient with a dual chamber pacemaker (DDD) is shown. In the first cardiac cycle, a normal activation is sensed by the pacemaker (P-QRS). In the second cardiac cycle, because of a transient loss of atrial sensing, the P wave is not sensed (Pns) and an atrial pacing (Ap) is delivered; the next spontaneous QRS, originating from the non-sensed P wave, falls within the "window of detection of crosstalk" and such that gives origin to a ventricular safety pacing (Vp); in this "committed" pacing, typically the AV interval lasts 110 ms. Also, in the third cardiac cycle the P wave is not sensed and therefore an atrial stimulus is delivered (Ap). The subsequent spontaneous QRS falls in the blanking period and therefore is not perceived by the pacemaker; a ventricular stimulus (Vp) at the programmed AV interval (180 ms) is delivered.

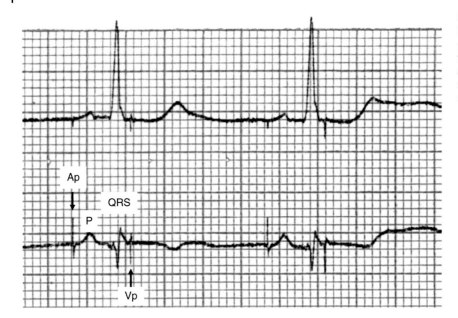

Figure 18.21 Ventricular under-sensing: loss of ventricular sensing in a DDD pacemaker. The ventricular channel lost the ability to sense the spontaneous activity of the ventricles: a ventricular stimulus (Vp) is delivered after the spontaneous QRS.

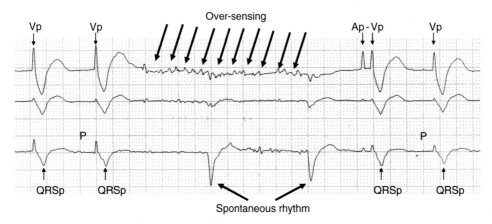

Figure 18.22 Ventricular over-sensing. Holter recording in patients with DDD pacemaker. Electrical signals of extracardiac origin (arrows) are able to inhibit the emission of the stimuli. An escape rhythm is present.

References

1 Trohman RG, Kim MH, Pinski SL. Cardiac pacing: the state of the art. Lancet 2004;364:1701–1719.
2 Vardas PE, Auricchio A, Blanc JJ, Daubert H, Ector H, Gasparini M, *et al.* Guidelines for cardiac pacing and cardiac resynchronization therapy. Europace 2007;9(10):959–998.
3 Bernstein AD, Daubert JC, Fletcher RD, Hayes DL, Luderitz B, Reynolds DW, *et al.* The revised NASPE/BPEG generic code for antibradycardia, adaptive-rate, and multisite pacing. PACE 2002;25:260–264.
4 Maisel WH, Moynahan M, Zuckerman BD, Gross TP, Tovar OH, Tillman DB, *et al.* Pacemaker and ICD generator malfunctions: analysis of Food and Drug Administration annual reports. JAMA 2006;295(16):1901–1906.

19

How to Perform Pacemaker Troubleshooting

Brian Olshansky[1,2] and Nora Goldschlager[3,4]

[1] *University of Iowa, Iowa, USA*
[2] *Mercy Hospital-North Iowa, Mason, Iowa, USA*
[3] *San Francisco General Hospital, San Francisco, CA, USA*
[4] *University of California, San Francisco, CA, USA*

Pacing can provide patients with adequate heart rates, when necessary, and, in some instances, the appropriate activation sequence (including atrial followed by ventricular depolarization with proper timing, and with both ventricles in synchrony) to optimize cardiac output and to meet the physiologic and metabolic needs of the body. When considering the practical aspects and management of the patient with a cardiac pacemaker and before considering the necessity for pacemaker troubleshooting, the first issue is to know the purpose of pacing for that patient and if the patient is pacemaker-dependent.

When it comes to troubleshooting, it is critical to define what the concern is and what unique pacemaker and programming characteristics are present. Oftentimes, the concern is observed pacing when pacing is not expected or, alternatively, no pacing when pacing is expected. Interrogation to assess electrogram characteristics and use of marker channels can generally provide an understanding of a problem or a perceived problem.

Pacemaker Options and Programming Characteristics

Various modalities of pacing are available (Table 19.1). Selection of the appropriate modality depends on the patient's clinical circumstances, including, but not limited to, heart rhythm abnormalities (indications), age, lifestyle, comorbidities, cardiac function, necessary medications, and other confounders. Pacemakers can be single chamber, atrial (AAI) or ventricular (VVI) based, dual chamber (DDD), or triple chamber (atrium and right and left ventricles – cardiac resynchronization therapy (CRT)) and may include rate-responsive capabilities using various

sensors (e.g., motion, ventricular contractility, body temperature, and minute ventilation) to guide increase or decrease in paced rate to meet metabolic demands.

Programmable pacemaker parameters, including timing intervals, are critical to optimize pacemaker function without incurring adverse parameter interactions or clinical problems and provide, in specific cases, atrioventricular (AV) synchrony, interventricular (VV) synchrony (CRT), or simply appropriate rate (Table 19.2). Some parameters are generally not programmable. Special programmable features can vary depending on the device (Table 19.3). Discussion of these timing parameters is beyond the scope of this chapter.

In addition to timing intervals and basic programmable parameters, accepted and standard sensing and pacing (capture) characteristics are expected to be understood. Intracardiac atrial electrical signals, generally representing atrial depolarization, should be expected to exceed 1.0 mV. Intracardiac right ventricular electrical signals, generally representing ventricular depolarization, should exceed 5.0 mV. Capture thresholds should generally be <1.0 V @ 0.5 ms in both the right ventricle and right atrium (but may be higher in the left ventricle).

In a normal situation, sensing and capture thresholds remain constant and fluctuate little. Despite the stability of intracardiac signal quality, sensing of the intracardiac electrical signals is generally programmed to be triple the sensed electrogram amplitude and pacing threshold is programmed at double the capture voltage or triple the pulse width to ensure consistent sensing and capture function, which can vary somewhat over time over time as a result of changes in myocardial function and anatomy, medications, autonomic tone, and electrolyte disturbances (particularly, potassium fluctuations).

How-to Manual for Pacemaker and ICD Devices: Procedures and Programming, First Edition. Edited by Amin Al-Ahmad, Andrea Natale, Paul J. Wang, James P. Daubert, and Luigi Padeletti.
© 2018 John Wiley & Sons, Inc. Published 2018 by John Wiley & Sons, Inc.
Companion website: www.wiley.com/go/al-ahmad/pacemakers_and_icds

Table 19.1 Common pacing modalities.

Chamber paced	Chamber sensed	Mode	Rate response
A	A	Inhibited – AAI Asynchronous – AOO	R
V	V, A	Inhibited – VVI Triggered – VAT (rarely used) Asynchronous – VOO	R
D (A + V)	D (A + V)	Inhibited/tracked – DDD Inhibited, no A pacing – VDD (rarely used) A + V pace, no A sense or track – DVI Inhibited – DDI Asynchronous – DOO	R

Table 19.2 Basic programmable parameters.

Mode of function
Lower rate limit (base rate)
Upper tracking rate (atrial-based)
Upper sensed rate (sensor-based)
Post-ventricular atrial refractory period
Ventricular refractory period
Atrial refractory period
Paced AV interval
Sensed AV interval
Dynamic AV interval
Sensitivity
Pacing output (voltage and pulse width)
Post-ventricular atrial blanking period
Ventricular blanking period
Post atrial ventricular blanking period

Table 19.3 Special programmable (often proprietary) features.

AV search hysteresis – lengthening of the AV interval to search for intrinsic AV conduction at AV intervals > the programmed interval

Rate-drop response – a faster rate programmed to occur (above the lower rate limit) if there is an abrupt drop in spontaneous rate

Rate smoothing – a gradual acceleration or deceleration in pacing rate in response to abrupt changes in intrinsic rate

MVP – (AAI ↔ DDD mode change) – AAI pacing unless there is AV block and then the mode switched to DDD

Hysteresis – the escape interval exceeds the pacing interval to allow for emergence of native rhythm

Mode change ("mode switch," "atrial tacking response") – when a specific atrial tachycardia occurs (usually atrial fibrillation) occurs, the DDD mode is automatically changed to DDI or VVI avoid tracking the atrial rate

Noise response – a feature that prevents inappropriate inhibition by electrical noise. Often this mode is DOO or VOO

Autocapture – lowering pacing output based on autodetection of an evoked potential

Table 19.4 Rate-response parameters.

Rate-adaptive pacing
Maximum sensor rate
Activity threshold
Response factor (magnitude of rate change for a given activity)
Reaction time (the interval of time for the rate to change)
Recovery time (the interval of time for heart rate to return to baseline)

The most complex pacemakers, those that involve leads in the atria and the ventricles, including dual and triple chamber pacemakers, have timing characteristics that include rate response using various sensors and programmed features (Table 19.4), sensed and paced AV intervals that vary with atrial-driven or sensor-driven rate to mimic normal AV conduction physiology and upper-rate (mode-switching) timing characteristics to prevent inappropriately rapid ventricular pacing in response to atrial sensing (tracking) such as might occur in atrial fibrillation, atrial flutter, or atrial tachycardias. Mode switching is an algorithm that can be programmed "on" to change a DDD mode of function to one in which atrial electrical signals are not tracked (DDI or, much less commonly, VVI in dual or triple chamber systems). Finally, refractory periods, independently programmable for atrial and ventricular sensed or paced events, prevent inappropriate and/or unnecessary detection of electrical signals that could inhibit needed pacing and/or prevent

inappropriate and unwanted pacing (such as tracking at the upper rate limit in pacemaker-mediated tachycardia or inappropriately mode switching on sensing far-field signals that mimic rapid atrial rates).

It is important to recognize that special features of a pacing system (including pulse generator and leads) can influence the analysis of the data. Therefore, before considering any pacemaker troubleshooting, it is important to understand the following:

1) The type of pacemaker and its capabilities;
2) The manufacturer and model of the pacing system with its specific intricacies and complexities;
3) Programming options and characteristics (such as rate-drop response, rate smoothing, AV search hysteresis, AAI ↔ DDD mode switch function when needed, mode switch);
4) Specific unipolar and/or bipolar lead-related issues including recalls or warnings; and
5) Specific interventions that can affect pacemaker function (including electromagnetic interference (EMI) in medical and non-medical environments (Table 19.5).

Table 19.5 Sources of electromagnetic interference (EMI).

Endogenous – myopotentials
Medical equipment

- Electrocautery
- Magnetic resonance imaging
- Cardioversion, defibrillation
- Transcutaneous pacing
- Electrotherapy
- Transcutaneous nerve stimulation
- Implanted neuromuscular stimulators
- Ionizing radiation
- Lithotripsy

Table 19.6 Interrogatable parameters.

Arrhythmia burden
Impedance
Rate histogram
Sensing
Pacing output
Lower rate limit
Upper rate limit
Trends (impedance, capture threshold, sensed signal voltage)
Activity level

Besides knowledge of the make and model of the pacemaker and leads involved, specific issues or problems arising at the time of system implant (such as central venous obstruction and anomalous central veins), the precise reason(s) for pacemaker implantation, prior programmed parameters including those obtained at implant, and known device and lead recall issues must be known.

It is best to store records of and choices for (and prior) programmed parameters in a given individual and why specific parameters were chosen, chest X-rays performed, electrograms recorded, timing cycle recordings, and any trans-telephonic monitoring data. If the make and model of a pacing system are unknown and/or records are not available, databases retained by manufacturers are repositories of this information. Obviously, much of the information necessary to manage specific patients properly is obtainable by pacing system interrogation, so it is essential that the proper programmers be applied to the correct pacing systems.

From this starting point, a practical approach to troubleshooting can be undertaken. The first step in troubleshooting any pacemaker is to obtain the correct programmer for a specific pacemaker, after which, the "interrogate" button is pressed. When the programmer's screen opens, the programmed parameters, trended information, such as lead impedances, sensed electrical events and capture thresholds, rate histograms, stored high rate episodes with their accompanying electrograms, and timing markers will be displayed (depending on the device) or can be obtained by pressing the relevant buttons (Tables 19.2, 19.3, and 19.6).

It is expected that the operator understands each of these parameters and understands that inhibiting the pacemaker in a dependent patient is a substantial problem. It is not essential to determine pacemaker dependence at each visit, although in many facilities this is carried out to ascertain the natural history of the rhythm for which the pacemaker was implanted and to assess the

nature and stability of the underlying native rhythm (if present) as well as the native P-QRST morphology.

It is important to know the reason for the pacemaker interrogation. Is it for an abnormality found at remote monitoring? Is it for symptoms from suspected pacemaker malfunction? Is it for a perceived abnormality observed on an ECG? Is it for a routine evaluation? Although a complete evaluation may be the best policy, focused interrogation will help address the needs of the patient.

The First Step: Interrogation

Before interrogating the pacing system, a 12-lead electrocardiogram (ECG) should be recorded to ascertain the patient's rhythm and other characteristics such as native or paced QRST morphology. This recording should be followed by a second 12-lead ECG with the magnet applied to the pulse generator. The magnet rate and function can provide a clue as to battery function. It is important to know the manufacturer's magnet rate, AV interval if applicable, and any specific function. Magnet rate and function are not programmable. We prefer to run the ECG as a 12-lead rhythm strip so that paced and spontaneous PQRST complexes can be visualized in all leads.

After establishing that the correct programmer for the implanted pacing system is being used, ensure good communication between the programming head and the pulse generator and press "interrogate." Unless there is a specific problem with communication (e.g., an incorrect programmer, pulse generator end-of-life or pacemaker location in an unexpected position such as the epigastrium), interrogation should not be problematic. It is important to be aware of any "red flag" messages that the programmer's screen shows as this will provide a clue to pacing system function, including end-of-life. If the pulse generator is at end-of-life, interrogation may not be possible as it requires battery energy; this information is generally available from the programmer screen.

After "interrogate" is pressed, a screen will arise showing the programmed parameters of the pacemaker. All information should be recorded, printed and all final information printed and saved on a disc. Most modern pacemakers have algorithms to check the pacemaker systematically. This includes checking sensing characteristics, lead impedances, capture thresholds, paced and sensed rates, and the percentage of time pacing and sensing in both chambers is occurring. Several pacemakers provide trended information of the above parameters, as well as activity levels of the patient. Often, rate response parameters, detection of stored arrhythmia episodes, and battery voltage, current, and impedance need to be interrogated independently. Tachycardia episodes can often be retrieved for analysis. Real time and stored electrograms are available in most modern pacemakers, allowing analysis of the electrograms, the timing measurements and how the pacemaker "thinks."

Sensing Thresholds

To check sensing thresholds in any given chamber, the base rate needs to be programmed temporarily or permanently below the rate of the spontaneous rhythm. Tracking function must be disallowed (i.e., the mode of function must be programmed out of DDD mode) in order to check for the spontaneous ventricular rhythm and rate. It is important to know whether the patient is pacemaker-dependent. It is not possible to test sensing without a spontaneous QRS rhythm >30/minute (the lowest programmable rate of all pacemakers) or if lowering the base rate is not tolerated by the patient when the pacemaker is programmed to allow the spontaneous rhythm to become manifest.

"Inhibit pacing" is a function that can be programmed temporarily, but this is not advised because asystolic pauses without a spontaneous escape rhythm can occur. In most instances, it is possible to check sensing. We recommend that lowering the base rate to check for native rhythms be carried out decrementally, at intervals of 5–10 pulses per minute. It is usually necessary to allow 10–20 s at a given low base rate to observe the emergence and warm-up of the native rhythm. Programming from a base rate of, for example, 75–30 pulses/minute in a single step often causes unnecessary discomfort and even fear in the patient.

To start, with a spontaneous rhythm present in the chamber tested, sensitivity is programmed to detect the rhythm and inhibit pacer functioning. Then, sensitivity is decreased gradually until the electrical activity is no longer sensed and asynchronous pacing occurs. It is also possible to record the sensed electrogram amplitude in millivolts. It is important to note exactly where in the surface P wave or QRS complex that the electrical signal generated by chamber depolarization is sensed. This is often distinctly after its inscription on the body surface ECG recording because of the time it takes for the depolarization wave front to reach the sensing electrode; this can cause confusion when measuring intervals or trying to understand pacemaker activity. By checking sensitivity, other signals that could be sensed, including T waves, muscle potentials, electromagnetic interference, or noise generated by a faulty lead can be understood. Appropriate measures must be taken to avoid this latter problem of "oversensing."

Pacing (Capture) Threshold

Ventricular and atrial pacing thresholds can be determined by starting at a high or programmed voltage output and gradually decreasing the output until the pacemaker does not capture (depolarize) the chamber tested. If there is any question about intermittent detection and pacemaker inhibition or loss of capture, simultaneous recording of the local intracardiac electrograms and marker channel annotation can help distinguish sensing inhibition from lack of pacer capture (the codes for the annotations are available in the "help" section of each programmer). This annotation is accomplished through the "markers" that specific devices use to indicate sensed events (e.g., "As" for atrial sense). A pacing stimulus output (e.g., "Ap" for atrial pace) does not indicate capture, only that the stimulus has been delivered. Chamber capture, and its loss, must therefore be documented by the surface ECG displayed on the programmer screen and/or an independent ECG recording. An independent ECG recording is not infrequently preferred, as the surface ECG displayed on the programmer screen does not always clearly show loss of capture in the atrium.

Rate-Response Parameters

Rate-response parameters and other characteristics can be determined and, for many pacemakers, projected rate response, in lieu of patient activity, can be determined. Rate response can be programmed "on," "off," and "passive," in which the sensor(s) monitor patient activity but are not used in device performance. Rate-response sensors include body motion and vibration, accelerometers and minute ventilation. The interrogated rate histogram allows appropriate programming changes to be made that affect better patient performance during activities of daily living.

AV Interval

The AV interval can be programmed to be fixed or vary by atrial- or sensor-based rate. There can be a sensed offset of the AV interval. In patients who have intact AV conduction, it is often best to minimize right ventricular pacing and adjust the AV interval for this purpose. However, specific adjustments, such as a very long programmed interval, may also affect hemodynamics and need to be considered.

AV interval adjustments are dependent upon the total atrial refractory period (TARP); in other words, the post ventricular atrial refractory period (PVARP) must be considered (AV interval plus PVARP = TARP). For patients who have AV block, it is important to adjust the AV interval such that it does not impinge upon the TARP at the programmed upper rate limit (URL) or when the spontaneous atrial rate exceeds the URL; should this be done inadvertently, 2 : 1 AV block with abrupt slowing in rate and symptoms may occur. If the TARP = URL (in milliseconds), 2 : 1 AV block will occur just above the URL and abrupt ventricular rate slowing at faster atrial rates are expected to be problematic. If not, a programmed pacemaker Wenckebach cycle will be present if TARP < URL. This is preferred for dependent patients with AV block but the settings of the AV interval are dependent upon the PVARP, the URL, the underlying rhythm, and the presence of retrograde conduction which can lead, potentially, to pacemaker-mediated tachycardia.

The Second Step: Pacemaker Troubleshooting

Prior to performing troubleshooting, the first critical question is: Why? Is the patient being seen simply for a routine follow-up visit or is a casual interrogation being performed simply because the patient is being seen for some other reason? In these instances, troubleshooting may uncover a problem that has little, if any, clinical significance or, on the contrary, may uncover a problem that is a "tip of the iceberg" in pacemaker function and malfunction.

More commonly, troubleshooting needs to be undertaken when a specific abnormality is observed or documented on a rhythm strip. Multiple simultaneously recorded ECG leads help validate these issues. Examples include: the pacemaker does not appear to activate the chamber paced when expected, pacing occurs when it should not be, or there is an irregularity in the rhythm or pacing stimulus output. Pacemaker interrogation will generally resolve confusions.

Requests for interrogation and evaluation of patients' pacemakers are appropriate if there are symptoms that could be explained by episodic bradycardias or unexpected tachycardias, in which case stored arrhythmia data might explain the clinical problem. Similarly, if patients are not regularly followed in a specialized clinic, pacemaker evaluation should be accomplished prior to operative procedures.

With trans-telephonic monitoring, lack of effective rate-response or episodic asymptomatic atrial tachyarrhythmias, especially atrial fibrillation, can precipitate a clinic visit. In some cases, patients with worsening symptomatic systolic heart failure may be found to be pacing too frequently in the right ventricle (usually pacing >25% of the time), which causes functional left bundle branch block with consequent ventricular desynchronization (i.e., the left and right ventricles do not depolarize and contract in a synchronous fashion). This specific problem may require reprogramming of the lower rate to a lower rate or extending the AV interval to reduce right ventricular pacing. Pacemaker troubleshooting is also required for patients with symptoms of syncope or near syncope that have not been ameliorated by the pacemaker or have begun after the pacemaker was implanted.

Defining Pacemaker and/or Lead Problems

It is not uncommon for clinicians to blame the pacemaker for any arrhythmia abnormality seen. Most of the time, the problem is not a result of pacemaker malfunction but to a lack of understanding of the timing and programming characteristics of the device. Interrogation allows recording of electrograms and recognition of how the pacemaker is "thinking" (timing cycle characteristics).

Atrial or Ventricular Non-capture

If, on a rhythm strip, or, preferably, a 12-lead ECG, pacemaker stimuli are seen but there is no apparent depolarization of myocardial tissue (capture) of a cardiac chamber, the failure to capture could reflect a problem with the lead as it is inserted into the pacemaker header, as is seen with loose connections, lead dislodgment from the heart, lead fracture or insulation breach with insufficient current reaching myocardium, myocardial tissue refractoriness or programmed outputs that are sub-threshold (Figures 19.1 and 19.2; Table 19.7) but apparent lack of capture may require observation of several ECG leads (Figure 19.3).

In the case of a recently implanted pacing system in which there is loss of capture, consideration must be given to the possibility of an acute rise in pacing threshold because of local inflammation at the tissue–myocardial interface (less likely with the current use of steroid-tipped

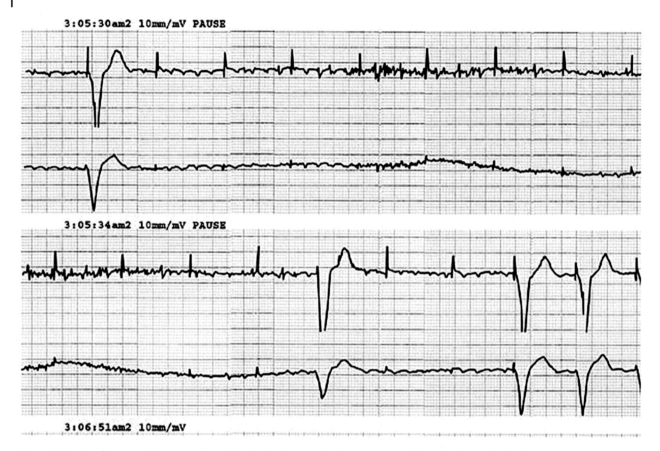

Figure 19.1 Simultaneous Holter recording strips illustrating ventricular non-capture. The atrial rhythm is fibrillation. Note the pacing stimulus with ventricular capture for the first QRS complex and the multiple pacing stimuli with no resulting QRS complex because of loss of ventricular capture.

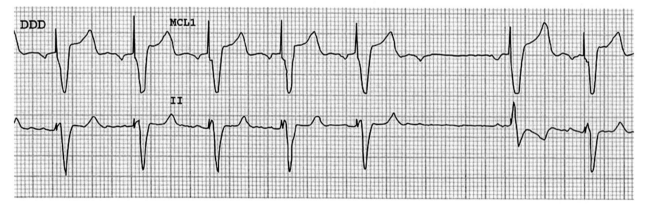

Figure 19.2 Lead MCL1 and V1 rhythm strips recorded in a syncopal patient. Note the 6th native P wave with no ventricular pacing stimulus after it. This patient had a lead fracture. No visible ventricular output was caused by oversensing and inhibition of ventricular stimuli from noise from a make–break conductor wire fracture was confirmed by intracardiac electrograms and marker channel.

leads), and to micro- or macro-dislodgment or perforation of the lead (Figure 19.4). Occasionally, loose connections between the lead(s) and the pulse generator header or inadvertent insulation breach occurring during implantation is the cause.

Acute Implantation

If the patient has a recently implanted lead and there appears to be intermittent or complete lack of capture, increasing the voltage output makes sense as the initial maneuver. However, there needs to be a check of lead

Table 19.7 Causes of pacemaker non-capture.

Tissue refractory (functional non-capture)
(e.g., prior depolarization)
Lead dislodgement
Increase in myocardial stimulation threshold
Lead insulation break
Conductor wire fracture
Inappropriately low programmed output
Generator end-of-life
Output programmed below threshold

position to exclude migration (dislodgement) on a highly penetrated chest PA and lateral chest X-ray, lead impedance measurements to exclude insulation breach or breakage, and careful and consistent follow-up of lead sensing and pacing thresholds, which are expected to remain stable (Figures 19.5 and 19.6). Micro-dislodgment can resolve. If there is concern for lead perforation, especially in the ventricle, programming lead function from bipolar to unipolar, thus pacing only from the lead tip or ring can be more successful than for bipolar capture as either the tip or ring of the lead would not necessarily be juxtaposed against the myocardium. Unipolarization of a lead, even if successful in the short term, not infrequently mandates revision or replacement to ensure permanent normal function.

A 12-lead ECG compared with the immediate post-implant recording can provide insight into positioning of the ventricular lead as the paced QRS morphology and axis resulting from pacing from the right ventricular apical area should result in a left bundle branch block pattern with a superior axis; if there is a new right bundle branch block morphology seen lead V_1 or a change in paced QRS complex axis, the lead has likely moved (Figure 19.4). On rare occasions, a transthoracic echocardiogram is needed to exclude pericardial effusion resulting from lead perforation. Cardiac tamponade diagnosed clinically or by echocardiography is an unexpected complication in today's practice.

Chronic Implantation

Non-capture in chronic pacing systems can be a result of a gradual increase pacing thresholds because of drugs (e.g., class I antiarrhythmic drugs, particularly flecainide), hyperkalemia, heart failure, or a slow change in lead impedance, with low impedances representing insulation breach and high impedances indicating lead fracture. However, the increase in capture thresholds can be abrupt. Gradual increases in thresholds are more likely caused by fibrosis at the lead tip while abrupt changes are more common in lead-related problems, such as those caused by fracture or insulation breaks. Abnormal lead impedance measurements will be present only during the actual occurrence of the pacing problem, but can be normal if pacing system function is normal at the time of interrogation. Although generally accurate, with autocapture turned on, it is possible that noise (EMI) or stimulus artifact could inhibit appropriate output for myocardial capture.

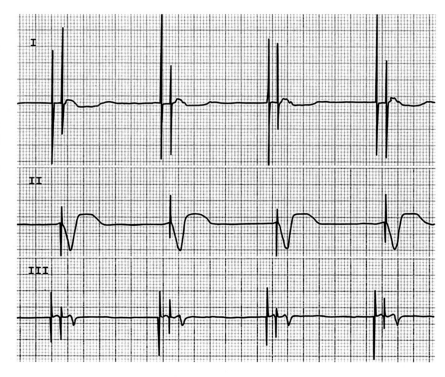

Figure 19.3 In lead I, the QRS complex occurs after the pacing stimulus but no P wave can be seen after the atrial stimulus. In lead II, no atrial stimulus or P wave can be seen. In lead III, there all P waves are clearly paced but it appears that there is lack of ventricular capture and a narrow conducted QRS complex. In reality, there is appropriate AV capture seen by looking in all three leads recorded simultaneously. These rhythm strips illustrate the value of obtaining simultaneously ECG recordings.

MCL 1

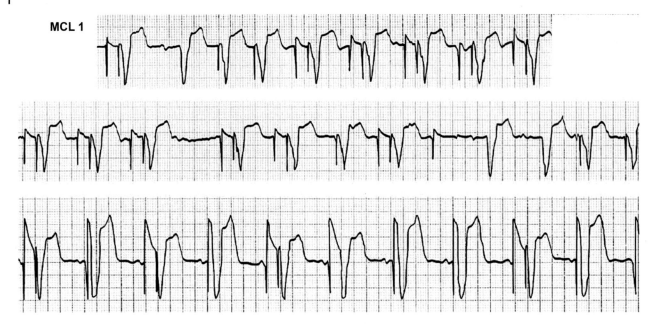

Figure 19.4 On this MCL1 rhythm strip, there is evidence for attempted atrial pacing and apparent ventricular pacing with different QRS morphologies. There may be intermittent atrial capture but in the middle strip it appears that the patient is in atrial flutter or fibrillation. There is an atrial lead dislodgment as can be seen in the lower strip. The atrial pacing stimulus is seen to capture the ventricle and alter the morphology QRST complex. Following this, there is no ventricular pacing stimulus because it is inhibited by the sensed portion of the QRS complex.

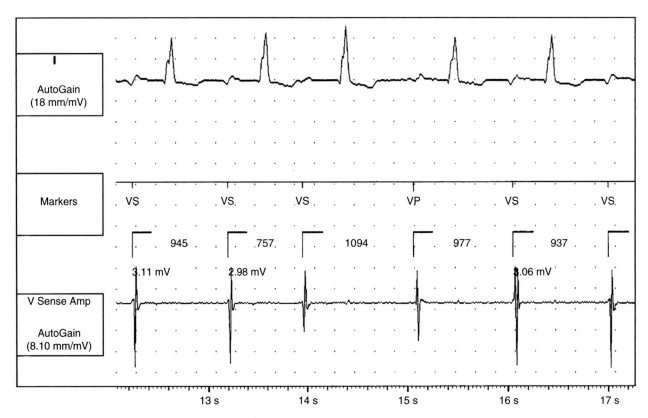

Figure 19.5 In this recording with body surface ECG (top), marker channel, and ventricular electrogram, the ventricular sense markers are sensing native P waves. There is no evidence for QRS sensing or pacing. This recording illustrates dislodgement of the ventricular lead into the atrium.

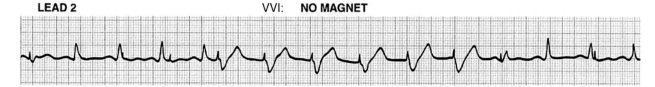

Figure 19.6 In this patient with a VVI pacing system, the rhythm strip (lead II) illustrates effective ventricular pacing except when the stimulus occurs in the ventricular refractory period but no evidence of sensing the native QRS complexes (undersensing). There are fusion QRS complexes (1st and 12th complexes).

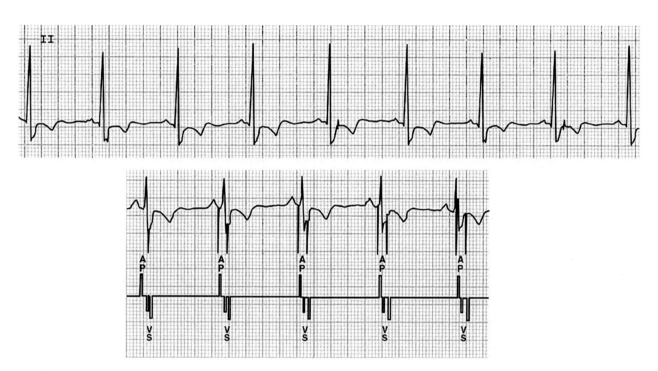

Figure 19.7 The underlying rhythm appears to be sinus. In the top strip, there is an occasional pacing stimulus that occurs after the QRS complex, during the ventricular refractory period. In the bottom strip (not simultaneously recorded with the top strip), native P waves are not sensed and all atrial stimuli appear to be pacing the ventricle. The ventricular sense marker (Vs) re-sensing that portion of the QRS complex which falls in the safety pace interval. Hence, there is a short AV interval.

Undersensing

When the intracardiac electrical signal is expected to be sensed and the pacemaker is expected to either inhibit or trigger but this does not occur, undersensing is often the explanation (Figures 19.7, 19.8, and 19.9; Table 19.8). However, before any intracardiac electrical signal is considered undersensed, it must be determined that it occurs outside the refractory (or blanking) period of the specific cardiac chamber or that the myocardium is refractory because of a prior depolarization. For example, an ectopic atrial depolarization occurring early after a paced (or sensed) QRS complex may occur in the PVARP and will not be acted upon. Competing rhythm disturbances may result in pacing in the atria or ventricles around the time of an electrical signal arising from that specific chamber. A pacing stimulus may occur within a P wave that is recorded earlier on the total body ECG, or within a QRS complex that similarly is seen to begin earlier on the body surface ECG (Figure 19.10). It is important to recognize that this phenomenon can be appropriate as it can take some time (several milliseconds) for the electrical signal generated by the depolarization wave front to propagate to the site of the lead electrode in that specific chamber. This is not undersensing, inasmuch as the escape interval of the system elapses before the electrical signal can be sensed. The resulting complex is termed "pseudo-fusion."

Apparent undersensing can also be a characteristic of a specific mode of function. For example, AOO or VOO (magnet mode) do not detect any atrial or ventricular signal, respectively. Similarly, AAI mode is not expected to sense ventricular events. Sensing of the electrical

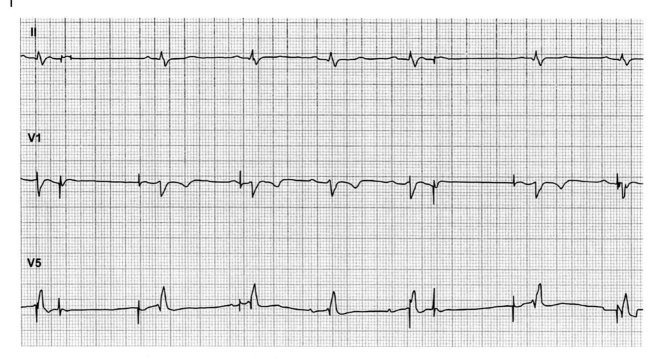

Figure 19.8 In this rhythm strip of leads II, V1, and V5, the atrial stimulus is falling on the onset of the QRS complex (pseudo-pseudofusion complex). The programmed AV interval is about 300 ms. Safety pacing is not occurring (the AV interval is the programmed one) because the QRS complex is occurring during the blanking period and thus there is no response to it. The ventricular stimuli do not capture the ventricle because they fall in its refractory period (functional non-capture).

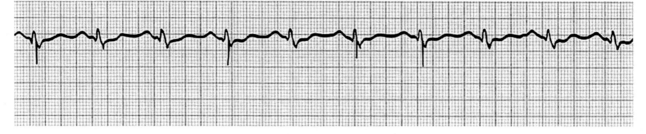

Figure 19.9 In this patient with a VVI pacing system there are pacing stimuli that occur near, and at the end of, the QRS complexes but do not change the QRS complex morphology. The QRS complexes thus represent pseudo-fusion complexes. The reason for this is that the detection of the ventricular electrical signal by the ventricular electrode is dependent on the sensing at the local dipole and there is delay at that spot relative to the inscription of the QRS complex on the body surface ECG. Although not evident in this lead, this patient had a right bundle branch block and thus had delay in activation to the right ventricular apex during the conducted beats. This could appear to be undersensing but instead it is appropriate behavior of the pacemaker.

Table 19.8 Causes of undersensing and apparent undersensing.

Poor intracardiac signal
Lead dislodgement
Insulation failure
Conductor wire fracture
Apparent undersensing – signal occurs in refractory or blanking period

signal generated in one chamber by the lead electrode in the other chamber is termed crosstalk and is not pacemaker malfunction. Crosstalk inhibition can follow. It can result from a high amplitude electrical signal and/or from lead locations that are near each other. Crosstalk can generally be treated by programming changes (decreasing sensitivity, extending the refractory periods, or programming "safety pace" on, in which crosstalk inhibition is avoided by deliberate delivery of a stimulus within the electrical signal generated in the opposite chamber).

True undersensing can be caused by lead dislodgment or change in electrical signal amplitude. If the signal amplitude is less than the programmed sensitivity, programming an increasing sensitivity may terminate undersensing but can cause oversensing. Furthermore, some electrical signals, such as those generated by

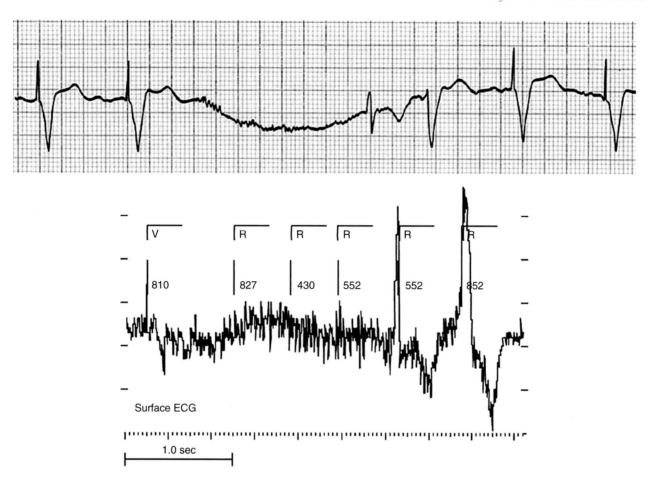

Figure 19.10 In this patient with a VVI pacing system, note the inhibition of pacing with sensing of "noise" (as seen on the marker channel on the strip below). This is caused by myopotential signals during arm movement. The pacing system designates these signals as sensed signals (R in this device). Myopotential oversensing is more common with a unipolar lead configuration.

ventricular tissue (PVCs), can be undersensed even though normally conducted ventricular depolarizations would not be. This undersensing can be a result of slowing in the slew rate (rate of change of voltage) at the lead electrode site even if the signal amplitude is large. Filters built in to the pacemaker may exclude detection of signals with slow rate of rise of electrical activity. Similarly, electrical signals generated during atrial fibrillation or other atrial tachyarrhythmias may not be detected as easily as sinus P waves from fluctuating amplitudes and slew rates.

Oversensing

Oversensing occurs when an apparent ("artifactual") electrical signal detected by the atrial or ventricular electrode is brought about by a signal originating in the same chamber (such as T waves or double counting of a QRS complex by a ventricular lead), a signal originating in the other chamber (crosstalk), sensing of electrical signals extrinsic to the body (environmental "noise" or

electromagnetic interference (EMI)) or intrinsic within the body such as that caused by fracture of a lead ("make–break" circuit) or insulation break in which short-circuiting of current exists (Table 19.9).

Oversensing by the ventricular lead can inhibit stimulus output, causing bradycardia or asystole. It is one of several causes for no stimulus output (Table 19.10). Oversensing by the atrial lead can cause bradycardia in an AAI device or, in a DDD system inappropriate tracking of the sensed signal leading to rapid ventricular pacing rates as well as loss of AV synchrony (Table 19.11).

Oversensing in the atrium does not apply to rhythm disturbances such as atrial fibrillation. In that case, if the "mode-switch" function does not occur, either because it has not been programmed "on" or because of underdetection of atrial electrical signals because of change in amplitude, apparent oversensing which in fact is undersensing can lead to inappropriately rapid ventricular paced rates because of normal tracking function of the sensed fibrillatory waves. Electromagnetic interference can result in the same phenomenon of unwanted

Table 19.9 Causes of oversensing.

Physiologic intracardiac signals

- T waves (VVI systems)
- R waves (AAI systems, DDDR systems with mode switch)
- Concealed extrasystoles (rare)

Physiologic extracardiac signals

- Muscle potentials (diaphragm, pectoral, seizure, shiver)

Electromagnetic interference

- Electrocautery
- Catheter ablation
- Cardioversion and defibrillation
- Ionizing radiation
- Magnetic resonance imaging
- Cell phones
- Antitheft devices
- iPhones
- Tasers
- Transcutaneous nerve stimulators
- Automobile "smart key" systems
- Chiropractic message therapy devices

Table 19.10 Causes of no stimulus output.

Normal inhibition by native atrial/ventricular events
Electromagnetic inhibition
Loose lead–generator connections
Lead insulation break – oversensing
Conductor wire fracture
Low-amplitude stimulus not registered by recording equipment
Battery end-of-life
Component failure

Table 19.11 Rapid paced ventricular beats.

DDD systems	PMT
Normal tracking of rapid atrial rates	Sinus tachycardia
	Atrial fibrillation
	Atrial flutter
	Atrial tachycardia
Myopotential triggering	With subsequent PMT
	Without subsequent PMT
Electromagnetic triggering	Cautery
	Environmental examples

PMT, pacemaker-mediated tachycardia.

stimulus output inhibition or unwanted tracking due to detection of electrical "noise" (Table 19.6).

Similar to EMI originating from the external environment, myopotentials (electrical muscle signals) detected by the atrial lead can lead to inhibition of atrial pacing and/or tracking of the sensed signals, or, if detected by the ventricular lead, can lead to inhibition of ventricular output. Myopotential inhibition (Figure 19.11) and environmental EMI are more likely to occur with unipolar lead configuration as there is a wider "antenna" to pick up electrical signals.

In some pacemakers, and specifically in some individuals, T waves can be detected inadvertently and "designated" as R waves, leading to inhibition of stimulus output at the expected time. The escape interval of the pacing system will be timed from the detection of the sensed signal. Some pacemakers have less ability to filter out T wave signals than others.

Crosstalk oversensing of pacing stimulus outputs, with consequent inhibition of output, unwanted tracking, or false diagnosis of rapid atrial rates leading to inappropriate mode switch operation has led to pacing system design features of built in programmable blanking intervals. These prevent pacing stimuli from being detected as true electrical signals and thus prevent inappropriate responses.

Both undersensing and oversensing are treated effectively by programming changes of sensitivity. However, increasing sensitivity to treat undersensing can result in unwanted oversensing and decreasing sensitivity can lead to undersensing of actual atrial or ventricular electrical events.

Impedance Measurements

Especially with trans-telephonic monitoring, but also with enhanced detection and storage capabilities, pacemakers can now store trends in lead impedance over time. Small changes mean little clinically, but major changes, for example, a decrease to below 200 Ω, indicate disruption of insulation between the poles of the pacemaker (Figure 19.12).

Gradual increase in lead impedance can indicate development of fibrosis (unusual). Abrupt increase, especially if intermittent can indicate lead fracture ("make–break" fracture). Lead fracture can be related to body or upper torso position or arm movement. When the diagnosis is suspected, deliberate patient movements must be performed to bring out the resulting loss of pacing stimulus as recorded from the body surface. On occasion, as the pacing output from the pulse generator itself is not disturbed, complete lead fracture can present as absence of a visible stimulus but, when seen, is a multiple of the programmed pacing cycle length.

Rate-Response Issues

Interrogation of pacemakers can provide the percentage of atrial and ventricular pacing. Depending on the pacemaker, rate response can be programmed "on" or to monitor the intrinsic heart rate. For a patient who has a

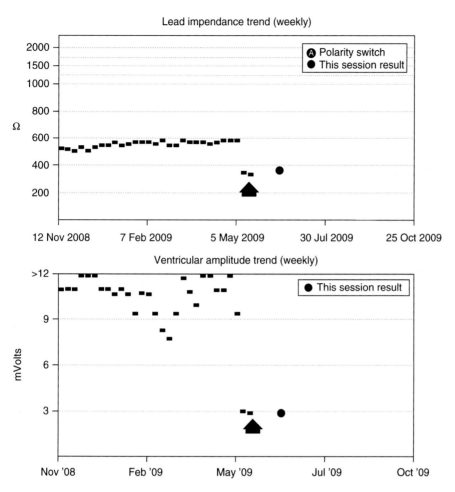

Figure 19.11 Following trends in electrical amplitude and lead impedance can indicate changes in the lead integrity. In this case, there is an insulation breach causing a marked and abrupt drop in impedance and signal size.

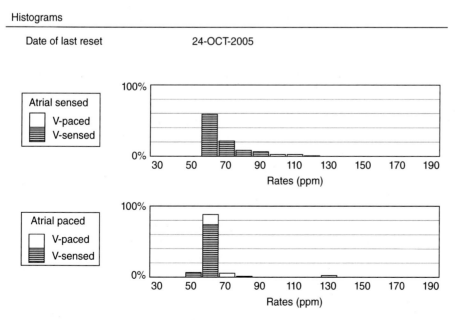

Figure 19.12 As indicated here, the distribution of atrial sensing with ventricular pacing or ventricular sensed events are seen at various rates. Similarly, during atrial pacing, ventricular paced and ventricular sensed events are seen. By observing a histogram such as this, one can determine if there is appropriate rate response and what the changes in rate are for a given patient. This information can helpful in the management of rate and interval adjustments.

pacemaker implanted for chronotropic incompetence and remains symptomatic, the rate histogram can be used to help determine need for rate response or its adjustment (Figure 19.12). The adjustment may involve a change in the lower rate, the degree of rate response or its threshold, or how much activity is required to activate the feature. Many devices provide a template of activity level to help optimize the rate response.

Other Specific Issues

Pacemaker-mediated tachycardia (PMT) is a specific arrhythmia that occurs in paced patients in which the ventricle tracks atrial events but the atrial events are caused by ventricular activation with retrograde (VA) conduction. This is most often a result of premature ventricular complex with retrograde atrial activation that is sensed and appropriately tracked, leading to a repetitive rhythm. PMT can be caused by a P wave that occurs after the PVARP that is sensed and then tracked (usually after a long P-V- paced interval such that the atria are no longer refractory after the ventricular stimulus is given), leading to another retrograde P wave and establishment of a repetitive rhythm. One way to prevent this type of tachycardia is to lengthen the TARP, which can be done by extending the PVARP automatically after a PVC. This design feature recognizes the fact that a PVC tends to initiate PMT. As noted earlier, long programmed AV or PV intervals that occur in order not to violate the upper rate limit are more likely to be associated with PMT as this allows for retrograde atrial activation when the AV node and atria are no longer refractory. Therefore, shortening the AV interval may also help avoid PMT, keeping in mind that more ventricular pacing than desirable may result from such a maneuver. It is important to recognize that changes in AV intervals and PVARP will affect upper tracking rates and ventricular paced rates when the atrial sensed rate exceeds the upper tracking rate limit. Most pacemakers have automatic algorithms to terminate PMT, including omission of a single ventricular stimulus in order to re-establish normally programmed AV or PV intervals.

Pacemakers can be used to detect specific rhythm disturbances. This is a feature that is being used increasingly in clinical practice. Pacemakers have most commonly been used to identify the amount and duration of atrial fibrillation episodes, the "burden of atrial fibrillation" (the percentage of time a patient is in atrial fibrillation). Devices differ in their ability to detect the burden of atrial fibrillation rather than simply number of fibrillation or mode-switch episodes. However, pacemakers are also important in the detection of ventricular tachycardias. Furthermore, pacemakers can be programmed to detect the amounts of atrial and ventricular

pacing to associate this with symptoms and distributions in heart rates (Figure 19.12).

Battery life can be detected by pacemaker interrogation. When the pacemaker reaches its elective replacement indicator, often at least 3 months of battery life are available but when the pacemaker reaches an end-of-life, programming and even interrogation become difficult or impossible because of the energy required for these processes. On occasion, the pacemaker near or at end-of-life can be so unstable that if it is exposed any external noise including electrocautery, it can immediately reprogram, sometimes even to a non-pacing mode. Part of the follow-up of any pacing system is to determine battery life and projected longevity; the longevity of the device depends on the percentage of pacing, and pacing voltage output as well as lead impedance because current flow (measured in coulombs) determines the battery drain.

A "power-on-reset" state can occur when pacemakers are exposed to EMI such as electrocautery. Pacemakers have zener diodes to protect their sensitive circuits from noise in the external environment including electromagnetic interference and DC shock used for external cardioversion. If these are sensed, the signals are blocked from going into the pulse generator and the voltage drops internally causing a potential power on reset. The pacemaker may be reprogrammed, often to a VVI mode that needs to be reset to the desired mode of function with reprogramming. Pacemakers that have low battery voltage are more susceptible to this phenomenon.

Conlusions

Pacemaker troubleshooting requires a stepwise approach:

1) Identification of the problem and the reason for evaluation.
2) Indications for the pacemaker, determination of pacemaker dependence and determination of the type of pacemaker and the programming characteristics, including unique features.
3) Interrogation of the device, and evaluation of marker channel information and stored intracardiac electrograms.
4) Relating the abnormalities seen on the surface electrocardiogram with potential issues with regard to programming characteristics and marker channel measurements.
5) Determination of problems resulting from electromechanical interference, inappropriate pacing and sensing.

Ultimately, with proper troubleshooting, a pacemaker can provide improved quality-of-life and functionality without danger.

20

How to Program an ICD to Program ATP, and Program for VT/VF Storm

P. Pieragnoli[1], G. Ricciardi[1], Margherita Padeletti[2], Stefania Sacchi[1], Alessio Gargaro[3], and Luigi Padeletti[4]

[1] Heart and Vessels Department, University of Florence, Florence, Italy
[2] Cardiology Unit, Borgo San Lorenzo Hospital, Florence, Italy
[3] Biotronik, Clinical Research Department, Vimodrone (MI), Italy
[4] IRCCS MultiMedica, Sesto San Giovanni, Milan, Italy

Anti-Tachy Pacing Therapy

An anti-tachy pacing (ATP) therapy is defined as a temporary high rate pacing delivered during a tachycardia. Ventricular ATP therapies automatically delivered by an implantable cardioverter-defibrillator (ICD) can terminate a relevant proportion of both slow and fast ventricular tachycardias (VT).

As these therapies are painless and require far less energy than a DC shock, each appropriate and successful delivery of an ATP therapy can significantly contribute to improving patient's quality of life and device longevity. In addition, as it has been shown that patients who receive shocks for any arrhythmia have a substantially higher risk of death than similar patients who do not receive such shocks [1], one may speculate that a fine tuning of ATP programming to maximize success rate and avoid shock delivery may also have a beneficial effect on mortality.

Pathophysiologic Background

Re-entry is one of the most common mechanisms that permit a VT to persist. Myocardial infarction (MI), arrhythmogenic disease of right ventricle VTs, dilated cardiomyopathy, and more rarely hypertrophic cardiomyopathy as well as post-surgical diseases are the basis of the most common forms of VTs requiring re-entry to initiate and persist.

Post-MI VTs comprise most of the VTs normally encountered in clinical practice and their re-entry mechanism is well understood. The anatomic substrate for re-entry is the interlacing of scar tissue and vital viable myocardium, which represent an anatomic barrier and an area of slow conduction, respectively. Areas with slow conduction can act as a corridor between at least two zones of normal conduction, favoring re-entry along with altered refractoriness and enhanced automaticity caused by the infarction.

A slowed conduction area may join proximally and distally a normally blocked pathway to form a closed circuit of conduction. When this happens, the slow pathway across the scar area can excite the alternative pathway distally, initiating a retrograde wavefront along the blocked pathway and establishing re-entry. This type of VTs is particularly prone to be terminated by rapid pacing.

Two important elements are necessary for an ATP therapy to terminate a VT: first, the VT cycle must be sufficiently regular; secondly, pacing should be critically timed with the VT cycle to induce the wavefront to enter the refractoriness. Both these characteristics are easily detected by modern devices, which are able to measure the VT cycle stability, calculating the exact programmed pulse coupling according to VT cycle length and delivering the pulse train automatically.

ATP Description

Theoretically, a single critically timed pulse can terminate re-entrant VTs but practically the efficacy is low. Multiple pulses delivered in the form of pacing drive trains more effectively interact with the VT circuit increasing the likelihood of termination.

There are several types of ATP therapy. In general, they consist of a sequence of one or more pulse trains, repeatedly delivered until episode termination is confirmed or high energy DC shock therapies are initiated. Pulses are delivered from the tip of the ventricular electrode, conventionally, but not necessarily, positioned in the apex of the right ventricle. To ensure local tissue capture and to generate wavefronts propagating through the myocardium of the left ventricle, maximum pulse amplitude and duration are applied during ATP.

More ATP sequences can be attempted before applying a DC shock in slow VTs, while one or very few pulse trains are recommended for faster and hemodynamically unsustainable VTs. Modern devices allow delivery of a single ATP sequence immediately before or during capacitor charging for the first shock therapy also in very fast regular VTs falling in the ventricular fibrillation (VF) detection zone.

ATP Therapies in the VT Detection Zones

ICD programming includes the definition of one or two VT detection zones programmed in terms of frequency or cycle length ranges. Typical settings are 360–300 ms (~167–200 bpm) for a first slow VT detection zone, with the addition of an optional 300–250 ms (200–240 bpm) fast VT zone, even if very recent evidence supports the view of even shorter cycle (higher rate) ranges. ATP therapies may be only programmed to precede shocks in the therapy sequence, after a predefined number of intervals (NID) have been detected within the respective VT detection zone. Each zone has its own NID counter which may be either sequential or forward–backward, depending on the device manufacturer. The most recent tendency is to prolong the detection process for VT as much as possible in order to permit self-termination; however, once the counter of a VT zone has reached the NID level, the first ATP therapy sequence (if programmed) is immediately initiated. The most common ATP types are burst and ramp pacing, even if there are different versions.

Burst

A single burst pacing pattern consists of a number of pulses (normally delivered at the maximum amplitude and duration output) with equal interstimulus intervals and a programmed coupling with the detected VT cycle length. For example (Figure 20.1), if a VT episode with an average cycle length of 340 ms is detected, a four-pulse burst with a 80% coupling implies the delivery of a first pulse with a $340 \times 0.80 = 272$ ms coupling with the last detected VT beat (R–S1 interval), followed by a sequence of further three pulses with a 272 ms mutual distance (S1–S1 intervals). If the first drive train is not effective and a VT is re-detected in the same detection zone, a second drive train may be automatically delivered, after recalculating an updated VT cycle length for a new R–S1 and S1–S1 coupling. Some changes in the second pulse sequences may be introduced in the therapy programming. For instance, a more aggressive S1–S1 interval may be required by introducing a decrement in the S1–S1 interval or an additional pulse may be appended to each repeated sequence. As very fast pacing can have a proarrhythmic effect, accelerating the arrhythmia rather than terminating it, a minimum pacing interval may be set up, preventing pulse trains with shorter cycle.

Ramp

A ramp stimulation pattern consists of a train of pacing pulses with an automatically decrementing interstimulus interval. Stimulation pattern is rate-adaptive for this form of ATP: the interval from the last sensed ventricular event during VT to the first pacing stimulus is a programmable percentage of the detected VT cycle length. Subsequent pulses within a pulse train are decremented by a fixed or adaptive quantity. As for burst pacing, a ramp therapy can consist of several repeated sequences, which may differ for the number of pulses, and the aggressiveness of VT cycle adaptation (Figure 20.1).

These patterns can be combined in a number of ways. For instance, in rare cases, an extra stimulus may be added to a burst train with a different (generally shorter) coupling (S1–S2 interval). All these variations on a theme probably have little clinical benefit.

Figure 20.2 shows a typical programmer panel where ATP therapy detail can be set up in detail.

ATP Therapies in the VF Detection Zone

Many tachycardias have a fairly regular cycle while falling in the VF detection zone generally programmed below 300–270 ms (above 200–220 bpm). They are VTs in all respects, even if VF therapies are associated. Even for these very fast VTs, modern devices allow delivery of at least one burst attempt, immediately before or during capacitor charging for a high energy shock.

Basically, when a ventricular episode reaches the NID for VF detection, a stability criterion is applied on the last ventricular intervals. A typical criterion may be that none of the last four intervals differed more than 12% of the average cycle. If the stability criterion has passed a burst pacing with programmable number of pulses and adaptive coupling is immediately delivered. During

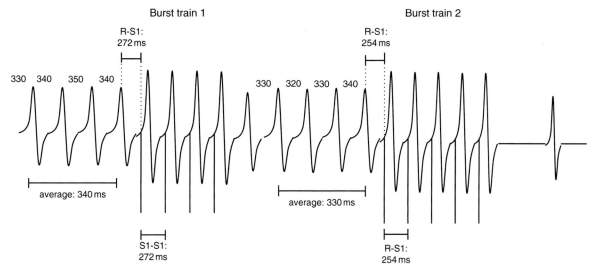

Burst train 1

R-S1:
272 ms

330 340 350 340

average: 340 ms

S1-S1:
272 ms

330 320 330 340

average: 330 ms

Burst train 2

R-S1:
254 ms

R-S1:
254 ms

VT average cycle: 340 ms

Burst train 1:
R-S1: 80% = 340 x 0.80 = 272 ms
N x S1-S1: 4 x 272 ms

VT average cycle is updated: 330 ms

Burst train 2:
R-S1: 80% – 10 ms = 330 ms x 0.80 – 10 ms = 254 ms
Add S1: ON
N x S1-S1: 5 x 254 ms

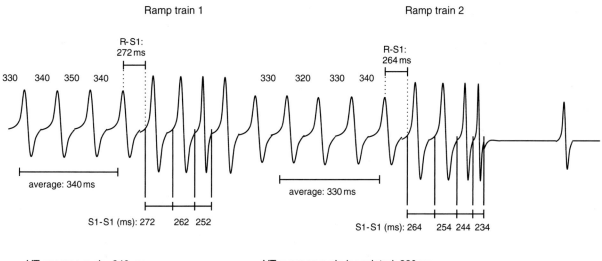

Ramp train 1

R-S1:
272 ms

330 340 350 340

average: 340 ms

S1-S1 (ms): 272   262 252

330 320 330 340

average: 330 ms

Ramp train 2

R-S1:
264 ms

S1-S1 (ms): 264   254 244 234

VT average cycle: 340 ms

Ramp train 1:
R-S1: 80% = 340 x 0.80 = 272 ms
S1 decrement: 10 ms
N x S1: 4

VT average cycle is updated: 330 ms

Ramp train 2:
R-S1: 80% = 330 ms x 0.80 = 264 ms
Add S1: ON
S1 decrement: 10 ms
N x S1: 5

Figure 20.1 (Top) Simple burst-pacing scheme. (Bottom) Simple ramp-pacing scheme. See text for details.

sequence delivering or upon the last train pulse capacitor charging for a subsequent programmed shock is initiated without waiting for outcome of the pacing therapy (Figure 20.3).

This single ATP "one-shot" has recently raised interest, as the benefits are multiple and obtained for little or no disadvantage. The advantages are that avoiding unnecessary shocks can have a positive impact on mortality as

	Rate	1. ATP	2. ATP	1. shock[
VT2	182	2*Burst	1*Ramp	40

Number S1	8		8		
Add S1	ON		ON		
R-S1 interval	80	%	80	%	
S1 decrement		ms	10	ms	
S1-S2 interval		%		%	
Scan decrement	20	ms	OFF	ms	
Minimum interval		200		ms	
ATP optimization		OFF			
ATP timeout		OFF		mm:ss	

Figure 20.2 Typical screenshot of an anti-tachy pacing (ATP) therapy programming in an implantable cardioverter-defibrillator (ICD). Both for a burst and a ramp pacing, the following programming parameters are displayed: number of sequences, the number of pulses within a sequence (Number S1), whether or not an incremental pulse will be added to the sequence at each repetition, the coupling interval of pulses (R–S1 interval) and their reciprocal decrement (S1 decrement for a Ramp), the progressive decrement of couplings of each subsequent sequence and minimum pacing interval S1–S2 interval.

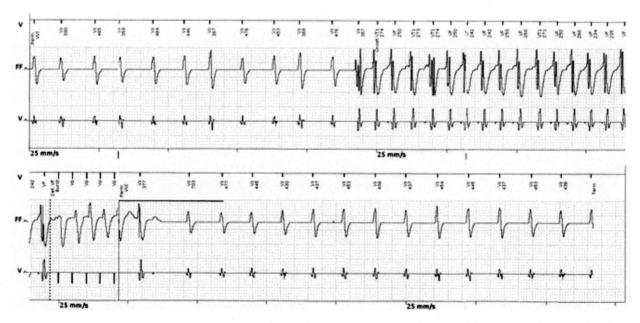

Figure 20.3 An example of one ATP "one-shot" delivered during a fast and regular ventricular tachycardia (VT) episode detected in the programmed ventricular fibrillation (VF) zone. In this case, the therapy consisted of a burst of 5 pulses with an 85% coupling, effective in terminating the arrhythmia. The ATP therapy lasted less than a second, and immediately upon the last pulse capacitor charging (represented by the horizontal black solid line) was initiated. After three intervals outside the VT detection zone, charging was interrupted, saving the energy for an unnecessary full capacitor charging cycle.

well as on the patient's comfort and acceptance of ICD therapy. In addition, some ICD models are able to monitor the patient's rhythm during the capacitor charging period and to abort it in situations of recovery of sinus rhythm, with an intuitively clear benefit for battery preservation. Potential downsides of this therapy are negligible: an irrelevant potential second delay of shock delivery (around 1 s) and acceleration or disorganization of the VT rhythm during (however, the programmed DC shock is committed in this case).

ATP Therapy Efficacy and Programming Recommendation

Slow VTs

ATP efficacy in terminating slow VT episodes (cycle length >300–320 ms) was studied as soon as the pacing feature was made available in the first implantable defibrillators in the early 1990s. Burst and ramp pacing schemes were reported to terminate 70–80% of both spontaneous episodes and monomorphic VTs induced during electrophysiologic studies. Spontaneous VTs appeared more prone to ATP termination then induced VTs. Also, burst and ramp showed similar VT termination rates, with the ramp being relatively less effective in fast VTs <300 ms.

Fast VTs and the Pain FREE Trials

Since then much has changed in general agreement about how and when to deliver ATP therapy. Rhythm acceleration is a possible outcome of ATP therapy, resulting in painful shock delivery and in hemodynamically unstable tachycardia with such potentially important clinical consequences as syncope. It was initially recognized that the probability of ATP failure and acceleration increases as VT cycle length decreases. Therefore, there was a common reluctance to program repeated ATP trains, especially ramp schemes, to treat fast VTs with cycle lengths below 300–290 ms. This view has been overtaken by the results of the most recent trials which consistently showed high success rates and low acceleration rates even in fast VTs.

The PainFREE trials were the first to address these issues. The first pilot study PainFREE Rx [2] was an initial registry applying standardized VT detection and ATP regimen to 220 patients with 1100 spontaneous episodes of VT. ATP success rate was 92% for slow VTs (cycle length ≤320 ms) and 89% for fast VTs. Later, the PainFREE Rx II trial used a randomized design to make a direct safety comparison between shock and ATP therapies for fast VT >188 bpm. It included 634 patients with either ischemic or non-ischemic cardiomyopathy. During a follow-up of 1 year, 1760 episodes of slow VT, fast VT, and VF were collected. The results showed that a single burst sequence of 8 pulses at 88% VT cycle length could safely terminate 77% of fast VTs and 90% of slow VTs. Consequently, shocks were reduced by 70% compared to the control group. ATP was not associated with any increase in sudden death, syncope, or even arrhythmia acceleration compared to the control group. The quality of life of the ATP group was also found to be superior to the control group. This evidence represents a solid basis to recommend programming a single burst train during or immediately before capacitor charging for shock delivery in fast and regular 200–250 bpm VT, as this feature is normally available in modern devices.

Detection Count to Initiate ATP Therapy in Slow and Fast VT

An important finding of the PainFREE Rx II trial was that prolonging the counter to 18 for the first fast VT detection markedly reduced the number of delivered therapy compared with the 12 count detection of the first PainFREE study. This suggested that a relevant proportion of spontaneous episodes self-terminate and should not be treated. This first hint was subsequently investigated by other studies. In the ADVANCE III study, the intervention counter was further prolonged to 30 out of 40 intervals and the rate of delivered therapies was compared with 18 of 24 interval count setting [3]. Simply waiting 12 more beats prior to ICD intervention could induce a 37% reduction in the incidence of ATPs. The ADVANCE III trial did not find significant effects of prolonged detection count on mortality and syncope. However, the MADIT RIT trial [4] was a three-arm study which randomly assigned primary prevention patients to: (i) high-rate therapy (with a 2.5 s delay before the initiation of therapy at a heart rate of ≥200 bpm); (ii) delayed therapy (with a 60 s delay at 170–199 bpm, a 12 s delay at 200–249 bpm, and a 2.5 s delay at ≥250 bpm); (iii) conventional programming (with a 2.5 s delay at 170–199 bpm and a 1.0 s delay at ≥200 bpm). The trial showed that programming strategies (i) and (ii) were associated with a significant reduction of the hazard ratio of inappropriate therapy and even all-cause mortality during long-term follow-up. Nevertheless, the striking importance of this result was counterbalanced by the apparent inconsistency that the huge reduction of therapy incidence was mostly driven by fewer ATP deliveries rather than shocks, raising questions concerning the cause–effect relationship between ICD therapy delivery and mortality.

Selection of ATPM Type and Programming

When compared on the basis of VT cycle length, burst pacing was more likely to terminate fast VTs (cycle length >300 ms) than ramp pacing, while no differences were detected for slower VTs. The incidence of rhythm acceleration was low but more likely with the ramp pacing in fast VTs. More recently, the randomized controlled PITAGORA study directly compared the efficacy in terminating fast VTs (cycle length of 320–240 ms) between one single sequence of burst (8 pulses at 88% coupling interval) and ramp (8 pulses at 91% coupling interval). Burst pacing proved more effective in

Table 20.1 Scheme for antitachycardia pacing therapy programming.

	Detection ranges		Detection duration	Antitachy pacing scheme	
	(bpm)	(ms)		Burst	Ramp
VF	≥240	≤250	9–12 s (30–40 intervals)	None	None
Fast VT	200–240	300–250	9–12 s (30–40 intervals)	No of sequence: 1 8 S1 × 85% CL	None
Slow VT	~167–200	370–300	>12 s* (>30–40 intervals)	No of sequence: 2* 8 S1 × 80% CL (add 1)	No. of sequences: 1* 8 S1 × 85–90% CL

CL, detected average cycle length; S1, sequence pulse; VT, ventricular tachycardia.
*For slower VTs, longer detection durations (e.g., 60 s) and multiple combinations of individually tailored antitachy pacing sequences may be considered.

terminating 75% of spontaneous fast VTs compared with a 54% efficacy obtained with the ramp [5].

The number of pulses within a burst sequence has also been investigated comparing 8 with 15 pulse trains with comparable results, although 15 pulses proved significantly better in patients without a previous history of heart failure and in patients with a preserved ejection fraction.

To sum up, ATP therapies effectively terminate most of the spontaneous slow and fast monomorphic VTs, and the efficacy is not impaired by prolonged detection durations or empirical programming. On this basis, the following ATP programming recommendation appears reasonable (Table 20.1):

- For VTs between 170 and 200 bpm, 2–3 ATP attempts (preferably two bursts and one ramp);
- For faster VTs up to 250 bpm, one single burst immediately before or during capacitor charging;
- For slow VTs below 170 bpm, more ATP attempts may be considered depending on individual patients; programming should be tailored on a patient-by-patient basis and no recommendations can be given based on current evidence.

ATP Therapy in Cardiac Resynchronization Therapy Defibrillators

As biventricular devices are able to deliver pacing pulses either from right ventricle, left ventricle, or both, ATP efficacy was also investigated in relation to the stimulation site of origin. However, it is important to note that the pathophysiologic mechanism of re-entrant VT is not dependent on, or influenced by, the site of origin of the VT circuit. The randomized, controlled ADVANCE CRT-D trial compared the efficacy of biventricular with right ventricular ATP therapies in terminating all kinds of ventricular tachycardias. Although ATP confirmed their efficacy also in patients implanted with a cardiac resynchronization therapy defibrillator (CRT-D) device, no significant differences emerged between biventricular and right ventricle delivered ATPs in the general population. A trend toward a lower acceleration rate during fast VT was observed in the patients group assigned to biventricular ATPs.

ATP Therapies in Electrical Storms

Patients with an ICD, especially the subgroup implanted for a secondary prevention indication, have a high risk of developing electrical instability manifested by repeated stable VTs in a short period. This condition is generally referred to as electrical storm (ES), even if definition varies remarkably among authors. Nowadays, the most widely used definition is ≥3 appropriate VT detections within 24 hours that result in ICD therapy (antitachycardia pacing or shocks) or are sustained (>30 s). Of note, the definition neither mentions hemodynamic instability of VTs nor the number of shock discharges and inappropriate detections. In addition, VT episodes must be separate, meaning that a sequence of unsuccessful ATP or shock therapies is not part of this definition. In contrast, incessant VT (i.e., VT continuously re-initiating within a few seconds after termination) should be considered as a particularly severe form of ES.

Incidence of ES has been reported in the range of 10–28% in 12–36 months, with a relatively lower rate for primary prevention patients. A definitive explanation of what triggers ES is still unknown. Nevertheless, it seems well established that the sympathetic tone has an impact on ES elicitation, as indirectly shown by the finding of a decreased baroreflex sensitivity, therapeutic effect of beta blockers, and a peak incidence during the morning hours.

Whatever the cause, 86–97% of ES consist of monomorphic VTs, revealing the presence of re-entry and electrophysiologic substrate in most cases. Therefore, detection and therapy programming in ICD is critical. First, shocks should minimize or even avoid, in slow incessant VTs, as sympathetic stress is an important trigger. Secondly, ATP therapies can terminate the majority of re-entry monomorphic VTs and should be used to delay or even replace high energy therapies, whenever possible. Some devices provide algorithms enabling shock discharge only when irregular VT cycles are detected. This feature could be usefully exploited during ES.

Detection duration certainly is another important parameter to be carefully programmed. Based on recent evidence, detection should be as long as possible to allow spontaneous termination, specially in hemodynamically tolerated VTs. It is unknown how many treated VTs would remain sustained if therapies were delayed further. It is even unclear what the duration cutoff is beyond which a VT becomes persistent and needs treatment. It should also mentioned that, at least in patients for whom ES is not a sporadic episode triggered by reversible causes, ICD therapies should be considered as an ultimate back-up. Radiofrequency catheter ablation can suppress incessant VTs and prevent ES recurrences. There is also increasing evidence that prophylactic catheter ablation of native VT forms can prevent ICD interventions.

References

1 Poole JE, Johnson GW, Hellkamp AS, Anderson J, Callans DJ, Raitt MH, *et al*. Prognostic importance of defibrillator shocks in patients with heart failure. N Engl J Med 2008;359(10):1009–1017.

2 Wathen MS, DeGroot PJ, Sweeney MO, Stark AJ, Otterness MF, Adkisson WO, *et al*; PainFREE Rx II Investigators. Prospective randomized multicenter trial of empirical antitachycardia pacing versus shocks for spontaneous rapid ventricular tachycardia in patients with implantable cardioverter-defibrillators: Pacing Fast Ventricular Tachycardia Reduces Shock Therapies (PainFREE Rx II) trial results. Circulation 2004;110(17):2591–2596.

3 Gasparini M, Proclemer A, Klersy C, Kloppe A, Lunati M, Ferrer JB, *et al*. Effect of long-detection interval vs standard-detection interval for implantable cardioverter-defibrillators on antitachycardia pacing and shock delivery: the ADVANCE III randomized clinical trial. JAMA 2013;309(24):2552.

4 Moss AJ, Schuger C, Beck CA, Brown MW, Cannom DS, Daubert JP, *et al*; MADIT-RIT Trial Investigators. Reduction in inappropriate therapy and mortality through ICD programming. N Engl J Med 2012;367(24):2275–2283.

5 Gulizia MM, Piraino L, Scherillo M, Puntrello C, Vasco C, Scianaro MC, *et al*; PITAGORA ICD Study Investigators. A randomized study to compare ramp versus burst antitachycardia pacing therapies to treat fast ventricular tachyarrhythmias in patients with implantable cardioverter defibrillators: the PITAGORA ICD trial. Circ Arrhythm Electrophysiol 2009;2(2):146–153.

21

How to Troubleshoot An ICD

Advay G. Bhatt, Santosh C. Varkey, and Kevin M. Monahan

Boston Medical Center, Boston University School of Medicine, Boston, MA, USA

Implantation of implantable cardioverter-defibrillators (ICDs) has dramatically increased over the last 20 years because of large clinical trials supporting improved mortality in secondary and primary prevention populations. As a result of progressive advances in medical therapy for ischemic heart disease and congestive heart failure, patients requiring ICDs are living longer. It is estimated that over 150 000 ICDs are implanted annually in the USA with three-quarters for primary prevention and one-quarter for secondary prevention. Concomitantly, it is increasingly recognized that although ICDs save lives, those receiving ICD therapies are at increased risk of mortality, hospitalizations, and declining quality of life when compared with those not receiving therapy.

First-generation ICDs were non-programmable and required surgical implantation. The devices have quickly evolved to be easily implanted endovascularly and highly programmable with the ability to deliver multi-tiered therapy coupled with extensive diagnostic or monitoring options. Each device manufacturer has proprietary diagnostic and treatment algorithms, which may perform differently in similar clinical circumstances. Furthermore, the complex engineering decisions and rigorous testing needed to design, manufacture, gain regulatory approval, and implant these devices safely are enormous and electromechanical failure remains a problem.

It is highly important for the general cardiologist, heart failure specialist, or electrophysiologist to have a thorough understanding of the algorithmic approach to tachyarrhythmia detection and therapy as well as common points of failure in order to be able to evaluate and recognize appropriate and inappropriate ICD function.

Basics of Ventricular Tachyarrhythmia Detection

Despite the sophistication and configurability of the current generation of ICDs, the central parameter to assess the presence of ventricular tachyarrhythmias (VT/VF) remains dependent on the sensed heart rate. Appropriate detection and avoidance of inappropriate detection of ventricular tachycardia/ventricular fibrillation (VT/VF) depends on two factors:

1) Ability of the device to filter or reject all signals that do not represent ventricular depolarization [1,2];
2) Establishing appropriate rate cutoffs for VT/VF zones [1,2].

It is essential the device sense physiologic signals of interest (i.e., ventricular depolarization) to monitor and deliver life-saving therapies while rejecting all other extraneous physiologic or non-physiologic signals. In order to distinguish a ventricular depolarization properly, the raw electrical signal is sequentially passed though an amplifier, band pass filter, rectifier, and level detector (sensitivity) [1]. The band pass filter allows a narrow frequency range of signals to pass while attenuating the remaining signals. The frequency range of ventricular and atrial depolarizations tend to overlap within this band; T waves are generally low frequency and myopotentials high frequency [1].

Reliable detection of VF requires the ability to sense signal amplitudes over a wide and rapidly changing dynamic range. For example, the device needs to be able

How-to Manual for Pacemaker and ICD Devices: Procedures and Programming, First Edition. Edited by Amin Al-Ahmad, Andrea Natale, Paul J. Wang, James P. Daubert, and Luigi Padeletti.
Companion website: www.wiley.com/go/al-ahmad/pacemakers_and_icds

to distinguish between ventricular pauses necessitating pacing and fine VF. This is accomplished with automatic gain control (AGC) where the peak or average signal amplitude is used to adjust the gain (sensitivity) dynamically [1,3]. The programmed sensitivity sets a minimum amplitude or floor below which the device will not sense. AGC dynamically decreases the sensitivity with fixed or programmable decay rates in order to be able to avoid crosstalk, oversensing of repolarization, and at the same time avoid undersensing VF. The need for high sensitivity in an ICD increases the risk of oversensing thereby inhibiting pacing or inappropriate detection of VT/VF.

In general, VT/VF zones are programmed with high rate cutoffs to avoid overlap with sinus tachycardia or atrial tachyarrhythmias. Inappropriately programming low rate cutoffs or multiple zones increases the likelihood of inappropriate ICD therapy.

The other programmable factor that affects whether ICD therapy is delivered depends on the detection interval needed to establish the presence of VT/VF. VT detection is based on the concept that VT generally is regular with a rate slower than VF [1]. If the ICD is sensing events with intervals within the designated VT zone, it counts them consecutively until the programmed number of intervals to detect (NID) or duration is met. VF detection is based on a probabilistic counter given that VF has very fast and irregular intervals with marked variation in the amplitude of the fibrillatory waves. A probabilistic counter allows utilizing AGC to reduce oversensing and tolerate intermittent dropout because of fine low-amplitude fibrillatory waves [1].

Implant-Related Problems

During device implant, the reasons for acute failure are technical or related to the skill and experience of the implanting physician. The most common issues are related to lead dislodgement, perforation, and connections. These factors are readily evaluated with routine post-implant interrogation and chest radiographs. All of these issues will require lead revision to correct the problem.

Lead dislodgement in single- or dual-chamber ICDs can be inferred from loss of capture, loss of sensing, inappropriate shocks for sinus tachycardia or supraventricular tachycardia (SVT), or undersensing of VT/VF. The implant techniques to minimize dislodgement include ensuring the lead tip is embedded in the myocardium fluoroscopically, with gentle traction, or assessing injury current; presence of sufficient slack to accommodate cardiac motion and inferior displacement when standing; and anchoring the leads in the pocket with suture sleeves.

Patients with lead perforation can present dramatically with hypotension or shortness of breath related to cardiac tamponade which is most safely dealt with in the operating theatre with cardiothoracic (CT) surgery. Patients with lead perforation may also present subacutely with pericardial pain, diaphragmatic capture, or intercostal muscle capture that would require lead revision. In the presence of an effusion, the risk of tamponade may be higher and lead revision should be undertaken with CT surgical back-up. An acute impedance rise raises the possibility of perforation. However, lead impedance and threshold may be unchanged if the ring electrode remains in contact with myocardium. The implant techniques to minimize perforation include avoiding having the stylet fully advanced into the lead when deploying the screw, over-torqueing the screw, assessing for out of range impedances, or diaphragmatic stimulation.

A loose set-screw or reversal of the right ventricular (RV) and superior vena cava (SVC) coil pins in the header of the device would result in oversensing from electromechanical interference (EMI) or myopotential sensing leading to inhibition of pacing or delivery inappropriate therapy, respectively. Low high-voltage (HV) impedance or ineffective defibrillation at the time of defibrillation threshold testing (DFT) may indicate reversal of the coils in the header of the device. Other considerations for elevated DFT at the time of implant include suboptimal lead position or pneumothorax. RV and SVC coil pin reversal would lead to pectoral myopotential or EMI oversensing (see Myopotentials and Electromechanical Interference).

Clinical Reasons to Assess ICD Function

The most common reasons patients present for ICD evaluation include shocks, presyncope, syncope, palpitations, audible alerts, perioperative management, or routine device follow-up.

Presyncope, syncope, and palpitations can be caused by a myriad of reasons including VT below the detection zone, VT falling in and out of the zone, VT/VF undersensing, non-sustained VT, frequent premature ventricular contractions, or SVT. Audible or haptic alerts are programmable parameters for battery depletion, prolonged charge time, magnet application, electrical reset, lead impedance warning, and intrathoracic impedance change. There is variability in whether the alerts are activated and educating patients in regards to the nature and implications of an alert. The tones or vibrations used for alerts may increase patient anxiety and are of decreasing utility as remote monitoring is adopted more widely.

A thorough history should be taken, including medications and recent procedures; physical examination to assess for trauma or signs of infection; electrocardiogram; chest radiograph to evaluate for dislodgement, fracture, or other lead abnormalities; and interrogation allow for comprehensive device evaluation. The goal is to evaluate battery status, lead integrity with close attention to the high-voltage components, programming characteristics, stored tachyarrhythmia episodes, and appropriateness and effectiveness of delivered therapies.

The most common diagnostic issue is distinguishing appropriate from inappropriate ICD therapy (each are managed differently) and effectiveness of antitachycardia pacing (ATP) or defibrillation.

ATP or shocks may be delivered for monomorphic or polymorphic VT, ventricular flutter, or VF. Delivery of ICD therapy needs careful evaluation for the presence of ischemia, decompensated heart failure, polypharmacy, and metabolic abnormalities. The presence of these triggering factors should prompt admission with goal of medical stabilization, optimization, and evaluating need for ablative therapies to reduce future shocks. Device optimization can be performed after assessing sensing of VT/VF, response to ATP, effectiveness of the first shock, presence of unwanted pacing, or ineffective cardiac resynchronization (CRT).

ATP or shocks may be inappropriately delivered as a result of oversensing extraneous physiologic signals; non-physiologic signals from EMI or device malfunction; or SVT, most commonly atrial fibrillation (AF).

Inappropriate ICD Therapy for Oversensing

Oversensing is the misinterpretation of voltage deflections not related to a QRS complex as ventricular depolarization, resulting in perception of a falsely elevated ventricular rate. This leads to inappropriate inhibition of pacing, ATP, or shock if sufficiently fast to be detected in the VT or VF zones.

The most common causes of oversensing can be classified as physiologic or non-physiologic signals. Physiologic signals may be intracardiac or extracardiac in origin and include T-wave oversensing, P-wave oversensing, R-wave double counting, and myopotentials [1–4]. Non-physiologic signals or EMI (noise) are exclusively extracardiac in origin and are related to lead malfunction, electrocautery, or other external sources (see Electromechanical Interference and Lead or Connector Failure) [1–3].

Oversensing can be caused by the sensing circuit or configuration, true bipolar or integrated bipolar. In general, integrated bipolar leads are more prone to oversensing because of a wider field of sensing between the cathode and anode. It is reported that oversensing occurs more frequently when there is a lead and pulse generator manufacturer mismatch.

T-wave Oversensing

T-wave oversensing (TWOS) is the most clinically relevant cause of oversensing from intracardiac signals. In general, TWOS is avoided in ICDs based off of the AGC sensitivity and decay delays as well as the ventricular blanking period. If the initial threshold is too high, the decay delay too long, or the blanking period too long, VF detection will be delayed. TWOS therefore occurs in settings with increased T-wave amplitude, low R-wave amplitude relative to T-wave, or when the QT interval is prolonged beyond the ventricular blanking period.

The common clinical settings this may be encountered is in hypertrophic cardiomyopathy, long QT syndrome, short QT syndrome, Brugada syndrome, hyperkalemia, and hyperglycemia. T-wave amplitude also varies with positional changes and alterations in autonomic tone (Figure 21.1) [1–3]. The other issue to remember is that each device manufacturer has different proprietary algorithms to avoid TWOS that perform differently in clinical practice.

When TWOS occurs, the ICD may interpret the events as VT/VF if the sensed R-wave to T-wave interval falls within the VT or VF detection zones. This is characterized by alternating electrogram (EGM) morphologies and less often with two distinct populations of V-V intervals, one short and one long.

The ability to effectively manage TWOS primarily relies on the relative difference in R and T-wave amplitudes. If R-wave amplitude is significantly greater than T-wave then a simple approach is to decrease ventricular sensitivity. Care must be taken that VF is adequately detected by reassessing sensing with DFT testing. Theoretically, increasing the ventricular blanking period would correct the problem. However, not all manufacturers support programmable ventricular blanking periods given that increasing the blanking period would lead to undersensing of VF. Medtronic now allows switching sensing between true and integrated bipolar configurations, which may rectify the problem given that this phenomenon is more frequently observed with true bipolar leads. St. Jude Medical devices allow programmable threshold start and decay delays, which may allow a programming solution. Other considerations include raising the detection zones for VT and VF, increasing the number of intervals to detect, or treating with beta blockers to lower sinus rates. In cases where T-wave oversensing is caused by a specific metabolic derangement, correction of the underlying abnormality will rectify the problem.

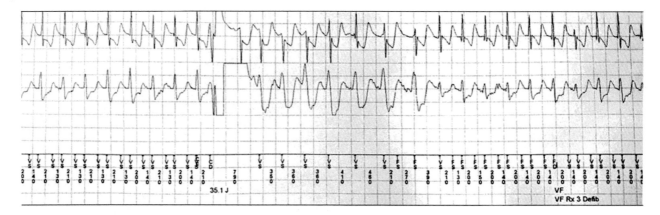

Figure 21.1 T-wave oversensing in the setting of sinus tachycardia and marked hyperglycemia that results in inappropriate shock. The tachycardia continues post-shock but T-wave oversensing is transiently not seen because of post-shock repolarization abnormalities. T-wave oversensing resumes after repolarization abnormalities resolve and VF is re-detected. With correction of hyperglycemia, T-wave oversensing was no longer appreciated. This may also be seen in hyperkalemia.

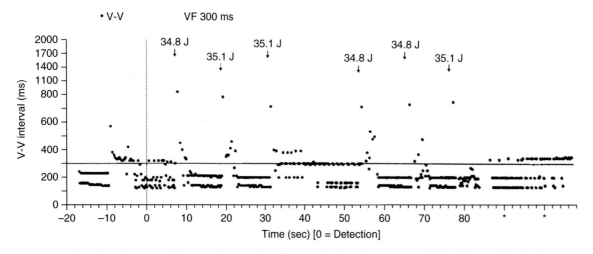

Figure 21.2 Transient R-wave double counting revealing classic railroad track appearance led to delivery of multiple inappropriate shocks.

These approaches will fail and endanger appropriate defibrillation if T-wave amplitude is nearly equal to or greater than the R wave. In these patients, the defibrillation lead may need to be repositioned or pace/sense lead implanted to obtain greater R-wave amplitude or, rarely, try a different filtering algorithm by exchanging the pulse generator to that of a different manufacturer.

R-wave Double Counting

R-wave double counting occurs with a multifaceted EGM and duration that exceeds the ventricular blanking period. This is now rare because of changes in devices. This problem may arise in the setting of marked intraventricular conduction delay, exacerbated in the setting of hyperkalemia or toxicity with sodium channel blocking agents, and is more common with integrated bipolar leads [1–3]. This was encountered more frequently in earlier generations of CRT-D devices that allowed for bipolar sensing between the right and left ventricular electrodes.

R-wave double counting results in two distinct populations of V-V intervals, one short and one long, which characteristically give a "railroad track" appearance on the interval plot (Figure 21.2).

Increasing the ventricular blanking period can rectify the problem but only St. Jude Medical devices have this support. Older CRT-D devices can be exchanged for newer models, which no longer have the extended bipolar sensing configuration.

P-wave Oversensing

P-wave oversensing is most frequently seen if the RV coil of an integrated bipolar lead does not fully cross the tricuspid annulus, thus allowing sensing of far-field atrial activity and the PR interval exceeds the ventricular blanking period. This may lead to inappropriate detection of VT/VF during sinus rhythm and SVT. It is most commonly seen with atrial flutter with proximal lead placement. P-wave oversensing may be observed with true bipolar leads in the setting of lead dislodgement or if the lead is deployed in the region of the proximal septum [1–3]. Decreasing ventricular sensitivity would only lead to undersensing VF; most often lead revision is needed.

Myopotential Oversensing

Normal electrical activity of muscle in proximity to the ICD system may be sensed throughout or for a fraction of the cardiac cycle. The two sources of myopotentials are the diaphragm and pectoral muscles.

Diaphragmatic myopotential oversensing (DMO) is most commonly observed with systems that include an integrated bipolar lead or sensing configuration. The myopotentials are high frequency electrical activity most prominent on the near field EGM. DMO is most often seen after long diastolic intervals or after ventricular pacing when the ICD is most sensitive; oversensing stops once a true R wave is sensed given AGC will readjust to be less sensitive [1–3]. Additionally, diaphragmatic myopotentials exhibit a respiratory variation as small changes in lead position affect sensing. This may lead to syncope or inappropriate delivery of therapy for VT or VF. Diaphragmatic myopotentials may be reproduced with Valsalva. It is commonly seen during straining to defecate with constipation.

If myopotential sensing is discovered but does not result in inappropriate device therapy, then no programming modifications may be necessary unless it inhibits pacing in pacing-dependent cases or limits effective CRT

(Figure 21.3). Frequent monitoring of non-sustained events will accelerate battery depletion so extending the detection interval would be another consideration. If DMO leads to inappropriate shocks, ventricular sensitivity may be decreased to correct the problem assuming adequate sensing of VF is reassessed. Less commonly, a new rate sensing lead may need to be inserted or the chronic defibrillation lead may need to be repositioned away from the right ventricular apex. This is most commonly seen with Boston Scientific devices; generator exchange may resolve the issue if lead revision is not possible.

Pectoral myopotential oversensing may be seen with true or integrated bipolar leads with electrical activity being most prominent on the far field electrogram [1–3]. This may be reproduced with isometric exercise. Pectoral myopotentials do not lead to inappropriate device therapy given that the far field electrogram is not used for rate sensing and unipolar sensing is not an option. However, pectoral myopotentials may limit the effectiveness of morphology-based SVT discriminators.

Electromechanical Interference

EMI is the sensing of external electrical activity as ventricular events that leads to VT/VF detection and therapy. The common clinical scenario is to receive shock without any warning or preceding symptoms. High frequency electrical activity is typically sensed on both the near and far field EGM but with greater amplitude on the far field EGM. EMI will be detected in both the atrial and ventricular leads in dual-chamber systems. This distinguishes EMI from defibrillation lead failure, as EMI would be confined to the affected lead [1–4].

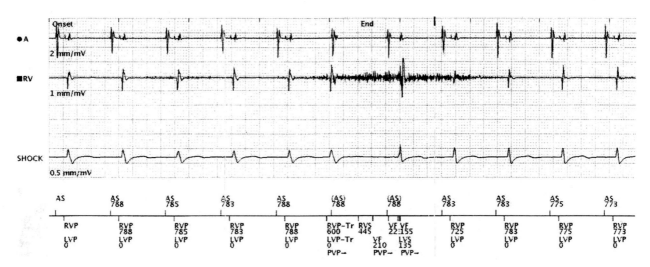

Figure 21.3 Intermittent diaphragmatic myopotential oversensing leading to detection of VF but did not result in shock. Reducing ventricular sensitivity led to improvement in oversensing without undersensing of VF.

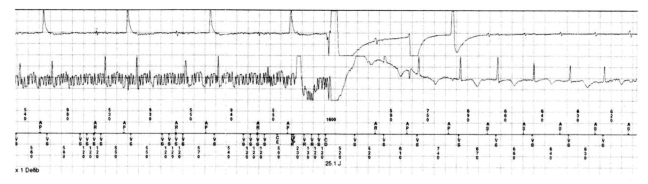

Figure 21.4 EMI caused by a poorly grounded pool filter that resulted in inappropriate shock.

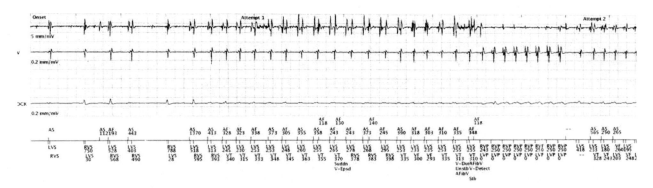

Figure 21.5 Phantom crosstalk caused by parasitic coupling that can lead to atrial sensing in a CRT device with an atrial port plug inserted. This was a CRT-D device in which the atrial port was plugged because of permanent AF. Oversensing in the atrial channel led to misclassification as SVT and to delay in VT/VF therapies.

These are not commonly encountered routinely but may be seen when in proximity to industrial electromagnets, magnetic resonance imaging equipment, and arc welding. Vibrating devices such as jackhammers and chainsaws are other sources of EMI leading to oversensing of VF detection. Another encountered source of EMI is a poorly grounded swimming pool filter. This may lead to VF detection and shocks when attempting to get out of the pool or touching something outside the water that then provides a means of grounding the source of EMI (Figure 21.4). Rarely, crosstalk is an internal source of EMI in otherwise normally functioning devices (Figure 21.5).

More commonly encountered sources of EMI are medical equipment including extracorporeal shockwave lithotripsy, radiotherapy, radiofrequency ablation, electrical nerve stimulation, MRI, or electrocautery. If electrocautery is used solely in short bursts, it is less likely to result in device therapy as detection criteria are often not met. Additionally, modern noise filtering on modern ICDs often limit inappropriate device therapy. Bipolar electrocautery, where both electrodes are located in close proximity of one another, is less likely to cause inappropriate detection and therapy.

Lead or Connector Failure

Despite extensive testing, the reliability and function of defibrillator leads are not known until deployed widely in clinical practice. Although the materials used by each of the major lead manufacturers are similar, there are differences in how these materials are applied.

The necessarily more complex design of ICD leads increases the probability of lead failure when compared with pacing leads. Longevity estimates for pacing leads suggests a very low rate a failure, whereas approximately 20% of ICD leads will develop defects necessitating intervention after 10 years.

Lead failure or recalls are inevitable. A clear understanding of the mechanisms of failure is essential. The etiology of lead failure includes:

1) Lead-related technical factors.
2) Patient-related factors:
   - Excessive upper-body activity;
   - Twiddling.
3) Implant-related factors:
   - Rough lead handling or endovascular trauma;
   - Subclavian rather than axillary/cephalic access;

- Positioning the lead with a stylet fully inserted;
- Over-torqueing of active-fixation mechanism;
- Excessive tightening of anchoring sleeve sutures;
- Kinking of the lead and connector in the pocket.

The modes of failure include insulation defect, lead fracture, abnormal impedance, and sensing failure. Disruption or abrasion of lead insulation typically occur as a result of rough handling, clavicular crush, or lead friction with other components of the device or anatomic structures, or inside out defects caused by the conductor. Fracture of the lead conductor tends to occur at points of mechanical stress such as points of component bonding, level of the clavicle, acute angulation with the suture sleeve, or elsewhere within the pocket.

The common signs of a breach in lead insulation include low impedance, sudden rise or loss of capture, and over- or undersensing [4,5]. The common signs of lead fracture are erratic sensing, oversensing, high impedance, or intermittent or loss of capture [4,5]. Abnormalities in pacing impedance, if present, are helpful in ascertaining the point of failure; however, they may be intermittent.

Oversensing because of lead or connector problems may be related to insulation breach, conductor fracture, loose set-screw, or header failure (Figures 21.6 and 21.7). The oversensing of non-physiologic signals with very short V-V intervals because of these problems tend to be intermittent and most frequently observed on the

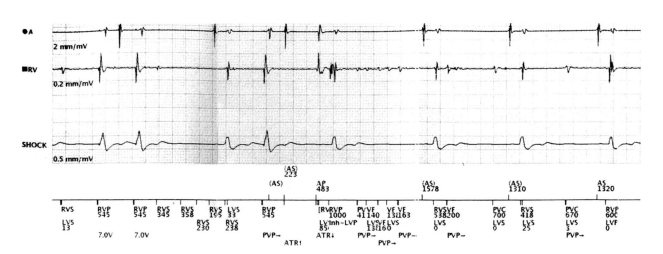

Figure 21.6 Oversensing leading to inhibition of pacing and inappropriate detection of non-sustained VF in the setting of a loose set-screw following CRT-D pulse generator change.

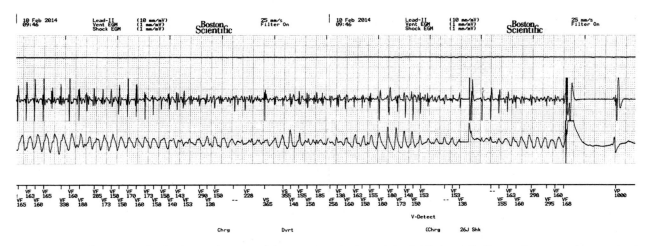

Figure 21.7 Undersensing of VF leading to diversion of therapy after which a 26 J shock failed to defibrillate and an external rescue shock was delivered. Increasing sensitivity reduced undersensing so that shock was not delayed and 26 J successfully terminated VF.

near field EGM. The exception is RV coil conductor failure in integrated bipolar leads; oversensing is on seen on both the near and far field EGM. Oversensing can reproduced with pocket manipulation or arm motion. A chest radiograph or fluoroscopy may allow visualization that the pin is proximal to the distal screw. Medtronic incorporates a Lead Integrity Alert (LIA) algorithm [2] that provides a repeating audible alert and automatically notifies the physician via remote monitoring if at least two of the following criteria are met:

1) Abrupt change in lead impedance when compared to a calculated baseline;
2) Two or more non-sustained high rate episodes with V-V intervals of less than 220 ms; or
3) 30 short V-V intervals in the preceding 72 hours.

LIA will automatically increase number of intervals needed to detect both VT and VF in order to try to minimize shocks. The algorithm provides advance warning, reduces shocks, and allows early intervention prior to complete lead failure.

Evaluation of Appropriateness of ICD Therapy for Tachycardia

ICDs deliver therapies for any tachyarrhythmia that falls within the predefined detection zones and meet detection criteria including VF, VT, SVT, and, rarely, double tachycardia. The most common SVT leading to inappropriate therapies is AF. Distinguishing between VT and SVT can be challenging, in particular when evaluating single-chamber ICDs compared to dual-chamber ICDs. A single-chamber ICD senses only ventricular events and the only stored data available are the near field and far field EGMs. A dual-chamber ICD senses both atrial and ventricular events. Inferences can be made based on the regularity, sudden onset, morphology, AV relationship, chamber onset, and response to premature beats or pacing as done via electrocardiography or electrophysiologic testing; the fundamental principles remain the same.

Both single- and dual-chamber ICDs have diagnostic algorithms, SVT discriminators, in order to distinguish between SVT and VT based on these fundamental principles. SVT discrimination is only applied within the VT zones, not VF zone, in order to minimize delays in detecting and treating VF. The algorithms can be helpful but over-reliance should be cautioned, as the algorithms are imperfect. SVT discrimination times out after a pre-specified time in order to avoid undertreating VT; however, SVT tends to be more stable and incessant than VT, which may result in inappropriate shocks.

The stored EGMs need to be reviewed systematically in order to determine whether the device correctly classified a tachyarrhythmia as SVT or VT.

Both single- and dual-chamber ICD SVT discrimination evaluates stability, sudden onset, and morphology [1–3]. Dual-chamber ICDs incorporate the ability to simultaneously evaluate atrial and ventricular electrograms, AV relationship, and chamber of onset [1–3].

Stability

The stability criterion is used to distinguish between VT and AF. VT generally starts suddenly with stable morphology and intervals. AF starts suddenly with variable morphology (because of rate-related aberrancy) and variable intervals. The effectiveness of the stability discriminator becomes less reliable with ventricular rates in excess of 180 beats per minute. AF with rapid conduction above this rate tends to be more regular. Transient organization into atrial flutter with regular ventricular conduction may result in reclassification as VT [1–3]. The stability criteria is programmable to allow for a greater degree of discrimination specificity. The most commonly encountered setting is variability of greater than 30 ms suggests AF. Triggered or automatic VTs are commonly seen with structural heart disease and may not meet stability criteria from acceleration, deceleration, or irregularity, which would inappropriately be classified as AF.

Sudden Onset

The sudden onset criterion is used to distinguish between sinus tachycardia and VT. VT starts abruptly whereas sinus tachycardia accelerates gradually. Similar to the stability, sudden onset becomes less reliable with ventricular rate in excess of 180 bpm. SVT starts abruptly and would be classified as VT should the rate fall within the VT zone [1–3].

Morphology

The morphology criterion is used to distinguish tachyarrhythmias from SVT and VT. A baseline sinus rhythm EGM template is required. Upon VT detection, the ICD in real-time will align and compare EGM morphology to the template. A quantitative assessment of match will be made differentiate between SVT and VT based on a pre-specified percentage match threshold. This feature is not programmable across all device manufacturers [1–3].

The key to proper function is to ensure an accurate template that is updated periodically given that EGM may change because of lead maturation, development of conduction disease, or antiarrhythmic agents. In the absence of native ventricular conduction, a template will not be able to be obtained. The other consideration is if the template was that of a premature ventricular beat or aberrated supraventricular beat. The effectiveness of morphology analysis will be negatively impacted based on alignment errors, truncation leading to loss of morphology information and misalignment, inclusion of far field EGM analysis would be affected by pectoral myopotentials, and rate-related aberrancy [1–3].

When visually assessing morphology, the near field EGM is typically used for analysis and, if different from that of sinus, then VT is diagnosed. However, use of the near field EGM alone may not be sufficiently powerful if the origin of VT is in proximity to the defibrillation lead; the use of the far field EGM may enhance discrimination. Another common error is to compare the tachyarrhythmia morphology to the post-shock morphology. Following a shock, EGM morphology remains significantly distorted compared to baseline because of transient local and global repolarization abnormalities.

AV Relationship

Dual-chamber ICDs first evaluate the AV relationship to evaluate for the presence of AV dissociation or association.

AV dissociation is present when there are more ventricular events than atrial events (V > A) resulting in classification as VT. A very rare exception that would be inappropriately classified as VT is a dual AV nodal response tachycardia [1–3].

AV dissociation or association cannot be fully evaluated when there are more atrial events than ventricular events (A > V) and as such discrimination of VT during AF, atrial flutter, or SVT is more difficult. Further discrimination relies upon factoring morphology, stability, and AV relationship, which are each weighted differently based on the manufacturer.

AV association is present when there are equal number of atrial and ventricular events, which may represent VT with 1:1 ventriculoatrial (VA) conduction, AV nodal dependent SVT, or sinus tachycardia. Sinus tachycardia is the most frequent 1:1 SVT and would have a gradual onset. VT with 1:1 VA conduction is infrequent. Transient AV or VA block supports the diagnosis of SVT or VT, respectively; AV block effectively rules out AV nodal dependent SVT. Further discrimination for 1:1 SVTs relies upon morphology, chamber of onset, and response ATP. A poor morphology match would necessarily be classified as VT. Initiation with short P-P interval or short V-V interval would support an atrial or ventricular origin, respectively. Atrioventricular nodal

re-entrant tachycardia (AVNRT) would have near simultaneous atrial and ventricular sensed events.

ATP may mimic ventricular overdrive pacing and entrain the atrium, thus allowing interpretation of the response following cessation of pacing (VAV and VAAV response). ATP often terminates VT and AV nodal dependent SVTs but termination of atrial tachycardia, atrial flutter, AF, and sinus tachycardia is very unlikely [1–3].

Theoretically, dual-chamber SVT discrimination should be superior in reducing delivery of ATP or shocks than single-chamber SVT discrimination. However, this remains unproven in clinical trials and remains controversial [1–3]. Dual-chamber SVT discrimination is limited by appropriate atrial sensing; P wave undersensing needs to be avoided but far field R wave sensing minimized. P wave undersensing can lead to inappropriate classification as VT and far field R wave oversensing would lead to inappropriate classification as SVT [1–3]. Programmable post-ventricular atrial blanking periods, thresholds, and decay rates offered by certain manufacturers may mitigate this problem.

Programming to Avoid Inappropriate Therapy

The common practice is to program multiple VT zones to facilitate delivery of ATP, which is effective for both slow and fast VT. Device programming in this manner allows for substantial overlap between sinus tachycardia, SVT, and VT that leads to inappropriate shocks. This drove the development SVT discrimination algorithms but remain unreliable. Aggressive programming may lead to overtreatment for events that may be self-limited. Furthermore, ATP may accelerate stable VTs into unstable rhythms requiring shock.

There is increasing recognition that delivery of ICD therapies are associated with poor outcomes and an ongoing debate continues of whether appropriate ICD therapies directly lead to excess morbidity and mortality or if it serves as a marker for poor outcomes.

The most important way to minimize delivery of inappropriate therapy is careful consideration of device selection (single- or dual-chamber ICD) and the programming parameters at the time of implant. Clinical trial data supports programming a single VF zone of greater than 200 bpm or multiple zones with marked prolongation in the detection time in order to reduce inappropriate shocks and mortality. This theoretically delays treatment of hemodynamically unstable VT.

Given these considerations, most primary or secondary prevention devices for VF arrest may best be served with programming a single VF zone with a prolonged detection time; ATP during charging may be enabled if needed. VT zones with delivery of ATP followed by shocks should only be programmed when there is documented sustained VT proven to be responsive to ATP.

Effectiveness of Shocks

The next step after determining that an ICD shock is appropriate is to determine the adequacy sensing and effectiveness of defibrillation.

Inadequate sensing of VF may lead to delays in detection, re-detection, and delivery of shock that may result in syncope, hemodynamic instability, or ineffective defibrillation [4,5]. A linear relationship exists between duration of VF and DFT. If encountered, the first approach is increase sensitivity and re-evaluate sensing. Another possibility is to change the sensing vector in systems that allow sensing both true bipolar and integrated bipolar configurations. If undersensing VF persists, then lead revision or a new rate sensing lead may be needed.

There are several patient-specific factors related to elevated DFT including dilated non-ischemic cardiomyopathy, infiltrative cardiomyopathy, obesity, pleural effusions, decompensated heart failure, and need for right-sided implant. Moreover, success of defibrillation is modified by ischemia, metabolic abnormalities, autonomic tone, and medications. In particular, chronic oral amiodarone is associated with an increase in DFT. Other medications associated with an increase in DFT include lidocaine, mexiletine, verapamil, propofol, anesthetic agents, cocaine, venlafaxine, and sildenafil.

Elevated DFT in the setting of reversible factors or medications should be managed with treatment of the underlying condition and medication cessation, respectively. DFT should be retested after an adequate period to allow washout. In the absence of a reversible cause, chest radiography should be obtained to confirm an appropriate apical lead position. Interrogation to evaluate HV system integrity may reveal impedance out of nominal range that may reflect a failing lead. In particular, sudden changes in impedances should suggest impending lead failure. Similarly, any lead with undersensing, oversensing, or changes in pacing impedances should prompt careful evaluation for lead failure.

In the absence of reversible causes or signs of lead failure a number of changes may be attempted to improve defibrillation with an adequate safety margin:

1) Change polarity;
2) Exclusion of SVC coil. HV impedance of less than 40 should prompt exclusion of the SVC coil;

3) Modification of tilt waveform on St. Jude Medical devices;
4) Medications that lower DFT (e.g., sotalol and dofetilide) may be attempted in select cases where other measures fail and an invasive approach is not desired.

Most cases of elevated DFT can be approached non-invasively. When there are no other alternatives, lead revision or implantation of additional shock electrodes (azygous, subclavian, coronary sinus, or subcutaneous array) or use of a high-energy device may be considered.

Battery Status

Modern ICDs are able to estimate longevity of the device at the current rate of usage. The rate at which batteries deplete is different for each manufacturer.

ICDs such as pacemakers establish two levels of battery depletion:

1) Elective replacement interval (ERI); and
2) End of life (EOL).

The ERI criterion indicates the device still has sufficient energy for full functionality for up to 3 months while device replacement is arranged. The EOL criterion indicates insufficient energy for full function and the device may function unpredictably. Device replacement should not be delayed as its ability to defibrillate is unclear.

Charge Time

Charge time, the time between arrhythmia detection and shock, depends on device and battery integrity. Longer charge time delays treatment which may lead to syncope, hemodynamic instability, or ineffective defibrillation.

Prolonged charge times indicate the need to reform the capacitor, component failure, battery failure, or battery depletion. The charge time gradually increases over time as a result of normal capacitor function. ICDs have programmable automatic capacitor reformation protocols to maintain appropriate function. As battery depletion progresses towards and reaches ERI, charge time will increase.

The first step when prolonged charge time is encountered is to check battery status and then to reform the capacitor. Charging the capacitors to full output and then maintaining the charge for 10 minutes reform the capacitor. The charge is dumped and the capacitor is recharged to reassess charge time.

References

1 Swerdlow CD, Gillberg JM, Olson WH. Sensing and detection. In Ellenbogen KA, Kay GN, Lau C, Wilkoff BL (eds). Clinical Cardiac Pacing, Defibrillation, and Resynchronization Therapy, 3rd edition. Saunders, 2007: 75–160.

2 Koneru JN, Swerdlow CD, Wood MA, Ellenbogen KA. Minimizing inappropriate or "unnecessary" implantable cardioverter-defibrillator shocks. Circ Arrhythm Electrophysiol 2011;4(5):778–790.

3 Swerdlow CD, Friedman PA. Advanced ICD troubleshooting: part I. Pacing Clin Electrophysiol 2005;28:1322–1346.

4 Swerdlow CD, Friedman PA. Advanced ICD troubleshooting: part II. Pacing Clin Electrophysiol 2006;29:70–96.

5 Epstein A. Troubleshooting of implantable cardioverter-defibrillators. In Ellenbogen KA, Kay GN, Lau C, Wilkoff BL (eds). Clinical Cardiac Pacing, Defibrillation, and Resynchronization Therapy, 3rd edition. Saunders, 2007: 1063–1086.

22

Management of ICD Device and Lead Failures and Recalls

Yousef Bader and N.A. Mark Estes III

Tufts University School of Medicine, Tufts Medical Center, Boston, MA, USA

As life-saving devices, implantable cardioverter-defibrillators (ICDs) and leads used with these devices require the highest possible standards of reliability. While numerous patients have benefited from these important technologies, these cardiac rhythm management systems are complex and have a finite rate of malfunction [1–5]. With meticulous design, careful manufacturing, rigorous testing, and robust monitoring cardiac rhythm devices and leads should continue to have a lower frequency of malfunction in the future. Timely detection, characterization, communication, and clinical management of product specific performance issues are critical to patient safety. While ICDs leads are designed to transfer information and life-sustaining therapy to and from the device in the hostile and mechanically stressful intravascular and cardiac environment of the human body, they are considered the weak link in cardiac rhythm management system. The high profile failure and recall of multiple ICDs and leads has served to undermine trust in the therapy. Recommendations for timely detection, characterization, communication, and correction of product performance issues have been developed to provide a systematic approach to clinical management and improvement in ICD and lead reliability [1–5].

Definitions of lCD lead malfunction, performance, and reliability are now standardized, thereby allowing evidence-based comparison of devices and leads [1]. Reliability represents the measure of freedom of a specific device or lead from structural or functional failure as a function of time. This time dependence of assessing ICD and lead performance makes it imperative that all devices and leads be followed over the entire duration of their functional life. Unfortunately, manufacturer product performance reports and independent registries are limited by underreporting of cardiac rhythm device and lead malfunction, insufficient patient follow-up, lack of uniform definitions, lack of returned product for failure analysis, and a passive monitoring system based on voluntary reporting [1].

Many recommendations related to device and lead performance, communication, premarket evaluation, post market surveillance, lead advisories, and clinical management are available [1,2]. The responsibilities of manufacturers, regulatory agencies, and healthcare providers in addressing acknowledged limitations of ICD and lead design, testing, manufacturing, surveillance, reporting, and improvement are clearly specified [1,2]. Among the many recommendations made for improving device and lead performance are registries reporting device and lead reliability in a logical and comprehensible manner. Independent analyses of prospective registry data provide the most credible, reliable, and trustworthy data [1,2].

Ensuring the clinical benefits of ICD systems established by numerous clinical trials is clearly in the best interests of patients with ICDs. Physicians and other healthcare professionals implanting or following ICDs and leads should remain mindful of their responsibility to report any lead failures to the Food and Drug Adminstration (FDA) and return any leads removed to the manufacturer, whether malfunctioning or not. Additional, all healthcare professionals involved with implanting or following ICDs and leads should be aware of the best management practices for reporting, communicating, monitoring, and managing ICD and lead recalls and failures [1,2].

Monitoring of ICD and Lead Performance

The function and longevity of ICD generators and leads is monitored by the companies that produce them, independent registries, and by the FDA. The manufacturers of pacemakers and ICDs report their device and lead reliability data on a publicly available website which is typically updated quarterly. However, the data is based on a passive monitoring system with reliance on returned product analysis and reports by healthcare professionals. Thus, it is likely that this represents significant underreporting. In the same fashion, the FDA Manufacturers and Users Device Experience (MAUDE) database relies on a passive monitoring system and as such there is significant underreporting [1,2]. The absence of mandatory post mortem pacemaker and ICD interrogation also represents a significant weakness of available databases.

Definition of Recall

When an ICD generator or lead appears to be failing with a frequency or failure mechanism that represents a clinically significant risk, the product may be recalled at the direction of the FDA [1]. When a device is recalled, the manufacturer and distributor of the device have an obligation to remove or correct the marketed product or the FDA can take legal action. Recalls are classified into three classes: I, II, and III. A class I recall represents the most serious and implies there is a reasonable probability that use of the product will result in serious adverse health consequences or death. Therefore, device and lead recalls and failures should be managed with great care and attention. ICDs and leads that have failed must be replaced and the mode of replacement should be at the discretion of the managing physician. Management of ICDs or leads that have been recalled function normally is more complex and requires a formal management strategy. Consensus documents related to ICD and lead reliability have been published and serve as a valuable resource [1,2]. These documents provide detailed information on management of advisory notifications, field action letters, technical notifications, performance updates, and other communications sent either by the FDA or manufacturers [1,2].

Management of ICD Recalls or Failure

The major objective of management of patients with recalled or malfunctioning ICDs is preventing any adverse patient outcome [1–4]. Despite increased awareness of device failures, device companies and the FDA do not make specific recommendations regarding management of these patients. Management decisions ultimately are left in the hands of physicians based on guidance from regulatory agencies, manufacturers, professional organizations, and patients. Consensus recommendations for the management of patients falling in this category have been developed (Table 22.1) [1,2]. Despite these recommendations, the management of recalled or malfunctioning ICDs varies considerably amongst physicians for the same clinical issue. In response to a recalled ICD with a low frequency of premature a battery failure, for example, overall 30% of recalled devices were replaced with the vast majority continuing to demonstrate normal function. The rate of replacement was physician dependent and varied from 0% to 100%.

When a clinician becomes aware of an ICD recall or failure, immediate assessment of the patient is essential with careful risk stratification of the patient for the potential for adverse outcomes related to the lack of proper device function (Table 22.2). Among the key clinical issues to address at the initial evaluation is the

Table 22.1 Considerations for implantable cardioverter-defibrillator (ICD) device replacement.

Consider device replacement if:

- The risk of malfunction is likely to lead to death or serious harm
- Patients are pacemaker dependent
- Patients with ICDs for secondary prevention of sudden death
- Patients with ICDs for primary prevention who have received appropriate therapy

Table 22.2 ICD device recall.

Clinical risk	Pacemaker dependent	Secondary prevention	Primary prevention with prior therapy	Primary prevention with no prior therapy
Risk of failure	High	High	Intermediate	Low
Management	Replace	Replace or monitor	Monitor	Monitor

current indication for defibrillation and pacemaker therapy. Generally, there is greater potential for harm because of the ICD not delivering therapy appropriately in individuals who have had the device implanted for secondary prevention of sudden death. Other patients who have had devices implanted for primary prevention with appropriate ICD therapy are also considered at higher risk that those without therapy. It is evident that ICD malfunction with failure to pace would put pacemaker-dependent patients at particular risk [3,4].

Rarely, the patient's initial indication for ICD placement no longer exists and it is clinically appropriate to program tachycardia detection and therapies off without replacing the device. When an indication for an ICD still exists, the ICD under advisory or recall should selectively be replaced based on several considerations. It is evident that the decision to replace an ICD or lead that is recalled but continues to function normally needs to be made on a case-by-case basis with careful consideration of the risks and benefits. Guidance from regulatory agencies, the device or lead manufacturer, and professional organizations is commonly provided [1–4]. However, in each patient the best available evidence, patient preference, and the risks and benefits of all management options need to be factored in to clinical decision-making.

In individuals with an ICD placed for secondary prevention or an ICD placed for primary prevention with a clinically appropriate shock, the probability of future device therapy for ventricular tachycardia or fibrillation is greater. This needs to be carefully considered in the decision to continue to monitor device function or replace the device [5]. In patients who are truly pacemaker dependent, failure of pacing can have life-threatening consequences. If a device has demonstrated failure and there is a continued indication for the ICD, replacement in a timely fashion is warranted. Any device or lead under advisory or recall or found to be functioning in an abnormal fashion should be returned to the manufacturer and reported to the FDA. This will allow investigation of the cause and frequency of failure. This information serves to improve monitoring strategies and improve future devices [1,2].

When an ICD or lead is subject to recall or is demonstrated to malfunction there are several other responsibilities of the physician including direct communication with the patient [1,2]. This should be carried out in a clear, concise, timely fashion. The communication should include explanation of the problem and provide guidance regarding management strategies. Manufacturers do contact patients independently of physicians. Accordingly, it is important to contact the patient directly with a discussion of their specific risk

and benefits of management strategies. A standardized Physician Device Advisory Notification form and Patient Device Advisory Notification letter provides guidance on the information that should be included in the letters regarding the lead recall [1].

Formal decision models to evaluate the risks and benefits associated with immediate device or lead replacement compared with continued monitoring have been developed and can be a useful resource [3,4]. The goal of these decision-making tools is to compare the risk of complications associated with device or lead replacement with doing nothing [3,4]. Several variables are considered including indications for device or lead implantation, anticipated course following device or lead failure, device failure rates from the recall ranging from 0.0001% to 1.0% per year. The device replacement mortality rates range from 0.10% to 1.00% per procedure [3,4]. The main factors influencing the decision to replace a device or lead were found to be the impact of device failure or lead estimated device failure rate [3,4]. The procedural mortality rate also marginally contributes but the remaining generator life and patient's age had no effect on the decision to replace a device [3,4]. For pacemaker-dependent patients, a failure rate in excess of 0.3% warrants device replacement and in all other patients, a failure rate of 3% is needed to favor device replacement [3,4]. In patients where device replacement can be avoided, physicians should increase follow-up monitoring in order to identify device failure early [3,4]. When appropriate, device reprogramming should be performed to minimize the risks associated with device failure including inappropriate ICD shocks [3,4].

Management of Lead Recall or Failure

There are many factors that merit consideration by the clinician when an ICD lead has been recalled or is not functioning normally (Table 22.3) [2–4]. Patients who have had a failed ICD lead should have tachycardia therapies deactivated if there is any risk of unnecessary or inappropriate shock or failure to detect and deliver appropriate therapy [2–4]. Typically, such patients are kept in an inpatient facility with continuous monitoring to ensure their safety until a final management strategy is developed and implemented. Decision-making with recalled or malfunctioning leads is more complex than with ICDs [2–4]. The options for patients with recalled but normally functioning leads are intensified monitoring of lead with remote monitoring, with activation of lead alerts that could identify a problem at an early stage [5]. Other options include replacement of

Table 22.3 Clinician recommendations for managing lead recall.

Clinician recommendations/implanting physician responsibilities

- Lead and generator longevity expectations and the potential for lead failure should be discussed with patients at the time of implant as a part of the consent process
- Implanting physicians must have a database of all patients with devices and leads implanted and model numbers
- Implanting facilities and physicians should monitor local outcomes and adverse events
- Implanting physicians must be able to maintain up to date with FDA recalls and advisories
- Implanting facilities should have the capabilities to perform remote monitoring, interpretation of data, and make device setting changes as necessary
- Implanting facilities should have the infrastructure and support to be able to contact each patient in the event of a lead recall. Communication with each patient should be performed verbally and in writing
- Healthcare professionals should report documented or suspected lead failures to the manufacturers and regulatory authority and all explanted leads or lead fragments should be returned to the manufacturer for analysis
- Direct physician patient contact should be performed via telephone, letter, or preferably in person when a lead recall has been established

Table 22.4 Patient and lead factors when considering lead revision.

Factors to consider in the risk–benefit analysis when managing normally functioning leads subject to advisory

Patient	Pacemaker dependence
	Prior history of ventricular arrhythmia
	Patient prognosis
	Risk of future arrhythmia
	Surgical risk of revision/replacement procedure
	Patient anxiety about lead failure
	Impending battery depletion
Lead	Rate of abnormal performance (observed or projected in advisory lead)
	Lead failure rates
	Malfunction characteristics (gradual vs. sudden, predictable vs. unpredictable)
	Identified lead subset with higher failure rate
	Malfunction mechanism known or understood
	Adverse clinical consequences of lead failure
	Availability of reprogramming to mitigate clinical risk
	Availability of algorithms for early detection of lead abnormality

the lead without extraction or extraction of the existing lead under recall and placement of a new lead. A final option includes placement of a pace/sense lead while leaving the high voltage shock lead in place. Recently, another option has evolved with placement of a subcutaneous ICD (S-ICD). While these devices do not have the capacity to provide pacing, they can be used safely with a pacemaker implanted with conventional transvenous bipolar leads. It is evident that for leads that are demonstrated to have a malfunction, the option of intensified monitoring is removed and the clinician should choose from among the other management strategies [1–5].

There are some clinicians who advocate extraction and replacement of all leads that are recalled or have demonstrated failure. Among the arguments advanced to support this practice is that the presence of multiple leads is associated with an increased risk of subclavian vein and superior vena cava obstruction, stenosis, or occlusion. Other arguments include an increased risk of infection and a risk of lead–lead interaction if the lead is abandoned and a second lead placed. Additionally, it is generally accepted that the risk associated with lead extraction increases with time with lead maturation in the vascular system. For every 3 years of implant duration, the risk of failed extraction increases twofold and the risk of major adverse outcome increases three- to fourfold if there are multiple RV leads or old leads. Lead extraction, however, is not a benign procedure.

Even when performed at high volume centers, the risk of major complication is approximately 2% and risk of death is 0.5%. Accordingly, decisions related to the strategy of lead extraction and replacement versus lead replacement without extraction need to be carefully considered. There should be particular emphasis on the expertise of the physician and experience of the center related to lead extraction. Other factors that should be considered in making clinical decision regarding how to best manage patients with recalled of malfunctioning leads are noted in Table 22.4. These include many of the same considerations for recalled or malfunctioned ICDs. However, lead characteristics merit careful consideration. These include the age and model of the lead, type of recall/failure mechanism, and failure rates.

The risk of adverse event as a result of this recall and the availability of monitoring techniques to detect early failure and reduce that risk of adverse patient outcomes [5]. When there is an option of following an ICD or lead that is functioning normally, a specific protocol for intensified monitoring should be developed and implemented [5]. Remote monitoring allows for frequent automated secure information retrieval thereby decreasing the necessity of frequent office visits. Manufacturer's recommendations should be followed carefully [5]. Examples of an algorithm developed to enhance monitoring include the Lead Integrity Alert (LIA) to detect early signals of failure of the Medtronic Fidelis lead. This algorithm is a software download into the ICD which recognizes lead failure early and minimizes the risk of shocks. For activation, two of three criteria need to be met within a 60 day period:

1) Abnormal RV lead impedance;
2) Two or more high rate sensed intervals shorter than 220 ms;
3) At least 30 short V-V interval counts within 3 days.

Once the criteria are met, the device will sound an alarm immediately from the ICD and every 4 hours. This notification and the device diagnostics will also be transmitted via remote monitoring for appropriate action by the following physician. In addition, the device will extend its detection algorithm by increasing the number of intervals needed to detect VT/VF to 30/40, therefore further minimizing inappropriate shocks. In a randomized prospective trial, when compared with standard monitoring, there was a 50% relative risk reduction in the number of patients receiving >5 shocks in the LIA group. Of patients in the LIA arm, 72% had no shocks or at least 3 days of warning before the first shock compared to 50% of those with standard monitoring.

Other device manufacturers have also developed similar programs to minimize the risk of shocks. St. Jude Medical has developed the SecureSense Lead Noise Discrimination algorithm, which provides the ability to withhold tachycardia therapy in the presence of lead noise for their Riata lead. This algorithm works by comparing the bipolar ventricular electrogram with the far field electrogram. If short cycle length events are present on the bipolar channel but not the far field channel, the algorithm classifies that as noise and delays or withholds therapy. An alert can also be programmed to notify the patient and physician if this occurs. When this algorithm was studied, with the algorithm on, 100% of true ventricular fibrillation episodes were detected, 97% of sustained RV lead noise was detected, and 90.5% of non-sustained RV lead noise was detected. The moment a device alert is activated, the patient should present for a thorough ICD interrogation to assess the integrity of the lead. Physicians undertake a comprehensive evaluation of the alert and determine whether there is true failure and the mechanism of failure. If lead or device failure is confirmed, tachycardia therapies should be deactivated and the patient monitored until a disposition is determined.

Routine fluoroscopy of recalled leads has been recommended by some manufacturers to guide management decisions but remains controversial. The Riata lead has shown a tendency to develop insulation defects and externalization of conductors. Not all leads with externalized conductors noted by flouroscopy demonstrate electrical abnormalities and some leads, which appear fluoroscopically normal, have failed. However, it has been demonstrated that leads with externalized cables have a 25% failure rate compared with only 6% in fluoroscopically normal leads. Therefore, in select cases where the risk of lead failure may alter the physician's management strategy, having fluoroscopic data can be valuable. Decisions regarding normally functioning leads which demonstrate externalized conductors assume particular importance at the time of device replacement.

To determine if lead revision is appropriate, one must balance the risk of lead failure in each individual patient with the risk of revising a lead. Patients should be categorized as high, intermediate, or low risk (Table 22.5). The main factors contributing to the decision-making should be pacemaker dependence and ICD placement for sudden cardiac death. Other patient factors include prior tachyarrhythmia therapy, patient's preference, and the patient's surgical risk. Lead characteristics are also important, including the rate and mechanism of failure, the clinical consequences of failure, and the presence of programs and algorithms to detect failure early and minimize adverse events [2]. For example, in the case of the Fidelis lead, there have been several reports indicating a high failure rate at the time of or soon after ICD generator change, with 21% failure rate within 1 year of generator change. This may argue for prophylactic revision of the lead at the time of generator change, but all patient and lead factors should be carefully considered before a management decision is made. If a decision to revise the lead is established, the managing physician should decide between several management options based on his or her individual and center's expertise [2].

Table 22.5 Recommendations for managing lead advisories.

Conservative non-invasive management with periodic device monitoring should be strongly considered particularly for:

- Patients who are not pacemaker dependent
- Patients with an ICD for primary prevention of sudden cardiac death who have not required device therapy for a ventricular arrhythmia
- Patients whose operative risk is high or patients who have other significant competing morbidities even when the risk of lead malfunction or patient harm is substantial

Lead revision or replacement should be considered if in the clinician's judgment:

- The risk of malfunction is likely to lead to patient death or serious harm; *and*
- The risk of revision or replacement is believed to be less than the risk of patient harm from the lead malfunction

Reprogramming of the pacemaker or ICD should be performed when this can mitigate the risk of an adverse event from lead malfunction

Conclusions

ICD and lead failures and recalls represent a clinical challenge for manufacturers, regulatory agencies, professional organizations, physicians, and patients. While there is a shared responsibility of manufacturers, regulatory agencies, and healthcare professionals participating in the care of patients with these cardiac rhythm management devices, ultimately management decisions are made by the physician. Recent recommendations for timely detection, characterization, communication, and correction of product performance issues serve to guide the management process. While a systematic approach should be taken to ICD and lead recalls and failure, the physician must remain mindful that every patient is unique and an individualized management strategy is important. Robust ICD software algorithms now allow early detection of performance problems with recalled ICDs or leads through remote monitoring. Physicians and other healthcare professionals participating in the care of patients with ICDs have responsibilities related to communication with the manufacturers, regulatory agencies, and patients. Reporting all relevant data related to ICD and lead malfunction and recall data in their patients is a responsibility that will improve future management decisions and ICD and lead reliability.

References

1 Carlson M, Wilkoff B, Ellenbogen K, Carlson MD, Ellenbogen KA, Saxon LA, *et al.* Recommendations from the Heart Rhythm Society Task Force on Device Performance Policies and Guidelines. Heart Rhythm 2006:10;1250–1273.

2 Maisel W, Hauser R, Hammill S, Hauser RG, Ellenbogen KA, Epstein AE, *et al.* Recommendations from the Hearth Rhythm Society Task Force on Lead Performance Policies and Guidelines. Heart Rhythm 2009;6:869–885.

3 Amin M, Matchar D, Wood M, Ellenbogen K. Management of recalled pacemakers and implantable cardioverter-defibrillators. JAMA 2006;296;4:412–420.

4 Burri H, Combescure C. Management of recalled implantable cardioverter-defibrillator leads at generator replacement: a decision analysis model for Fidelis leads. Europace 2014;16(8):1210–1217.

5 Resnic FS, Gross TP, Marinac-Dabic D, Loyo-Berrios N, Donnelly S, Normand SL, *et al.* Automated surveillance to detect postprocedure safety signals of approved cardiovascular devices. JAMA 2010;304:2019–2027.

23

How to Program an ICD to Minimize Inappropriate Shocks

Paul J. Wang and Winston B. Joe

Stanford University School of Medicine, Stanford, CA, USA

Implantable cardioverter-defibrillators (ICDs) have become a dominant strategy in the prevention of sudden cardiac death. While there is substantial evidence supporting the benefit of ICD implantation in patients at high risk for sudden cardiac death, there is also evidence to suggest that ICD shock therapy may have adverse effects on health outcomes, quality of life, and mortality. To optimize the risk–benefit ratio of ICD therapy, it is essential to minimize ICD shocks for rhythms other than clinically relevant ventricular tachycardia (VT) or ventricular fibrillation (VF). A meta-analysis of large clinical trials identified high rates of inappropriate shock (10–24% during 20–45 month follow-up) [1]. Recent expansion of ICD indications to include primary prevention may increase the proportion of inappropriate shocks to appropriate shocks.

This chapter describes strategies for prevention of inappropriate ICD discharge, including optimization of programmable settings, pharmacologic suppression of arrhythmias, and prophylactic catheter ablation. The most common causes of so-called inappropriate therapy include sinus tachycardia or supraventricular arrhythmias above the rate cutoff, oversensing of lead noise, electromagnetic interference, T waves, and QRS double counting. There are steps that address many of these causes collectively or individually. Programming options such as increasing the rate cutoff and increasing duration, for example, can be used to prevent most of these causes. Other algorithms can be used to prevent T-wave oversensing or to reject lead related noise. A combination of these algorithms can be used to reduce the incidence of inappropriate therapy.

Programming

The fundamental criterion used by all ICDs is a detected rate above the programmed rate cutoff for the programmed duration. Other programmable features vary among single, dual, and subcutaneous ICDs [2].

Rate Cutoff and Duration

Selection of the appropriate rate for initial detection of VT is a balance between the potential to underdetect some slower VTs and the prevention of detecting and treating many of the causes of inappropriate therapy [3]. In addition, lengthening the detection duration may allow transient arrhythmias to self-terminate and reduce the likelihood of non-essential shocks. Supraventricular tachycardia (SVT) discriminators were included in these studies and thus the independent contribution of SVT discriminators is difficult to ascertain.

Multiple studies have investigated the effect of increasing the rate cutoff and extended duration on inappropriate therapy. The EMPIRIC (Comparison of Empiric to Physician-Tailored Programming of Implantable Cardioverter Defibrillators) trial, which compared standardized ICD settings to physician-tailored settings with respect to shock-related morbidity, illustrates the potential value of shorter cycle lengths for VT detection. In this study, the intervention arm utilized VT detection at 150 beats per minute (bpm) with 16 beat duration, a Fast VT detection at 200 bpm with 18 out of 24 intervals, and VF detection at 250 bpm with 18 of 24 intervals. The time to first shock was non-inferior in the intervention arm with a reduction of patients with five or more shocks. There was no significant difference in total mortality, syncope, emergency room visits, or unscheduled outpatient visits. There was a reduction in the number of the unscheduled hospitalizations in the intervention arm [4,5].

The ability of rate-cutoff settings to reduce inappropriate therapy was also investigated in the MADIT-RIT (Multicenter Automatic Defibrillator Implantation Trial to Reduce Inappropriate Therapy) study, a randomized prospective study in primary prevention ICD patients. In MADIT-RIT, patients were randomized to one of three groups:

1) High-rate therapy (detection at ≥200 bpm with a 2.5-s delay to therapy);
2) Delayed therapy (60-second delay at 170–199 bpm, 12-s delay at 200–249 bpm, and 2.5-s delay at ≥250 bpm); and
3) Conventional therapy (2.5-second delay at 170–199 bpm and 1-s delay at ≥200 bpm).

Groups with high rate-cutoff limits and longer delays to therapy were found to have lower incidence of inappropriate shock therapy and lower overall mortality [4,6]. A subanalysis of the MADIT-RIT trial also demonstrated high-rate cutoff and delayed VT therapy programming were associated with significant reductions in first and total inappropriate and appropriate ICD therapy in patients with ischemic and non-ischemic cardiomyopathy [7].

The PREPARE study was a prospective, cohort control study of 700 patients. The programmed settings in this study included VT monitor at 167 bpm for 32 intervals, Fast VT at 182 bpm for 30 out of 40 beats, and VF at 250 bpm for 30 out of 40 beats duration. ATP was used for regular rhythms from 182 to 250 bpm and SVT discriminators were used for rhythms less than 200 bpm. The comparison cohort consisted of the EMPIRIC trial and MIRACLE ICD. The PREPARE study patients had 8.5% shock rate compared to 16.9% shock rate in the control group [8].

The RELEVANT (Role of Long Detection Window Programming in Patients With Left Ventricular Dysfunction, Non-ischemic Etiology in Primary Prevention Treated With a Biventricular ICD) study randomized patients with non-ischemic cardiomyopathy and ICDs for primary prevention to short (12/16 interval) or long (30/40 interval) detection [9]. In the long detection window cohort, there was a decrease in overall ICD therapy incidence, with 90% of VT/SVT events self-terminating before the end of the detection window [9]. Similarly, the ADVANCE-III Trial found long detection times (30/40) were associated with a 37% reduction in shock and a lower incidence of ATP, but without any significant change in total mortality [10].

A summary of these studies and an additional randomized trial [11] investigating rate and duration settings is provided in Table 23.1.

Despite evidence in favor of longer detection windows, recent data from the US CareLink® Network have identified that 60% of ICDs are left with relatively short nominal number of intervals detected (NID) settings of 18/24 [12]. The above data suggest that selective lengthening of NID settings in these patients may significantly reduce non-essential shocks in the ICD population.

Optimizing SVT Discrimination Algorithms

Algorithms to differentiate SVT from VT have an important role in minimizing inappropriate therapy because arrhythmias may have a rate that exceeds the programmed detection rate [4]. Without such algorithms, therapy would be delivered whenever the rate criteria are met. Although increasing the rate cut and detection duration may decrease inappropriate therapy, frequently atrial fibrillation (AF) is conducted very rapidly. In fact, AF and other SVTs are responsible for up to 79% of inappropriate therapy [13]. SVT/VT discrimination algorithms are particularly important in secondary prevention ICD patients and those taking antiarrhythmic agents. In such patients, the rate cut may be set at a lower rate and thus SVT and VT rates are more likely to overlap [2].

These discrimination algorithms can decrease inappropriate therapy delivered for supraventricular arrhythmias [14]. There are a number of algorithms that can be used in all devices, including single and dual-chamber ICDs. The *sudden-onset* detection algorithm, for example, recognizes abrupt changes in RR interval that occur in VT but not in sinus tachycardia. While capable of differentiating sinus tachycardia from VT at the lower boundary of VT detection, sudden-onset differentiation has a number of associated shortcomings. VT events that occur during an episode of sinus tachycardia or SVT or in the presence of ventricular ectopy can inappropriately avert shocks by misidentifying them as SVT. Abrupt onset AF with rapid ventricular response may also be misclassified as VT and result in inappropriate shocks [2]. Sinus tachycardia is gradual in onset, so the sudden onset detection algorithm is quite effective in suppressing therapy for sinus tachycardia. However, as other rhythms are usually sudden in onset, additional algorithms are usually necessary.

One such algorithm, *stability*, relies on the stable RR interval associated with VT to discriminate VT from AF but is not generally useful in preventing therapy for other supraventricular arrhythmias. This algorithm is continually applied throughout the arrhythmia so that any VT without initial RR variability will still be classified as VT, so long as the RR interval stabilizes over time [2]. Therapy

Table 23.1 Summary of rate cut and duration optimization studies.

Trial name	Year results published	Study size	Study design	Investigated parameters	Findings
EMPIRIC	2006	900	RCT	Rate cut	Cohort with shorter rate-cutoff faired better with respect to avoidance of inappropriate shock in initial duration of 12 month follow-up
RELEVANT	2009	324	Observational	Duration	Fixed long detection windows reduced ICD therapy burden and HF hospitalizations without entailing additional syncope or death
ADVANCE-III	2013	1902	RCT	Duration	Extended detection windows led to lower rates of shock due to self-termination of non-sustained arrhythmias
MADIT-RIT	2012	1500	RCT	Rate cut, duration	Significant reduction in inappropriate therapy in high-rate and delayed-therapy groups. Additional reduction in all-cause mortality in the high-rate group and a reduction that trended toward significance in the delayed-therapy group
PROVIDE	2013	1670	RCT	Rate cut, duration, SVT discriminators, ATP for fast VT	Combination of high rate-cutoff, long detection duration, SVT discriminators, and aggressive ATP results in significant reductions in appropriate and inappropriate shock
PREPARE	2008	1391	Observational	Rate cut, duration, ATP for fast VT	Reduced therapy for NSVT, ATP eliminates 75% of shocks for fast VT

ADVANCE III, Avoid Delivering Therapies for Non-sustained Arrhythmias in ICD Patients III; ATP antitachycardia pacing therapy; EMPIRIC, Comparison of Empiric to Physician-Tailored Programming of ICDs; ICD, implantable cardioverter-defibrillator; MADIT-RIT, Multicenter Automatic Defibrillator Implantation Trial-Reduce Inappropriate Therapy; NSVT non-sustained ventricular tachycardia; PROVIDE, Programming Implantable Cardioverter-Defibrillators in Patients with Primary Prevention Indication to Prolong Time to First Shock; RCT, randomized controlled trial; RELEVANT, Role of Long Detection Window Programming in Patients With Left Ventricular Dysfunction, Nonischemic Etiology in Primary Prevention Treated with a Biventricular ICD; SVT, supraventricular tachycardia; VT, ventricular fibrillation.

may still be delivered for rhythms where RR interval variation is minimal such as rapid AF, atrial flutter, and regular SVTs despite the stability algorithm. While it is possible for episodes of VT with irregular RR intervals to have therapy withheld, this occurrence is not common.

There are several forms of the *morphology discrimination* (MD) algorithm. A real time electrogram morphology during the tachycardia is compared with a previously obtained sinus rhythm template. If the morphology of the complexes during the tachycardia differs from the sinus template by a programmed threshold or percentage, the rhythm is designated as VT. The MD algorithm generally is felt to have greater sensitivity (92–99%) and specificity (90–97%) than onset and stability algorithms [4]. Nevertheless, MD algorithms occasionally result in misclassification errors and unnecessary ICD shocks. For strategies to address these misclassification errors see Table 23.2.

Table 23.2 Correcting morphology discriminator misclassifications.

Origin of MD misclassification	Correction strategy
SVT with rate-related aberrancies	Set automatic template updating to "off" and acquire new template while pacing in the AAI mode at rate sufficient to capture any aberrancy. For non-reproducible aberrancies, reduce fraction of electrogram required to exceed match threshold [14]
EGM misalignment or truncation	May be avoided with appropriate electrogram source selection and gain adjustment [2]
Myopotential distortion	Near-field electrogram for MD prevents pectoral myopotential oversensing [14]
Lead maturation or bundle branch block	Acquire new templates periodically to update changes in sinus EGM, if automatic template updates cannot be obtained, avoid use of MD until completion of lead maturation (3 months post-implantation) [2,14]

AAI, atrial demand pacing; EGM, electrogram; MD, morphology discrimination algorithm; SVT, supraventricular tachycardia.

Single and Dual-Chamber ICDs

Single-chamber ICD algorithms rely on interval and morphology-based ventricular electrogram information to differentiate between SVT and VT [2,4]. Dual-chamber ICDs benefit from information gathered from the atrial channel. While a number of studies demonstrate that dual-chamber ICDs may result in a lower incidence

of inappropriate therapy, this effect is not uniform and may be relatively modest in size [15–18]. For example, Friedman *et al.* [19] found that routine implantation of dual-chamber ICDs for primary prevention increased cost without improvements in quality of life or reductions in inappropriate therapy. However, the OPTION (Optimal Anti-Tachycardia Therapy in Implantable Cardioverter-Defibrillator Patients Without Pacing Indications) study demonstrated that dual-chamber ICDs can reduce the risk for inappropriate shock when used in combination with algorithms for minimizing ventricular pacing [20]. Some of the factors that limit the benefit of dual-chamber algorithms include atrial undersensing or atrial signals falling in blanking periods. In addition, there may be episodes misclassified as atrial tachycardia events because of far-field sensing of the R wave on the atrial channel [2,4].

Programmable Therapeutic Settings

Anti-tachycardia Pacing

ATP terminates re-entrant ventricular tachycardia by pacing at faster than the VT rates, depolarizing re-entrant tissue in the excitable gap, and terminating re-entry [21]. ATP has been shown to terminate 60–90% of VT episodes and has displaced defibrillation as the primary therapy administered by ICDs [4,8,22,23]. Acceleration to fast VT (FVT) follows ATP in only 1–5% of episodes. VTs of short cycle lengths, the nature of the arrhythmogenic substrate, the use of anti-arrhythmic drugs, and the ATP protocol used are factors associated with acceleration to FVT [22].

ATP can be delivered as a train or burst, where the interval between consecutive stimuli is fixed, or as a ramp in which the interval between consecutive stimuli sequentially shortens. While burst and ramp settings appear to be equally effective for slow VT, burst pacing is less likely than ramp pacing to result in VT acceleration in the setting of FVTs [24].

Therapy Zones

Modern ICDs allow for the programming of one to three zones for VT detection and monitoring. A tachycardia must have a high enough rate to fall into these zones in order for the ICD to deliver ATP or shock. In the highest rate zone, there is usually only shock therapy, or shock therapy and one ATP train. If a second rate zone is used, more ATP trains may be employed. For patients with slower VTs (usually less than 240 bpm), more than one ATP trains are usually selected.

Recently, the RISSY-ICD (Reduction of Inappropriate ShockS bY InCreaseD zones) trial found that simple adjustments to zone boundaries could significantly diminish the likelihood of non-essential shock. In this study, Cay *et al.* [25] randomized 223 primary prevention patients into a three-zone programming group with conventional boundary programming, or a high-zone programming group in which the lower limit of each of the three zones was increased. High-zone settings were associated with reductions in non-essential shocks with no adverse effects on mortality.

Sensing Optimization

T-Wave Oversensing

T-wave oversensing (TWOS) can lead to inappropriate shock therapy. TWOS is most commonly associated with low amplitude R waves (<3 mV) as well as hypertrophic cardiomyopathy with resultant high-amplitude T waves, electrolyte abnormalities such as hyperglycemia and hyperkalemia, medications such as histamine-2 receptor blockers, injury current-related increase in the T-wave voltage, and changes in sympathetic tone [26]. Device-specific filtering characteristics and programmable settings can influence the occurrence of TWOS. Decreasing ventricular sensitivity to minimize TWOS is feasible only in patients with sufficiently large R : T ratios and adequate R-wave amplitude and is thus not the preferred strategy [2]. Both St. Jude and Biotronik ICDs allow for altering the initial value, onset time, and slope of sensitivity algorithm after a sensed QRS. Biotronik devices also increase high-pass filtering to decrease TWOS. The TWOS algorithm in Medtronic Protecta ICDs compares outputs from the standard sense amplifier with output using a differential high-pass filter [4].

Lead Fracture Surveillance

In some cases, lead fracture manifests as sudden changes in lead impedance and noise detection which may result in sensed VT. Early recognition of lead injury may therefore decrease the risk of inappropriate shock [4]. Medtronic's Lead Integrity Alert (LIA) and Lead Noise Oversensing Algorithms are capable of alerting patient and physician to the presence of lead failure. The efficacy of LIA in preventing unnecessary shocks has been validated in a number of studies [27,28]. Lead Noise Oversensing algorithms compare near and far-field electrogram amplitudes to help identify lead and connection problems. Incongruities in peak-to-peak amplitudes on far- versus near-field signals indicate that amplitude measurement windows are sensing both R waves and isoelectric potentials caused by lead or connection issues [4].

Noise Protection Algorithms

Noise protection algorithms distinguish electromagnetic interference from myocardial activation. The primary challenge is to continue to detect the rapid signal rates of VF. Boston Scientific's Dynamic Noise Algorithm uses noise frequency and power approximation to identify electromechanical interference. Once this determination has been made, the algorithm raises a dynamic sensing floor above the noise amplitude to prevent oversensing and likelihood of inappropriate ICD therapy [4].

Overall Reduction in Inappropriate Therapy

Using a combination of these algorithms, a significant reduction in inappropriate therapy can be achieved. In a series of over 2500 patients, the inappropriate shock rate at 1 year was 2.5% for single-chamber devices and 1.5% for dual or triple-chamber devices [23].

Pharmacologic Considerations

Antiarrhythmic medications can prevent both appropriate and inappropriate shock in ICD patients by suppressing atrial and ventricular arrhythmias, slowing the rates of VTs, and allowing for broader application of ATP [29]. In the OPTIC (Optimal Pharmacological Therapy in Implantable Cardioverter Defibrillator Patients) trial, combined beta blocker–amiodarone therapy in ICD patients resulted in a 75% reduction in number of patients experiencing ICD discharge at 1 year [30].

While tailored antiarrhythmic therapy may reduce ICD shock, the benefits of class III antiarrhythmic

therapy must be weighed against risks and adverse effects on a case-to-case basis. Interestingly, some studies have shown that sotalol does not significantly reduce the risk of shock when compared with other beta blockers alone [30,31]. In a sub-analysis of the MADIT-CRT Trial, carvedilol, as opposed to metoprolol, reduced the risk of inappropriate ATP and shock [32].

Catheter Ablation

Catheter ablation can minimize inappropriate shock therapy but the data are somewhat limited.

The frequent association between episodic SVT and inappropriate ICD shock suggests that prophylactic ablation of SVTs may be an important potential option for ICD patients. Mainigi *et al.* [33] found that 95% of ICD patients with SVT had no further inappropriate ICD shocks after catheter ablation of SVT. In patients who received multiple ICD discharges because of rapid AF or atrial flutter, successful AVN modification reduced shock frequency [34]. In a study of 22 patients with ICD discharge caused by atrial tachycardia, inappropriate shocks did not occur at a mean follow-up of 19 months after SVT ablation [35].

Table 23.3 Potential rate cut and duration programming.

MADIT-RIT Parameters

Arm	Zone	Rate/duration	Therapy
High-Rate Arm	1	$\geq$170 bpm	Monitor
	2	$\geq$200 bpm for 2.5 s	Shock + Quick Convert ATP
Duration-Delay Arm	1	$\geq$170 bpm for 60 s	ATP + Shock
	2	$\geq$200 bpm for 12 s	ATP + Shock
	3	$\geq$250 bpm for 2.5 s	Shock + Quick Convert ATP

PREPARE Parameters

Detection	Rate/duration	Therapy
VT (monitor)	$\geq$167 bpm for 32 beats	None
FVT (via VF)	$\geq$182 bpm for 30 of 40 beats	Burst (1 sequence), 30–35 J (max output) × 5
VF (on)	$\geq$250 bpm for 30 of 40 beats	30–35 J (max output) × 6

ATP, antitachycardia pacing; bpm, beats per minute; J, joules; VF, ventricular fibrillation; VT, ventricular tachycardia. Additional MADIT-RIT parameters: For Zones 1 and 2 of the duration-delay arm, set Rhythm ID Detection Enhancement ON; Additional PREPARE parameters: Supraventricular tachycardia criteria on (dual chamber, biventricular implantable cardioverter-defibrillator): atrial fibrillation/flutter, sinus tachycardia (1 : 1 VT-ST boundary = 66%), supraventricular tachycardia criteria on (single chamber): wavelet morphology discrimination (match threshold = 70%), supraventricular tachycardia limit = 300 ms, burst antitachycardia pacing: 8 intervals, pacing cycle length = 88% of tachycardia cycle length.

Subcutaneous ICD

The entirely subcutaneous implantable cardioverter-defibrillator (S-ICD) is a new alternative to transvenous implantable cardioverter-defibrillators (TV-ICDs). The EFFORTLESS (Boston Scientific Post Market S-ICD Registry) trial and the IDE (S-ICD System IDE Clinical Investigation) study showed that the incidence of inappropriate shocks is reduced with the addition of discriminators [36].

Conclusions

Inappropriate ICD shocks have a negative impact on quality of life. Increased rate-cutoffs with or without increased duration have been shown to reduce inappropriate therapy. Specific algorithms can be used to differentiate SVT from VT. ATP therapy may reduce overall shock incidence. A reduction in inappropriate shock therapy may decrease patient morbidity and mortality, and measures should be taken to minimize therapy unless absolutely necessary [29,37–41].

Guide to Programming

For primary prevention ICDs, select a rate-off and duration similar to that used in the MADIT-RIT trial or PREPARE study. These parameters are summarized in Table 23.3. SVT discriminators should be programmed on. ATP should be programmed on for the VT zone as well as for the VF zone if possible. Additionally, if available, lead integrity algorithms should be programmed on. If evidence of TWOS exists, program TWOS algorithm on.

References

1 Germano JJ, Reynolds M, Essebag V, Josephson ME. Frequency and causes of implantable cardioverter-defibrillator therapies: is device therapy proarrhythmic? Am J Cardiol 2006;97(8):1255–1261.

2 Madhavan M, Friedman PA. Optimal programming of implantable cardiac-defibrillators. Circulation 2013;128(6):659–672.

3 Mansour F, Khairy P. Programming ICDs in the modern era beyond out-of-the box settings. Pacing Clin Electrophysiol 2011;34(4):506–520.

4 Koneru JN, Swerdlow CD, Wood MA, Ellenbogen KA. Minimizing inappropriate or "unnecessary" implantable cardioverter-defibrillator shocks: appropriate programming. Circ Arrhythm Electrophysiol 2011;4(5):778–790.

5 Wilkoff BL, Ousdigian KT, Sterns LD, Wang ZJ, Wilson RD, Morgan JM. A comparison of empiric to physician-tailored programming of implantable cardioverter-defibrillators: results from the prospective randomized multicenter EMPIRIC trial. J Am Coll Cardiol 2006;48(2):330–339.

6 Moss AJ, Schuger C, Beck CA, Brown MW, Cannom DS, Daubert JP, *et al.* Reduction in inappropriate therapy and mortality through ICD programming. N Engl J Med 2012;367(24):2275–2283.

7 Sedlacek K, Ruwald AC, Kutyifa V, McNitt S, Thomsen PE, Klein H, *et al.* The effect of ICD programming on inappropriate and appropriate ICD therapies in ischemic and nonischemic cardiomyopathy: the MADIT-RIT trial. J Cardiovasc Electrophysiol 2015;26(4):424–433.

8 Wilkoff BL, Williamson BD, Stern RS, Moore SL, Lu F, Lee SW, *et al.* Strategic programming of detection and therapy parameters in implantable cardioverter-defibrillators reduces shocks in primary prevention patients: results from the PREPARE (Primary Prevention Parameters Evaluation) study. J Am Coll Cardiol 2008;12(52(7)):541–550.

9 Gasparini M, Menozzi C, Proclemer A, Landolina M, Iacopino S, Carboni A, *et al.* A simplified biventricular defibrillator with fixed long detection intervals reduces implantable cardioverter defibrillator (ICD) interventions and heart failure hospitalizations in patients with non-ischaemic cardiomyopathy implanted for primary prevention: the RELEVANT [role of long detection window programming in patients with left ventricular dysfunction, non-ischemic etiology in primary prevention treated with a biventricular ICD] study. Eur Heart J 2009;30(22):2758–2767.

10 Gasparini M, Proclemer A, Klersy C, Kloppe A, Lunati M, Ferrer JB, *et al.* Effect of long-detection interval vs standard-detection interval for implantable cardioverter-defibrillators on antitachycardia pacing and shock delivery: the ADVANCE III randomized clinical trial. JAMA 2013;309:1903–1911.

11 Saeed M, Hanna I, Robotis D, Styperek R, Polosajian L, Khan A, *et al.* Programming implantable cardioverter-defibrillators in patients with primary prevention indication to prolong time to first shock: results from the PROVIDE study. J Cardiovasc Electrophysiol 2014;25:52–59.

12 Medtronic CareLink Database. Accessed July 2012.

13 Daubert JP, Zareba W, Cannom DS, McNitt S, Rosero SZ, Wang P, *et al.* Inappropriate implantable cardioverter-defibrillator shocks in MADIT II: frequency, mechanisms, predictors, and survival impact. J Am Coll Cardiol 2008;51(14):1357–1365.

14 Gard JJ, Friedman PA. Strategies to reduce ICD shocks: the role of supraventricular tachycardia-ventricular tachycardia discriminators. Card Electrophysiol Clin 2011;3:373–387.

15 Kuhlkamp V, Dornberger V, Mewis C, Suchalla R, Bosch RF, Seipel L. Clinical experience with the new detection algorithms for atrial fibrillation of a defibrillator with dual chamber sensing and pacing. J Cardiovasc Electrophysiol 1999;10:905–915.

16 Deisenhofer I, Kolb C, Ndrepepa G, Schreieck J, Karch M, Schmieder S, *et al.* Do current dual chamber cardioverter defibrillators have advantages over conventional single chamber cardioverter defibrillators in reducing inappropriate therapies? A randomized, prospective study. J Cardiovasc Electrophysiol 2001;12:134–142.

17 Theuns DA, Klootwijk AP, Goedhart DM, Jordaens LJ. Prevention of inappropriate therapy in implantable cardioverter-defibrillators: results of a prospective, randomized study of tachyarrhythmia detection algorithms. J Am Coll Cardiol 2004;44:2362–2367.

18 Friedman PA, McClelland RL, Bamlet WR, Acosta H, Kessler D, Munger TM, *et al.* Dual-chamber versus single-chamber detection enhancements for implantable defibrillator rhythm diagnosis: the Detect SupraVentricular Tachycardia study. Circulation 2006;113:2871–289.

19 Friedman PA, Bradley D, Koestler C, Slusser J, Hodge D, Bailey K, *et al.* A prospective randomized trial of single- or dual-chamber implantable cardioverter-defibrillators to minimize inappropriate shock risk in primary sudden cardiac death prevention. Europace 2014;16(10):1460–1468.

20 Kolb C, Sturmer M, Sick P, Reif S, Davy JM, Molon G, *et al.* Reduced risk for inappropriate implantable cardioverter-defibrillator shocks with dual-chamber therapy compared with single-chamber therapy: results of the randomized OPTION study. J Am Coll Cardiol 2014;2(6):611–619.

21 Sweeney MO. Antitachycardia pacing for ventricular tachycardia using implantable cardioverter defibrillators. Pacing Clin Electrophysiol 2004;27(9):1292–1305.

22 Arias MA, Puchol A, Castellanos E, Rodriguez-Padial L. Anti-tachycardia pacing for ventricular tachycardia: good even after being bad. Europace 2007;9(11):1062–1063.

23 Auricchio A, Schloss EJ, Kurita T, Meijer A, Gerritse B, Zweibel S, *et al.* Low inappropriate shock rates in patients with single- and dual/triple-chamber implantable cardioverter-defibrillators using a novel suite of detection algorithms: PainFree SST trial primary results. Heart Rhythm 2015;12(5):926–936.

24 Gulizia MM, Piraino L, Scherillo M, Puntrello C, Vasco C, Scianaro MC, *et al.* A randomized study to compare ramp versus burst antitachycardia pacing therapies to treat fast ventricular tachyarrhythmias in patients with implantable cardioverter defibrillators: the PITAGORA ICD trial. Circ Arrhythm Electrophysiol 2009;2(2):146–153.

25 Cay S, Canpolat U, Ucar F, Ozeke O, Ozcan F, Topaloglu S, *et al.* Programming implantable cardioverter-defibrillator therapy zones to high ranges to prevent delivery of inappropriate device therapies in patients with primary prevention: results from the RISSY-ICD (Reduction of Inappropriate ShockS bY InCreaseD zones) trial. Am J Cardiol 2015;115(9):1235–1243.

26 Srivathsan K, Scott LR, Altemose GT. T-wave oversensing and inappropriate shocks: a case report. Europace 2008;10(5):552–555.

27 Gunderson BD, Swerdlow CD, Wilcox JM, Hayman JE, Ousdigian KT, Ellenbogen KA. Causes of ventricular oversensing in implantable cardioverter-defibrillators: implications for diagnosis of lead fracture. Heart Rhythm 2010;7(5):626–633.

28 Swerdlow CD, Gunderson BD, Ousdigian KT, Abeyratne A, Sachanandani H, Ellenbogen KA. Downloadable software algorithm reduces inappropriate shocks caused by implantable cardioverter-defibrillator lead fractures: a prospective study. Circulation 2010;122(15):1449–1455.

29 Borne RT, Varosy PD, Masoudi FA. Implantable cardioverter-defibrillator shocks: epidemiology, outcomes, and therapeutic approaches. JAMA Intern Med 2013;173(10):859–865.

30 Connolly SJ, Dorian P, Roberts RS, Gent M, Bailin S, Fain ES, *et al.* Comparison of beta-blockers, amiodarone plus beta-blockers, or sotalol for prevention of shocks from implantable cardioverter defibrillators: the OPTIC Study: a randomized trial. JAMA 2006;295(2):165–171.

31 Lee CH, Nam GB, Park HG, Kim HY, Park KM, Kim J, *et al.* Effects of antiarrhythmic drugs on inappropriate shocks in patients with implantable cardioverter defibrillators. Circ J 2008;72(1):102–105.

32 Ruwald MH, Abu-Zeitone A, Jons C, Ruwald AC, McNitt S, Kutyifa V, *et al.* Impact of carvedilol and metoprolol on inappropriate implantable cardioverter-defibrillator therapy: the MADIT-CRT trial (Multicenter Automatic Defibrillator Implantation With Cardiac Resynchronization Therapy). J Am Coll Cardiol 2013;62(15):1343–1350.

33 Mainigi SK, Almuti K, Figueredo VM, Guttenplan NA, Aouthmany A, Smukler J, *et al*. Usefulness of radiofrequency ablation of supraventricular tachycardia to decrease inappropriate shocks from implantable cardioverter-defibrillators. Am J Cardiol 2012;109(2):231–237.

34 Korte T, Niehaus M, Meyer O, Tebbenjohanns J. Prospective evaluation of catheter ablation in patients with implantable cardioverter defibrillators and multiple inappropriate ICD therapies due to atrial fibrillation and type I atrial flutter. Pacing Clin Electrophysiol 2001;24(7):1061–1066.

35 Miyazaki S, Taniguchi H, Kusa S, Komatsu Y, Ichihara N, Takagi T, *et al*. Catheter ablation of atrial tachyarrhythmias causing inappropriate implantable cardioverter-defibrillator shocks. Europace 2015;17(2):289–294.

36 Burke MC, Gold MR, Knight BP, Barr CS, Theuns DA, Boersma LV, *et al*. Safety and efficacy of the totally subcutaneous implantable defibrillator: 2-Year results from a pooled analysis of the IDE Study and EFFORTLESS Registry. J Am Coll Cardiol 2015;65(16):1605–1615.

37 Tan VH, Wilton SB, Kuriachan V, Sumner GL, Exner DV. Impact of programming strategies aimed at reducing nonessential implantable cardioverter defibrillator therapies on mortality: a systematic review and meta-analysis. Circ Arrhythm Electrophysiol 2014;7(1):164–170.

38 Mark DB, Anstrom KJ, Sun JL, Clapp-Channing NE, Tsiatis AA, Davidson-Ray L, *et al*. Quality of life with defibrillator therapy or amiodarone in heart failure. N Engl J Med 2008;359(10):999–1008.

39 Schron EB, Exner DV, Yao Q, Jenkins LS, Steinberg JS, Cook JR, *et al*. Quality of life in the antiarrhythmics versus implantable defibrillators trial: impact of therapy and influence of adverse symptoms and defibrillator shocks. Circulation 2002;105(5):589–594.

40 Poole JE, Johnson GW, Hellkamp AS, Anderson J, Callans DJ, Raitt MH, *et al*. Prognostic importance of defibrillator shocks in patients with heart failure. N Engl J Med 2008;359(10):1009–1017.

41 Moss AJ, Greenberg H, Case RB, Zareba W, Hall WJ, Brown MW, *et al*. Long-term clinical course of patients after termination of ventricular tachyarrhythmia by an implanted defibrillator. Circulation 2004;110(25):3760–3765.

24

How to Perform CRT Optimization

Kevin P. Jackson and James P. Daubert

Division of Clinical Cardiac Electrophysiology, Duke University Medical Center, Durham, NC, USA

Congestive heart failure (CHF) is a resource-intensive and costly chronic disease. Current indications for implantation of cardiac resynchronization therapy (CRT) include the presence of severe cardiomyopathy and evidence of ventricular conduction delay on ECG with symptoms of CHF despite medications. Numerous studies have demonstrated the benefit of CRT in improving cardiovascular hemodynamics, functional capacity, and decreasing mortality. However, up to one-third of patients do not experience any improvement. Patients classified as non-responders to CRT are frequently sent for echocardiographic optimization of the device's atrioventricular (AV) and interventricular (VV) intervals. This chapter reviews the data behind and techniques for CRT optimization.

Defining Response to CRT

The definition of response to CRT has varied across clinical trials and in clinical practice. This has led to a broad range of reported response rates. In one of the early randomized controlled trials of CRT, 34% of patients felt moderately or markedly improved in the control arm compared with 60% in the CRT arm [1]. Improvements in the three co-primary endpoints of New York Heart Association (NYHA) functional class, 6-minute hall walk, and heart failure quality of life (HF QOL), were all superior in the CRT arm but improvement also occurred in these subjective measures in the "placebo" arm. For more objective secondary endpoints such as maximal oxygen consumption (peak VO$_2$) or reduction in left ventricular (LV) end-systolic dimension by echocardiography, the mean improvement in the control arm was negligible. In the MADIT-CRT trial, the non-CRT control group had a mean reduction in LV

echocardiographic end-systolic volume (18 mL), though it was far less than the CRT arm (57 mL) at 1 year compared to the baseline echo [2]. Nevertheless, the placebo effect of CRT and ongoing effects of beta blockers and other medical therapy must be accounted for when considering the response rate attributable to biventricular pacing. When considering the response rates from the large randomized trials of CRT, the percentage non-response varies from about 20–30% for subjective measures as opposed to 30–50% for echocardiographic measures (Figure 24.1) [3,4].

Unfortunately, trials of CRT rarely use the same criteria for response to therapy and agreement is poor amongst the various measures [5]. In a prospective trial of 426 patients undergoing CRT implantation, there was particularly poor agreement of response criteria between subjective or effort-dependent measures (NYHA class or 6-minute walk time) and echocardiographic measures (ejection fraction or LV chamber volumes). Of the 15 most frequently used response criteria in the published literature, the range of reportable response rates was from 32% to 91% depending on the criteria used. Short-term measures associated with long-term survival or a reduction in "hard endpoints" such as heart failure hospitalization or other significant cardiovascular events are most useful in assessing true "response" to CRT. Several studies have shown that evidence of LV reverse remodeling after CRT, measured as a >10% reduction in LV end-diastolic volume, predicts improved long-term survival [6]. As such, many centers use repeat echocardiography at 6 months post-CRT implantation with careful comparison of LV dimensions compared to baseline as a reliable indicator of response to CRT.

A number of factors can contribute to the lack of improvement after CRT, whether defined as persistent advanced heart failure symptoms or lack of ventricular remodeling. Broadly, these may be grouped into issues

How-to Manual for Pacemaker and ICD Devices: Procedures and Programming, First Edition. Edited by Amin Al-Ahmad, Andrea Natale, Paul J. Wang, James P. Daubert, and Luigi Padeletti.
© 2018 John Wiley & Sons, Inc. Published 2018 by John Wiley & Sons, Inc.
Companion website: www.wiley.com/go/al-ahmad/pacemakers_and_icds

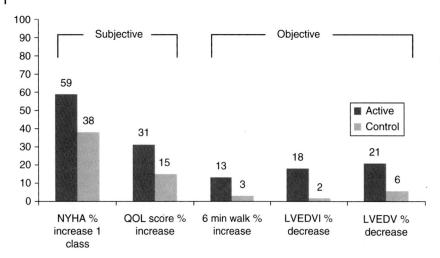

Figure 24.1 Response rates in the active (CRT) and control (non-CRT) arms of major clinical trials. Considerable placebo effect is observed for subjective compared with objective measures of response. [Data adapted from references 1–4].

Table 24.1 Approach to optimization of cardiac resynchronization therapy at each stage of care.

Pre-operative	• Patient selection
	• Dyssynchrony echocardiogram to identify latest activated LV segment
	• Cardiac MRI to identify transmural scar
Intraoperative	• Lead placement on latest mechanically activated LV segment
	• Lead placement on latest electrically activated LV segment (QLV)
	• Acute hemodynamic evaluation (dP/dt max)
Postoperative	• Titration of evidence-based medications
	• Exercise training/cardiac rehabilitation
	• Management of arrhythmias (atrial fibrillation, PVCs) resulting in suboptimal BiV pacing percentage
	• Echocardiographic-based optimization of device timing
	• Lead revision
	• Investigational approaches including: multiple site LV pacing, endocardial LV pacing

BiV, biventricular; LV, left ventricular; MRI, magnetic resonance imaging; PVC, premature ventricular contraction.

pertaining to patient selection, device implantation technique, and postoperative programming and patient management. The most common causes of poor response to CRT include improperly programmed AV intervals, arrhythmias (especially premature ventricular contractions or atrial fibrillation), poor lead position, an insufficient percentage of biventricular pacing, inadequate medical therapy, and lack of underlying wide QRS. A multidisciplinary approach to the identification and correction of these underlying conditions has been shown to improve the frequency of CRT response [7]. In managing a patient with CRT, optimization of each of these factors and corrective action where possible may improve outcomes (Table 24.1).

Pre-Implant Optimization

Guidelines for CRT implantation were updated in 2012 by the governing bodies of the American College of Cardiology (ACC), American Heart Association (AHA), and Heart Rhythm Society (HRS), in large part to refine patient selection criteria. These updated guidelines reflect evidence from multiple randomized controlled trials that CRT is most beneficial in patients with underlying left bundle branch block (LBBB) and wide QRS (>150 ms). In a retrospective subgroup analysis of the MADIT-CRT trial, for example, 13% of subjects had right bundle branch block (RBBB) and 17% had non-specific intraventricular conduction delay (IVCD), however only patients with LBBB had a significantly reduced risk of death, heart failure event or ventricular tachycardia [8].

Measures of mechanical dyssynchrony, including echocardiogram-based LV strain analysis have been studied in patients with marginal (120–150 ms) or narrow (<120 ms) QRS durations. In several single-center studies, the presence of significant mechanical dyssynchrony by various echocardiographic measures was associated with improved CRT response; however, randomized controlled trials using these techniques failed to show benefit [9]. While the use of echocardiographic dyssynchrony analysis to select patients appropriate for CRT implantation is not indicated, evidence suggests that pre-procedure dyssynchrony evaluation can be used to target the LV lead and improve the response rate to CRT. In the TARGET (Left Ventricular Lead Placement to Guide Cardiac Resynchronization Therapy) study, 220 patients were randomized to either standard LV lead placement or targeted placement based on the latest wall of activation on echocardiographic speckle-tracking analysis. More patients with an LV lead placed on or near the wall with latest activation had LV reverse remodeling after CRT than those with standard (unguided) LV lead placement (70% versus 55%; p = 0.031) [10]. Similarly, the STARTER (Speckle Tracking Assisted Resynchronization Therapy for Electrode Region) study found a reduction in heart failure hospitalization in patients with guided LV lead placement versus those without (11% versus 22%; p = 0.031) [11].

In patients with ischemic cardiomyopathy, placement of the LV lead on an area of transmural myocardial scar has been associated with worse outcomes. Contrast-enhanced MRI (cMRI) offers excellent spatial resolution and is the most validated modality for scar detection prior to CRT implant. Echocardiographic strain analysis has been compared to cMRI and may allow adequate determination of scar location, thereby eliminating the need for multiple imaging studies pre-CRT implant [12].

Implant Optimization

Measurement of Left Ventricular Electrical Activation

During the early era of CRT implantation, measurement of the electrical delay at the final implant location of the LV lead was common practice. With data that

posterolateral or lateral LV sites were generally preferable, however, a strictly anatomic implant strategy became commonplace. Given the underwhelming response rates to CRT with current implant strategies, there is renewed interest in measurement and placement of LV leads at sites of delayed electrical activation. Comprehensive mapping of electrical activation in patients with LBBB shows significant heterogeneity in the location of the line of functional block [13]. By measuring the electrical activation from the QRS onset on the surface ECG to the local activation on the LV lead, the implanting physician can optimize the lead location based on the site of latest electrical delay (QLV) (Figure 24.2). Placement of the LV lead on sites of significant electrical delay measured either as an absolute value (QLV >95 ms) or as a percentage of the QRS duration (>50%) results in improvements in both acute hemodynamic response and long-term clinical outcomes, although randomized controlled trial data are lacking [14,15].

Acute Hemodynamic Response to CRT

Another method of "fine-tuning" the LV lead position during CRT implantation involves placement of an open-lumen catheter or pressure wire into the LV chamber,

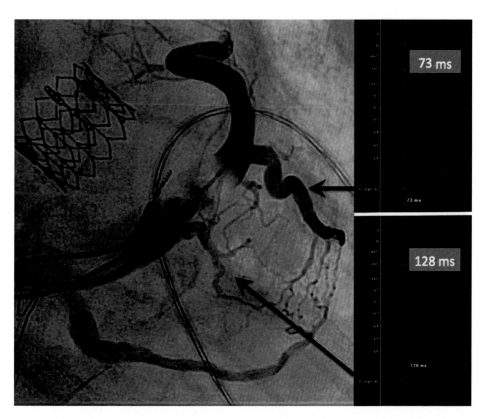

73 ms

128 ms

Figure 24.2 Example of measurement of QLV. Two potential target branches are identified. A 0.014 inch wire capable of unipolar sensing (VisionWire, Biotronik, Berlin, Germany) is advanced into each branch and measurements are made from the onset of the QRS to the initial, rapid deflection on the unipolar signal (IC EGM). The posterolateral branch is found to have a significantly prolonged QLV (128 ms) compared to the high lateral branch (73 ms) and is targeted for LV lead implantation.

thereby allowing real-time assessment of hemodynamics with biventricular pacing, including measurement of stroke work and the maximum rate of left ventricular pressure (dP/dtmax). In small studies, positioning the LV lead in regions demonstrating maximal acute improvement in LV hemodynamics from baseline has translated to improved long-term clinical response rates [16]. Non-invasive measures of hemodynamic changes during CRT implantation are possible using standard echocardiography; however, technical considerations including procedure sterility and maintaining adequate imaging windows during prolonged implant procedures limit this technique.

Post-Implant Optimization

Ensuring Biventricular Capture

One of the simplest and most important assessments of patients after CRT implantation is a careful examination of the percentage of biventricular pacing. Studies have shown that biventricular pacing percentage should be as close to 100% as possible in order to achieve an optimal response. In a large observational database of over 80 000 patients, 40% of patients had <98% biventricular pacing, and 11% had <90% pacing [17]. Atrial fibrillation (AF) is the most frequent cause of loss of CRT; however, multiple other causes of decreased biventricular pacing percentage must be considered (Table 24.2).

In order to accurately assess adequate LV capture, 12-lead electrocardiography is essential. A baseline ECG for future comparison should be established intraoperatively or at device follow-up when capture is confirmed by device interrogation. Analysis of the frontal plane axis as well as the R-wave pattern across the precordial leads

Table 24.2 Causes of loss of biventricular pacing.

Cardiac arrhythmia	Atrial fibrillation
	Ventricular ectopic beats
	Sinus tachycardia (causing upper rate behavior)
Mechanical factors	Lead dislodgement
	Late exit block
	Inoperable LV lead due to phrenic nerve stimulation
Programming factors	Excessively long AV interval programming
	Fusion or pseudo-fusion of native conduction
	Excessive inter-atrial conduction delay with inadequate AV delay

AV, atrioventricular; LV, left ventricular.

can help identify proper LV pacing. In one algorithm proposed by Ammann *et al.* [18], the presence of either an R/S ratio ≥1 in V1 or an R/S ratio ≤1 in lead I confirms the presence of LV capture with sensitivity and specificity of nearly 95%. This algorithm works best when the LV lead is in a lateral position; however, as pacing from an inferior or posterior LV lead location results is absence of an R/S ratio ≤1 in lead I in a significant proportion of patients (24–36%). In addition, if the RV lead is placed in the outflow tract, biventricular capture may demonstrate a mostly negative QRS complex in V1 with a right inferior frontal plane axis.

Arrhythmia Management

If a decrease in biventricular pacing percentage is determined to be secondary to the presence of atrial or ventricular arrhythmias, prompt management is essential to restore effective CRT. Several device-based algorithms have been developed to mitigate the loss of biventricular pacing including ones that deliver biventricular or LV pacing upon sensed intrinsic ventricular activation. Although a small study showed favorable acute hemodynamic changes during this type of triggered pacing, long-term studies have not been performed [19]. It is also important to realize that counts of biventricular pacing through the device may overestimate fully paced complexes because of unrecognized fusion beats during AF (Figure 24.3). In a study of 19 patients with CRT and permanent AF in which device counters showed >90% LV pacing, analysis of continuous Holter monitor tracings revealed complete biventricular capture in only 76% [20]. Therefore, in patients with AF where response is poor after CRT implant, device counters reporting an adequate biventricular pacing percentage may be unreliable and AV node ablation or sinus rhythm restoration should be considered.

The presence of AF potentially reduces the benefit of CRT because of the competition of rapid, natively conducted beats. Among patients with standard CRT implantation criteria and a history of atrial arrhythmia, the percentage biventricular pacing is a strong predictor of HF hospitalization and all-cause mortality [21]. In this study of over 1800 patients, those with >92% biventricular pacing had a 66% reduction in HF hospitalization or all-cause mortality compared to patients with <92% biventricular pacing (p <0.001). Slowing intrinsic conduction to allow adequate CRT pacing may require high-doses or multiple AV nodal agents that may have deleterious effects.

In patients with AF who otherwise meet criteria for CRT implantation, adequate rate control and therefore maximal CRT pacing percentage is best achieved with AV node ablation. Although the major randomized

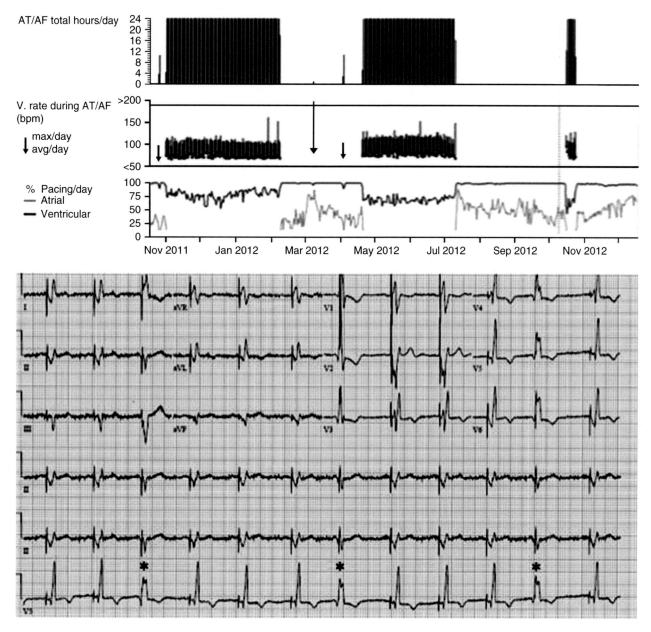

Figure 24.3 Example of loss of biventricular pacing in a patient with underlying atrial fibrillation. Top panel shows device interrogation demonstrating inadequate cardiac resynchronization therapy during prolonged periods of atrial fibrillation. Bottom panel shows 12-lead ECG with loss of biventricular pacing due to natively conducted beats (asterisk) during atrial fibrillation.

controlled trials of CRT largely excluded patients with AF, data from observational studies supports CRT implantation in this population with adjunct AV node ablation. Gasparini *et al.* [22] showed that overall mortality was equivalent at 3 years in patients with CRT and AF who underwent AV node ablation versus patients with CRT in sinus rhythm. Similarly, a meta-analysis of three studies comparing patients with permanent AF and CRT who underwent AV node ablation, mortality was decreased 58% in comparison to patients who did not undergo AV node ablation [23].

Similar to AF, frequent premature ventricular contractions (PVCs) are suspected to reduce the effectiveness of CRT by reducing the percentage of biventricular-paced beats and by causing fusion of some additional percentage of paced beats [24]. Although a high burden of PVCs is relatively common in CRT recipients, little work has been done to investigate the role of PVC burden in predicting response to CRT therapy. In a prospective study assessing the effect of PVC ablation in CRT non-responders, subjects were included if they had no clinical or echocardiographic response to CRT 1 year after

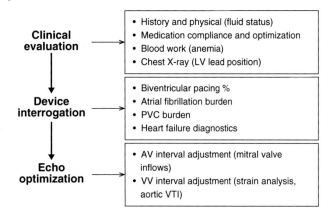

Clinical evaluation
- History and physical (fluid status)
- Medication compliance and optimization
- Blood work (anemia)
- Chest X-ray (LV lead position)

Device interrogation
- Biventricular pacing %
- Atrial fibrillation burden
- PVC burden
- Heart failure diagnostics

Echo optimization
- AV interval adjustment (mitral valve inflows)
- VV interval adjustment (strain analysis, aortic VTI)

Figure 24.4 Step-wise evaluation for CRT non-responders.

implantation and had >10 000 PVCs per day on Holter monitoring [25]. Sixty-five patients underwent PVC ablation and follow-up echocardiography after 6 months showed improvements in mean LV ejection fraction (LVEF; 26.2–32.7%; p <0.001), LV end-systolic volume (178–145 mL; p <0.001), and median NYHA class (3.0–2.0; p <0.001). Whether use of anti-arrhythmic medications would be as effective as ablation for PVC suppression in CRT has not been studied.

Adjunct Heart Failure Treatment

Optimization of heart failure medications, including neurohormonal blockers and diuretics, is often easier after CRT implantation because of improved hemodynamics and less concern for medication-induced bradycardia. A systematic approach to medication titration, utilizing a heart failure specialist in a protocol-driven clinic, has been shown to improve clinical and echocardiographic outcomes in a prospective study [26]. Similarly, structured exercise training after CRT implantation results in further response to CRT, although the durability of this over the long-term has not been studied [27]. Prior to consideration of echocardiographic-based optimization, a thorough analysis of all factors contributing to CRT non-response is warranted (Figure 24.4).

Echocardiographic-based CRT Optimization

An optimally programmed A-V delay allows adequate atrial diastolic filling (E wave) without truncation of atrial systole (A wave). Echocardiography allows direct visualization and real-time adjustment of intervals to maximize LV filling with confirmation of beneficial effects via non-invasive hemodynamic measures. Newer

echocardiographic techniques including speckle tracking strain analysis may aid in the programming of optimal V-V intervals as well.

A-V Interval Optimization

To ensure proper AV interval programming a number of different methodologies have been proposed. The most common technique is the iterative method, which utilizes visual examination of the mitral inflow pattern to optimize the timing of left atrial systolic and diastolic events. In CRT, the AV interval must be short enough that biventricular pacing is uniformly delivered, yet not so short that left atrial contraction is pre-empted. Using the iterative method, the first step is to determine the longest AV interval still providing ventricular capture; this will often result in fusion of E and A waves because of shortening of the time of atrial diastole. Next the AV interval is shortened in 20 ms increments until truncation of the A wave is seen on the mitral inflow pattern. The AV interval is then increased in 10 ms increments until the E and A waves are distinct (no fusion) and there is no evidence of A wave truncation (Figure 24.5).

An alternative echocardiographic approach to AV interval optimization examines LV ejection rather than filling, comparing the aortic velocity time integral (VTI), a surrogate for stroke volume, at different programmed AV intervals. This method is limited by technical factors (i.e., transducer angle) and has poor intra- and inter-observer variability [28]. Measurement of the mitral inflow VTI correlated better with invasively measured LV dP/dT in a small study compared to aortic VTI [29]. Measurement of cardiac output by mitral or aortic VTI may also be used to complement or verify iterative evaluation of the mitral inflows as well.

Several small studies have demonstrated that echo-based CRT optimization results in improvement of acute hemodynamic measures and short-term functional outcomes. Optimization of the AV interval by the aortic VTI method, for example, was compared in a small (n = 40) randomized study to an empiric AV interval of 120 ms. Interestingly, the mean optimal AV delay was 119 ms; however, the range of optimal delays was 60–200 ms. After 3 months, NYHA functional class and QOL score significantly improved in the optimized group versus the control group and there were trends toward improvement in echocardiographic remodeling [30]. Larger trials with longer follow-up have been disappointing, however. In the SMART-AV (SmartDelay Determined AV Optimization) trial, 980 patients were randomized 1 : 1 : 1 to fixed AV delays, echo-optimized AV delays (via the iterative method), or device-based optimization using intracardiac electrograms. At 6 month follow-up, there was no difference

Figure 24.5 Steps for AV interval optimization using iterative analysis of mitral valve inflows. Upper panel demonstrates fusion of the E and A waves with an AV interval extended to 200 ms. Progressive shortening of the AV interval in 20 ms increments results in truncation of the A wave at a delay of 120 ms (middle panel). The AV interval is increased in 10 ms increments until no A-wave truncation is seen and there is no evidence of E/A wave fusion. Mitral valve velocity-time integral (MV VTI) values confirm hemodynamic improvement using this method.

Step 1
➤ AV interval is extended until biventricular pacing is lost
➤ AV interval is shortened 30 ms to ensure complete biventricular capture

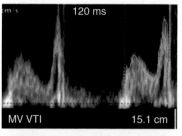

Step 2
➤ AV interval is shortened in 20 ms intervals until truncation of the A wave is noted

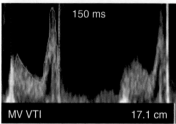

Step 3
➤ AV interval is extended 10 ms until E and A waves are distinct and there is no evidence of A wave truncation

between groups in the primary outcome of reverse remodeling or secondary outcomes of NYHA class, QOL score, or 6-minute walk time [31].

An important aspect of AV interval optimization relates to whether the atrium is tracked or paced. Right atrial pacing may induce significant interatrial conduction delay depending on the location of the right atrium (RA) lead. Pacing from the RA free wall or appendage can augment the delay between the activation time at the RA lead and left atrium (LA) mechanical events. In acute hemodynamic studies, atrial pacing during CRT has been found to have detrimental effects on dP/dT compared to atrial tracking using a VDD mode [32]. However, in a randomized study comparing atrial sensed programming (DDD-40 or DDDR-40) with atrial paced programming (DDD-70), no significant clinical difference was seen at 1 year [33]. When atrial pacing is utilized, nominal or "out-of-box" offsets for paced AV delays appear inadequate and may need to be programmed >70 ms longer than optimized sensed A-V delays [34].

V-V Interval Optimization

All current CRT devices allow sequential activation of the right and left ventricles via adjustment of the V-V interval. Normally, pre-excitation of the RV should be avoided, as this may result in worsening LV function [35].

The simplest echocardiographic method of V-V interval optimization involves sequential analysis of aortic VTI as a surrogate for maximizing cardiac output. Newer techniques incorporate analysis of LV strain patterns by speckle tracking analysis to guide the need for V-V interval adjustment (Figure 24.6).

While V-V interval optimization may result in acute hemodynamic improvement, long-term clinical benefit is less clear. In the RHYTHM II ICD study, despite short-term hemodynamic improvement, optimization of the V-V interval conferred no additional clinical benefit at 6 months compared with simultaneous biventricular stimulation [36]. Similarly, DECREASE-HF compared simultaneous, sequential, and LV-only pacing in 306 patients and found no difference in outcomes between the biventricular-paced cohorts [37]. While routine V-V optimization for all recipients of CRT does not appear warranted, preliminary data from the RESPONSE-HF trial suggests that VV interval adjustment in clinical non-responders to CRT may yield some benefit [38].

The American Society of Echocardiography recommends routine echocardiographic assessment after CRT; however, based on currently available evidence, routine optimization of the AV interval for all recipients of CRT devices is not justified [39]. In addition, echo-based optimization techniques are time consuming and labor intensive. Whether patients who are deemed to be

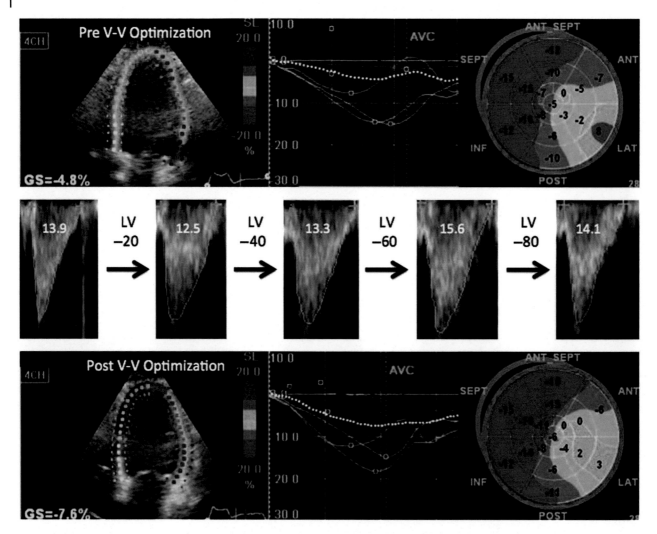

Figure 24.6 Optimization of the VV interval using speckle tracking strain analysis of longitudinal left ventricular contraction. Pre-optimization images (upper panel) demonstrate pre-stretching and delayed contraction of the basal and mid lateral wall with a regional strain of −4.8%. With pre-excitation of the left ventricular lead by 60 ms, maximal cardiac output as determined by LVOT VTI (middle panel) was achieved. Post-optimization images (lower panel) demonstrate improved contraction of the lateral wall with an increase in regional strain to −7.6%. Note that mid and apical lateral segments remain grossly unchanged due to transmural infarct in these regions.

non-responders to CRT should undergo echocardiogram-based optimization is still unclear. Using a protocol-driven approach, one study of 75 CRT non-responders found poor timing resulting from improperly programmed A-V delays was present in nearly 50% of patients. Patients who were felt by the investigators to have had a "favorable intervention" by AV optimization had improved survival compared to patients without AV optimization (Table 24.3) [7].

Device-based CRT Optimization

Device-based algorithms to find and program optimal AV delays eliminate the need for echocardiography and have other potential advantages, including automation of

the process to allow more frequent adjustments. The SMART-AV trial compared outcomes in over 1000 patients randomized to three different optimization methodologies: a device-based electrogram approach, an echo-based mitral inflow iterative approach, and a fixed AV delay of 120 ms [31]. The device-based electrogram approach had been validated against LV dp/dt and was found to outperform echocardiogram-based optimization techniques. However, in SMART-AV, no significant differences were found in the primary endpoint (LV end systolic volume 6 months after implant) or other echocardiographic or clinical secondary outcomes. Similarly, the FREEDOM trial compared a device-based A-V optimization performed every 3 months with standard of care (echo-based optimization at investigator discretion) in 1647 patients [40]. Similar to SMART-AV, there was no

Table 24.3 Randomized, controlled trials of A-V and V-V interval optimization.

Trial	AV/VV	Optimization Technique	Outcome
Sawhney *et al.* [30]	AV	Echocardiogram (aortic VTI)	No improvement in NYHA class ≥1
RESPONSE-HF [38]	VV	Device (QuickOPT™)	No improvement in composite endpoint (NYHA class ≥1 and ≥10% increase in 6MWT
RHYTHM ICD II [36]	VV	Echocardiogram (LVOT VTI)	No improvement in NYHA class ≥1
DECREASE-HF [37]	VV	Device (Expert Ease™)	No difference in LV reverse remodeling
Abraham *et al.* [41]	VV	Echocardiogram (SPWMD)	11% increase in clinical HF composite score
CLEAR [42]	AV + VV	Device (SonR™)	No improvement in composite endpoint (survival + HF hospitalization + ≥10% increase in QoL + NYHA class ≥1)
SMART-AV [31]	AV	Device (SmartDelay™)	No improvement in NYHA class ≥1
FREEDOM [43]	AV + VV	Device (QuickOPT™)	No improvement in clinical HF composite score
ADAPTIV-CRT [44]	AV + VV	Device (AdaptivCRT) versus Echocardiogram (iterative)	Non-inferiority of device versus echocardiogram optimization for improvement in clinical composite score

AV, atrioventricular; HF, heart failure; LVOT, left ventricular outflow tract; 6MWT, 6-minute walk time; NYHA, New York Heart Association; QOL, quality of life; SPWMD, septal-to-posterior wall motion delay; VTI, velocity time integral; VV, ventriculo-ventricular.

significant difference between these groups for the primary endpoint of improvement in heart failure clinical composite score or secondary endpoints of heart failure class or 6-minute walk test.

More recently, the Adaptive-CRT trial reported the results of a novel device-based optimization algorithm compared with echo-based optimization. This algorithm seeks to reduce unnecessary RV pacing in patients with intact right bundle branch conduction while at the same time fuse LV pacing to natively conducted RV contraction. In addition, the device dynamically adjusts the AV and VV intervals based upon timing measurement of the intracardiac electrograms. The results of this study showed that the use of this automated algorithm was non-inferior to echo-based optimization; however, neither method was compared with nominal settings.

Further studies to determine the clinical benefit of this and other device-based optimization methods are underway.

Conclusions

Randomized controlled studies of routine echo-based optimization of AV and VV intervals after CRT implantation have not shown benefit over nominal or "out-of-box" settings. In patients deemed to be non-responders to CRT, device optimization may have a role as part of a comprehensive evaluation of possible contributing factors. In the future, device-based algorithms with the advantage of automatic, dynamic AV and VV interval adjustment may further improve response rates to CRT.

References

1 Abraham WT, Fisher WG, Smith AL, Delurgio DB, Leon AR, Loh E, *et al.* Cardiac resynchronization in chronic heart failure. N Engl J Med 2002;346(24):1845–1853.
2 Moss AJ, Hall WJ, Cannom DS, Klein H, Brown MW, Daubert JP, *et al.* Cardiac-resynchronization therapy for the prevention of heart-failure events. N Engl J Med 2009;361(14):1329–1338.
3 Bristow MR, Saxon LA, Boehmer J, Krueger S, Kass DA, De Marco T, *et al.* Cardiac-resynchronization therapy with or without an implantable defibrillator in advanced chronic heart failure. N Engl J Med 2004;350(21):2140–2150.
4 Cleland JG, Daubert JC, Erdmann E, Freemantle N, Gras D, Kappenberger L, *et al.* The effect of cardiac resynchronization on morbidity and mortality in heart failure. N Engl J Med 2005;352(15):1539–1549.
5 Fornwalt BK, Sprague WW, BeDell P, Suever JD, Gerritse B, Merlino JD, *et al.* Agreement is poor among current criteria used to define response to cardiac resynchronization therapy. Circulation 2010;121(18):1985–1991.
6 Solomon SD, Foster E, Bourgoun M, Shah A, Viloria E, Brown MW, *et al.* Effect of cardiac resynchronization therapy on reverse remodeling and relation to

outcome: multicenter automatic defibrillator implantation trial: cardiac resynchronization therapy. Circulation 2010;122(10):985–992.

7 Mullens W, Grimm RA, Verga T, Dresing T, Starling RC, Wilkoff BL, *et al*. Insights from a cardiac resynchronization optimization clinic as part of a heart failure disease management program. J Am Coll Cardiol 2009;53(9):765–773.

8 Zareba W, Klein H, Cygankiewicz I, Hall WJ, McNitt S, Brown M, *et al*. Effectiveness of cardiac resynchronization therapy by QRS morphology in the Multicenter Automatic Defibrillator Implantation Trial–Cardiac Resynchronization Therapy (MADIT-CRT)/Clinical Perspective. Circulation 2011;123(10):1061–1072.

9 Beshai JF, Grimm RA, Nagueh SF, Baker JH 2nd, Beau SL, Greenberg SM, *et al*. Cardiac-resynchronization therapy in heart failure with narrow QRS complexes. N Engl J Med 2007;357(24):2461–2471.

10 Khan FZ, Virdee MS, Palmer CR, Pugh PJ, O'Halloran D, Elsik M, *et al*. Targeted left ventricular lead placement to guide cardiac resynchronization therapy: the TARGET study: a randomized, controlled trial. J Am Coll Cardiol 2012;59(17):1509–1518.

11 Saba S, Marek J, Schwartzman D, Jain S, Adelstein E, White P, *et al*. Echocardiography-guided left ventricular lead placement for cardiac resynchronization therapy: results of the Speckle Tracking Assisted Resynchronization Therapy for Electrode Region trial. Circ Heart Fail 2013;6(3):427–434.

12 Delgado V, van Bommel RJ, Bertini M, Borleffs CJ, Marsan NA, Arnold CT, *et al*. Relative merits of left ventricular dyssynchrony, left ventricular lead position, and myocardial scar to predict long-term survival of ischemic heart failure patients undergoing cardiac resynchronization therapy. Circulation 2011;123(1):70–78.

13 Auricchio A, Fantoni C, Regoli F, Carbucicchio C, Goette A, Geller C, *et al*. Characterization of left ventricular activation in patients with heart failure and left bundle-branch block. Circulation 2004;109(9):1133–1139.

14 Gold MR, Yu Y, Singh JP, Stein KM, Birgerdotter-Green U, Meyer TE, *et al*. The effect of left ventricular electrical delay on AV optimization for cardiac resynchronization therapy. Heart Rhythm 2013;10(7):988–993.

15 Singh JP, Fan D, Heist EK, Alabiad CR, Taub C, Reddy V, *et al*. Left ventricular lead electrical delay predicts response to cardiac resynchronization therapy. Heart Rhythm 2006;3(11):1285–1292.

16 Duckett SG, Ginks M, Shetty AK, Bostock J, Gill JS, Hamid S, *et al*. Invasive acute hemodynamic response to guide left ventricular lead implantation predicts chronic remodeling in patients undergoing cardiac resynchronization therapy. J Am Coll Cardiol 2011;58(11):1128–1136.

17 Cheng A, Gold MR, Waggoner AD, Meyer TE, Seth M, Rapkin J, *et al*. Potential mechanisms underlying the effect of gender on response to cardiac resynchronization therapy: insights from the SMART-AV multicenter trial. Heart Rhythm 2012;9(5):736–741.

18 Ammann P, Sticherling C, Kalusche D, Eckstein J, Bernheim A, Schaer B, *et al*. An electrocardiogram-based algorithm to detect loss of left ventricular capture during cardiac resynchronization therapy. Ann Intern Med 2005;142(12 Pt 1):968–973.

19 Aktas MK, Jeevanantham V, Sherazi S, Flynn D, Hall B, Huang DT, *et al*. Effect of biventricular pacing during a ventricular sensed event. Am J Cardiol 2009;103(12):1741–1745.

20 Kamath G, Cotiga D, Koneru J, Arshad A, Pierce W, Aziz EF, *et al*. The utility of 12-lead holter monitoring in patients with permanent atrial fibrillation for the identification of nonresponders after cardiac resynchronization therapy. J Am Coll Cardiol 2009;53:1050–1055.

21 Koplan BA, Kaplan AJ, Weiner S, Jones PW, Seth M, Christman SA. Heart failure decompensation and all-cause mortality in relation to percent biventricular pacing in patients with heart failureis a goal of 100% biventricular pacing necessary? J Am Coll Cardiol 2009;53(4):355–360.

22 Gasparini M, Auricchio A, Metra M, Regoli F, Fantoni C, Lamp B, *et al*. Long-term survival in patients undergoing cardiac resynchronization therapy: the importance of performing atrio-ventricular junction ablation in patients with permanent atrial fibrillation. Eur Heart J 2008;29(13):1644–1652.

23 Ganesan AN, Brooks AG, Roberts-Thomson KC, Lau DH, Kalman JM, Sanders P. Role of AV nodal ablation in cardiac resynchronization in patients with coexistent atrial fibrillation and heart failure: a systematic review. J Am Coll Cardiol 2012;59(8):719–726.

24 Ruwald MH, Mittal S, Ruwald AC, Aktas MK, Daubert JP, McNitt S, *et al*. Association between frequency of atrial and ventricular ectopic beats and biventricular pacing percentage and outcomes in patients with cardiac resynchronization therapy. J Am Coll Cardiol 2014;64(10):971–981.

25 Lakkireddy D, Di Biase L, Ryschon K, Biria M, Swarup V, Reddy YM, *et al*. Radiofrequency ablation of premature ventricular ectopy improves the efficacy of cardiac resynchronization therapy in nonresponders. J Am Coll Cardiol 2012;60(16):1531–1539.

26 Mullens W, Kepa J, De Vusser P, Vercammen J, Rivero-Ayerza M, Wagner P, *et al*. Importance of adjunctive heart failure optimization immediately after implantation to improve long-term outcomes with cardiac resynchronization therapy. Am J Cardiol 2011;108(3):409–415.

27 Patwala AY, Woods PR, Sharp L, Goldspink DF, Tan LB, Wright DJ. Maximizing patient benefit from cardiac resynchronization therapy with the addition of structured exercise training: a randomized controlled study. J Am Coll Cardiol 2009;53(25):2332–2339.

28 Valzania C, Biffi M, Martignani C, Diemberger I, Bertini M, Ziacchi M, *et al.* Cardiac resynchronization therapy: variations in echo-guided optimized atrioventricular and interventricular delays during follow-up. Echocardiography 2007;24(9):933–939.

29 Jansen AH, Bracke FA, van Dantzig JM, Meijer A, van der Voort PH, Aarnoudse W, *et al.* Correlation of echo-Doppler optimization of atrioventricular delay in cardiac resynchronization therapy with invasive hemodynamics in patients with heart failure secondary to ischemic or idiopathic dilated cardiomyopathy. Am J Cardiol 2006;97(4):552–557.

30 Sawhney NS, Waggoner AD, Garhwal S, Chawla MK, Osborn J, Faddis MN. Randomized prospective trial of atrioventricular delay programming for cardiac resynchronization therapy. Heart Rhythm 2004;1(5):562–567.

31 Ellenbogen KA, Gold MR, Meyer TE, Fernndez Lozano I, Mittal S, Waggoner AD, *et al.* Primary results from the SmartDelay determined AV optimization: a comparison to other AV delay methods used in cardiac resynchronization therapy (SMART-AV) trial: a randomized trial comparing empirical, echocardiography-guided, and algorithmic atrioventricular delay programming in cardiac resynchronization therapy. Circulation 2010;122(25):2660–2668.

32 Bernheim A, Ammann P, Sticherling C, Burger P, Schaer B, Brunner-La Rocca HP, *et al.* Right atrial pacing impairs cardiac function during resynchronization therapy: acute effects of DDD pacing compared to VDD pacing. J Am Coll Cardiol 2005;45(9):1482–1487.

33 Martin DO, Day JD, Lai PY, Murphy AL, Nayak HM, Villareal RP, *et al.* Atrial support pacing in heart failure: results from the multicenter PEGASUS CRT trial. J Cardiovasc Electrophysiol. 2012;23(12):1317–1325.

34 Gold MR, Niazi I, Giudici M, Leman RB, Sturdivant JL, Kim MH, *et al.* Acute hemodynamic effects of atrial pacing with cardiac resynchronization therapy. J Cardiovasc Electrophysiol 2009;20(8):894–900.

35 Sogaard P, Egeblad H, Pedersen AK, Kim WY, Kristensen BO, Hansen PS, *et al.* Sequential versus simultaneous biventricular resynchronization for severe heart failure: evaluation by tissue Doppler imaging. Circulation 2002;106(16):2078–2084.

36 Boriani G, Muller CP, Seidl KH, Grove R, Vogt J, Danschel W, *et al.* Randomized comparison of simultaneous biventricular stimulation versus optimized interventricular delay in cardiac resynchronization therapy. The Resynchronization for the HemodYnamic Treatment for Heart Failure Management II implantable cardioverter defibrillator (RHYTHM II ICD) study. Am Heart J 2006;151(5):1050–1058.

37 Rao RK, Kumar UN, Schafer J, Viloria E, De Lurgio D, Foster E. Reduced ventricular volumes and improved systolic function with cardiac resynchronization therapy: a randomized trial comparing simultaneous biventricular pacing, sequential biventricular pacing, and left ventricular pacing. Circulation 2007;115(16):2136–2144.

38 Weiss R. V-V Optimization in cardiac resynchronization therapy non-responders: RESPONSE-HF trial results. Abstract AB12-5, HRS. 2010.

39 Gorcsan J 3rd, Abraham T, Agler DA, Bax JJ, Derumeaux G, Grimm RA, *et al.* Echocardiography for cardiac resynchronization therapy: recommendations for performance and reporting: a report from the American Society of Echocardiography Dyssynchrony Writing Group endorsed by the Heart Rhythm Society. J Am Soc Echocardiogr 2008;21(3):191–213.

40 Abraham WT, Gras D, Yu CM, Gupta MS: Freedom Steering Committee. Rationale and design of a randomized clinical trial to assess the safety and efficacy of frequent optimization of cardiac resynchronization therapy: the Frequent Optimization Study using the QuickOpt Method (FREEDOM) trial. Am Heart J 2010;159(6):944–948.

41 Abraham WT, Leon AR, St John Sutton MG, Keteyian SJ, Fieberg AM, Chinchoy E, *et al.* Randomized controlled trial comparing simultaneous versus optimized sequential interventricular stimulation during cardiac resynchronization therapy. Am Heart J 2012;164(5):735–741.

42 Ritter P, Delnoy PP, Padeletti L, Lunati M, Naegele H, Borri-Brunetto A, *et al.* A randomized pilot study of optimization of cardiac resynchronization therapy in sinus rhythm patients using a peak endocardial acceleration sensor vs. standard methods. Europace 2012;14(9):1324–1333.

43 Vanderheyden M, Blommaert D, Abraham W, Gras D, Yu CM, Guzzo L. Results from the FREEDOM trial: assess the safety and efficacity of frequent optimization of cardiac resynchronization therapy. Acta Cardiol 2010;65(5):589.

44 Martin DO, Lemke B, Birnie D, Krum H, Lee KL, Aonuma K, *et al.* Investigation of a novel algorithm for synchronized left-ventricular pacing and ambulatory optimization of cardiac resynchronization therapy: results of the adaptive CRT trial. Heart Rhythm 2012;9(11):1807–1814.

25

How to Manage Device Infections and When to Reimplant After Device Extraction

Giosuè Mascioli

Unit of Arrhythmology and Cardiac Pacing, Cliniche Humanitas Gavazzeni, Bergamo, Italy

In the last 50 years, the importance of cardiac implantable electronic devices (CIEDs) has increased as fast as their ability in improving the management of many serious cardiovascular diseases and patients' quality of life. This explains why the guidelines that rule their use are frequently updated and widened in scope. Between 1996 and 2004, the numbers of implanted pacemakers (PMs) and implantable cardioverter-defibrillators (ICDs) increased 19% and 60%, respectively. In the last 20 years, we can estimate that more than 4.5 million patients have been implanted with a CIED and that about 1 million new leads are implanted every year. Thus, it is easy to understand that such a high number of implants, in an aging population affected with several comorbidities, sustains a parallel increase in complications linked to these devices.

Device-related complications include malfunctioning (which affects almost 28% of PMs within 10 years after implant and 40% of ICDs within 8 years), venous thrombosis (15–40%), infections (0.5–12%), and recalls.

Among these complications, the incidence of cardiac device infection is underestimated but is associated with the worst prognosis. Unfortunately, some reports show that the incidence of infection is growing faster than the number of new implants, and in some centers the prevalence of CIED endocarditis has increased from less than 5% to more than 30% in the last 10 years.

In the LExICon trial [1], the mortality rate observed with any kind of infection dwarfs the rate associated with transvenous lead extraction. The authors showed that the in-hospital death rate in non-infected patients was 0.3%, but increased to 1.7% in patients with local infection (i.e., limited to the device pocket) and rose to 4.3% in patients with device-related endocarditis.

It is very important to remember that prophylaxis at the time of implant, a watchful eye for the early signs of infection, and prompt intervention after diagnosis are not only the right way to handle a CIED infection, but often the only way to give the patient a good chance of survival.

Nevertheless, there is still the need for official guidelines for the management of these complicated patients. The most recent document is the Heart Rhythm Society (HRS) expert consensus, endorsed by the American Heart Association and published in *Heart Rhythm* in July 2009 [2].

Risk Factors

Every patient implanted with prosthetic material could become a potentially infected patient, and CIEDs are no exception. This does not mean that there is no way to fight and prevent the problem, but identifying patients at higher risk is challenging. Risk factors linked to the patient's characteristics include any comorbidities, especially chronic kidney disease (defined as a glomerular filtration rate <60 mL/min) and diabetes mellitus, while chronic heart failure and chronic obstructive pulmonary disease (COPD) should only be considered as minor risk factors [3]. Furthermore, any factor that underlies a condition of immunosuppression (e.g., chronic therapy with steroids, neoplastic disease, or merely aging) [4], the presence of other focuses of infection (i.e., other infected prosthetic materials, infections of the oral cavity), having fever 24 hours before entering the operating room, and previous intervention related to the CIED, as in the case of replacement, upgrading, or revision of lead or device, should be regarded as potentially risky situations.

Other factors are related to the CIED itself.: ICD and cardiac resynchronization therapy (CRT) devices are more prone to infection, and – generally speaking – the

How-to Manual for Pacemaker and ICD Devices: Procedures and Programming, First Edition. Edited by Amin Al-Ahmad, Andrea Natale, Paul J. Wang, James P. Daubert, and Luigi Padeletti.

more complex the device, the higher the risk of infection, probably because procedures are longer and usually require more professionals in the operating room. Temporary pacing before the procedure (implant, replacement, or lead extraction) is another important risk factor, because it is allows easy venous access for microbes. Even the operator's experience seems to have a role in infections. Centers that perform more than 100 implant procedures per year seem to have a lower risk of infection.

Finally, one of the most important and controversial risk factors is the use of antiplatelet and/or anticoagulant therapy. In most of the trials, the use of these drugs, particularly if in association, is linked to an higher incidence of subcutaneous hematoma and this represents an optimal environment for microbial growth, delays the tissue healing, and may sometimes need an evacuation procedure that can be a source of infection.

Clinical Presentation of CIED Infection

A device infection can present in many different ways, but for the purposes of this chapter, we divide it into two groups: device pocket infection and endovascular infection without clear signs of pocket involvement.

In the first scenario, all the classic signs of inflammation can be observed: the skin can appear erythematous, warmer, flushed, swollen, and painful, sometimes with a dehiscence, secreting a serous, hematic, or purulent material. Occasionally, a low-grade fever is present and blood inflammatory indexes are elevated. It may happen that, at the first contact with a specialist, the generator or the leads have already eroded through the skin and appear on the surface, totally or in part. The cause of the erosion can be an infection or just skin fragility, as in the case of chronic steroid use, radiotherapy, or chronic diseases of the connective tissues. However, once exposed, the device inevitably becomes contaminated and must be considered infected.

In endovascular infection, the patient usually presents with fever that can be continuous or intermittent (it is not uncommon to record temperatures higher than 38°C). This condition can be associated with positive blood cultures. With negative blood cultures, usually the main reason is the use of an empiric antibiotic therapy. In some case, transthoracic or – even better – transesophageal echocardiography shows vegetations adhered either to the leads or to the cardiac valves; these vegetations are often longer than 1 cm, perhaps because the low pressures of the right district allows their growth

without damaging them. One of the worst presentations of infection is systemic embolism resulting from a friable cardiac vegetation: unfortunately, this can sometimes be the first expression of a vegetation and in many case it is crippling.

However, local infection is the most common presentation. If we consider both cases with and without bloodstream infection, it represents almost 70% of all instances [4].

Local infections usually appear within 6 months of the index procedure [3], while systemic infections are usually late complications; in the latter case, sometimes the source of infection is "outside" the CIED and this remote site should be identified and treated before or contemporaneously to device extraction.

Aetiology

Staphylococcus is the most common class of bacteria responsible for device infection, both systemic and restricted to the subcutaneous pocket (almost 70–80% of cases) [4]. Amongst this species, *Staphylococcus epidermidis* and other coagulase-negative staphylococci (CoNS) are the most frequent, followed by *Staphylococcus aureus*. The high incidence of CoNS infection is easy to understand, because the bacteria are part of the usual environment of our skin, and, moreover, can adhere to prosthetic materials and build a protective biofilm, which is able to protect them from the host defense system and from antibiotics. *S. aureus* is the most virulent bacteria; it is usually responsible for the majority of infections linked to central venous access and *S. aureus* bacteremia is harmful even if not originating by the CIED, because this bacteria is able to colonize the device even during other invasive procedures. This is the reason why a persistent occult gram-positive bacteremia has been proposed as an indication to promptly start specific antibiotic therapy and to remove the device, even before demonstration of its involvement in the infective process (class of recommendation I; level of evidence B) [2]. Methicillin-resistance prevalence, both for CoNS and *S. aureus*, as reported in several studies, can be as high as 50–60%. Other gram-positive bacteria, as Streptococci and Corynebacterium, are involved in less than 5% of infections. Gram-negative bacteria are involved in nearly 10% of device infections. Only a minority of patients are affected with mycotic infection, mainly by *Candida albicans*, but this happens almost exclusively in seriously immunocompromised subjects. Polymicrobial infections affect about 10% of patients and in another 10% both blood and pocket cultures are negative, usually for previous empiric antibiotic therapy.

Diagnosis

In case of suspected CIED infections, patients should be referred to a physician with specific experience in this setting, so that the diagnostic evaluation could be rapidly started. The first step is to obtain a complete blood count with differential white cells count, inflammatory markers (C-reactive protein, erythrocyte sedimentation rate, and procalcitonin), glycemia, and serum creatinine concentration (as markers of the most common risk factors). In the presence of purulent drainage from the generator pocket, swabs for bacterial cultures should be collected and sent for analysis. Needle aspiration from the pocket, even if swollen or fluctuant, should be absolutely avoided, because this can be a source of contamination. A culture from the inner pocket (and from the lead tips) can be taken only in the operating room, with the maximum level of asepsis.

At least two (three is better) sets of blood cultures (even without fever) should be obtained. Different modes of access must be used and, if the patient has a central venous catheter, blood cultures from the catheter should also be obtained because it can also be the source of infection. If blood cultures are taken during an empirical antibiotic therapy or in a very early phase of the infection, they can have a negative result, and therefore should be repeated after a few days, taking into consideration the possibility of withholding antibiotics. Two sets positive for the same bacteria (with same sensitivity and resistance to antimicrobial agent) is a diagnostic criteria of endocarditis, as well as the presence of a typical endocarditis bacteria (i.e., *S. aureus*) in just one set.

Echocardiography has a fundamental role in the diagnostic evaluation, in order to establish the presence and site of vegetations. Transesophageal echocardiography (TEE) is the gold standard to find vegetations (Figure 25.1), to establish their connections to leads, valves, and other cardiac structures, and to measure their dimensions. This aspect should not be neglected, because the larger the vegetation, the higher the embolic risk at the moment of lead extraction. TEE is also able to reveal the presence of cardiac abscesses, one of the most typical manifestations of *S. aureus* infection. However, it is important to remember that a negative TEE does not exclude the presence of a CIED infection. It is evident that even if TEE has a greater usefulness in the diagnostic iter, transthoracic echocardiography (TTE) plays an important part in monitoring the vegetations and cardiac function during antimicrobial therapy. After lead removal, both techniques can sometime show a characteristic find, described as a double rail image which stands on the lead way. This image, called "ghost" by some authors [5], is the fibrous sheath that previously covered the lead and seems to be associated with a worse prognosis.

There are many conditions that limit the resolution power of echocardiographic methods (i.e., valvular prosthesis or high thoracic impedance, as in case of obesity or emphysema), thus some authors suggest that other techniques, such as 3-D echocardiography, CT scan, intravascular ultrasound (IVUS), and ^{18}F-FDG positron emission tomography (PET) should be used to study of cardiac vegetations. IVUS in particular appears to be more accurate than TEE in determining the position of vegetations [6]. Among these techniques, ^{18}F-FDG-PET

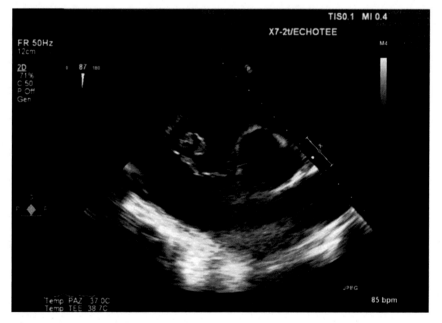

Figure 25.1 Huge vegetations on the tricuspid valve found at transesophageal echography in a patient with systemic infection of a single chamber implantable cardioverter-defibrillator (ICD). (Personal case)

(a)   (b)

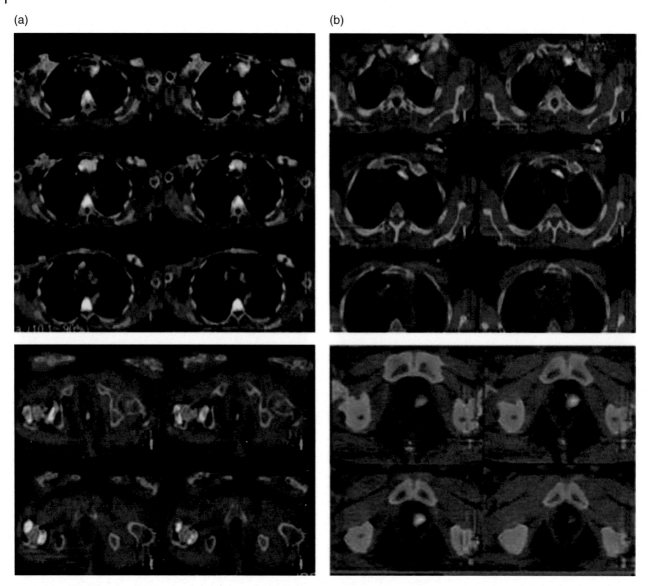

Figure 25.2 ^{18}F-FDG-PET. (a) A patient with an infection both of the pacemaker (PM) pocket and of the intravascular portion of the pacing system (see the gold spotting at these levels). In the lower part of the figure there is an uptake of ^{18}F-FDG also at the hip prosthesis, probable origin site of the infective process. (b) A patient who presented with mild swelling of the PM pocket, without erythema or pocket erosion and without any sign of systemic infection, in whom the ^{18}F-FDG uptake was only evident at the device pocket. In the lower part of the figure, there is uptake of ^{18}F-FDG also at the prostate; the patient underwent prostate biopsy 3 months before coming to our attention. (Personal cases)

(Figure 25.2) appears as the most promising, because of its high sensitivity and specificity (89% and 86%, respectively) in identifying CIED infections even in the initial phases. ^{18}F-FDG is a glucose analogue that is incorporated in cells with higher metabolic activity (e.g., neoplastic cells, leukocytes); it was initially used in oncology for the localization of metastatic lesions, but its utility was recognized in the diagnosis of osteomyelitis, to find unknown sites of infection. Recent studies have demonstrated the usefulness of ^{18}F-FDG-PET in the diagnostic iter of CIED infection, in order to find the original site of infection.

Therapy

Antibiotic Therapy

An empirical antibiotic therapy should always be administered in systemic signs of infection. Drug therapy should cover both gram-positive and gram-negative bacteria and methicillin-resistant *S. aureus*. In local infection, however, it is appropriate to wait until the immediate pre-operative period, unless the device will not be removed before 24 hours from the diagnosis [7]. In the choice of the most appropriate antimicrobial agent, help from an infectivologist should be obtained. The most often involved bacteria are staphylococci and streptococci (i.e., gram-positive bacteria), so the most effective antibiotics are oxacillin and amoxicillin/clavulanic acid for methicillin-sensitive (MS) strains, vancomicin for methicillin-resistant (MR); daptomicin is a reliable alternative for both species. Ceftazidime and piperacillin/tazobactam are extremely useful against gram-negative species. For critical patients, it is appropriate to include in the initial therapy one of these antibiotics too. The choice of drug therapy should be based both on the patient's characteristics, in order to avoid drug-related toxicity as much as possible, and on the antibiogram based on blood cultures. Unfortunately, there are only a few limited clinical trials that tested the minimal duration of antibiotic therapy or discovered when it is appropriate to switch from intravenous to oral treatment. However, many authors suggest referring to the same guidelines that are used to manage non-CIED-related endocarditis. The duration of antimicrobial therapy after device explantation should be decided on the basis of the results of blood cultures and TEE [7]. If blood cultures are positive (or negative, but after a period with empirical antimicrobial treatment), clinical signs and symptoms of systemic infection are present, and the TEE shows vegetations on the leads, antibiotics should be administered for a period of 2–4 weeks, and another 2 weeks of treatment should be provided if vegetations are associated with systemic complications such as osteomyelitis, septic venous thrombosis, and so on. If TEE is negative, 2 weeks of treatment are generally enough, but if the infection is determined by *S. aureus*, it should be prolonged for another 2 weeks. In negative blood cultures, the infection should be considered as confined to the generator pocket, and 7–10 days of antibiotics after complete removal of the PM or ICD system should be sufficient. The antibiotic therapy should be considered as effective after the blood culture, taken every 48 hours starting on the day after extraction procedure, becomes negative and systemic signs of infection (fever, C-reactive protein, leukocytes, procalcitonine) disappear. After the first negative sample, no other blood cultures are required.

Surgical Therapy

Before performing a CIED explantation, the operator must be aware of the clinical condition of the patient, of the risk factors and comorbidities and, moreover, of the presence and the position of all device and leads, including those previously abandoned. To this aim, a good anamnesis is fundamental and must be include all the steps of the device history: brand and model, indication to implant, eventual previous replacements, revisions

and up-gradings, and year of any procedure. The patient should be asked about previous use of antibiotic therapy, previous endocarditis or infection in other sites, and presence of other prostheses. A chest X-ray is mandatory before the procedure to assess the kind of leads involved if not known, and their number and position; even a device control is necessary to document the settings and to check if spontaneous rhythm is present, because in patients with PM dependency a temporary pacing is required as a bridge from explantation to replacement.

The estimation of vegetation size, assessed by TEE, is very important in this phase because it helps in determining the embolic risk we can derive from a transvenous approach for the extraction or if a surgical intervention is needed. The literature is not helpful in determining a cutoff for vegetations' dimensions, as there are reports of vegetations larger than 40 mm being removed percutaneously without any significant complications. It should be remembered that percutaneous lead extraction is a potentially lethal procedure and therefore should be performed only in hospitals with the appropriate experience. As stated in the HRS document [2], cardiac surgery standby and an intensive care unit are necessary to perform this procedure safely.

The current guidelines suggest the following situations in which the benefit of lead extraction overweigh the risk of the procedure and of infection [2]:

Class I: Complete device and leads removal is recommended in:
- Patients with definite CIED system infection, as evidenced by valvular endocarditis, lead endocarditis or sepsis (level of evidence B);
- Patients with definite CIED pocket infection, as evidenced by pocket abscess, device erosion, skin adherence, or chronic draining sinus without clinically evident involvement of the transvenous portion of the lead system (level of evidence B);
- Patients with definite valvular endocarditis without definite involvement of the lead/s and/or device (level of evidence B);
- Patients with occult gram-positive bacteremia (level of evidence B).

Class II: Complete device and leads removal is reasonable in:
- Patients with persistent occult gram-negative bacteremia (level of evidence B).

Class III: Complete device and leads removal is not indicated:
- For superficial or incisional infections without involvement of the device and/or the lead/s (level of evidence C);
- To treat chronic bacteremia from a source other than CIED (level of evidence C).

The extraction procedure in infection should always be performed as soon as possible; nevertheless, the timing should be decided on the basis of the clinical condition of the patient:

- In severe sepsis, even before microbial diagnosis, extraction should be considered as an emergency procedure;
- In the presence of vegetations, the procedure should follow a brief period of focused antibiotic therapy in order to reduce the bacterial charge and, possibly, the size of vegetations;
- In local infection, the procedure could be scheduled, without "losing time," once all the required professionals are present for a safe procedure.

Transvenous Lead Removal

In term of definition, there is a difference between lead "removal" and lead "extraction," the former being the removal of a lead from the heart without any special technical tool (i.e., with traction alone) and the latter is removal of the lead with specialized equipment. Even if the duration of implant does not play a part in this definition, lead removal is more frequent with recently implanted leads, usually less than 6 months.

The success of the procedure is based on the achievement of the desired clinical outcome. We can define a "complete procedural success" as removal of all targeted leads from the vascular space without any permanently disabling complication or death. A "clinical success" is the removal of all targeted leads with retention of a small portion (usually less than 5 cm) of the lead that does not negatively impact the outcome goal of the procedure.

A "failure" is defined as the inability to achieve either complete or clinical success, or the development of any permanently disabling complication or procedure-related death.

The procedure starts with the removal of the device and the debriding of the leads as close as possible to the entrance site. Once the leads have been insulated, a gentle traction can be applied, after having inserted an ordinary stylet, in order to try to remove the lead from the heart. Too much traction can result in damaging of the lead conductor, thus compromising the success of the procedure. If traction is unsuccessful, the lead must be prepared for the insertion of a locking stylet: the connector is cut and the conductor insulated. The two most common kind of locking stylet (Figure 25.3) are those with an anchor at the distal tip or with a kind of stent that runs all along the stylet itself. The aim of this tool is to allow one to pull directly on the distal tip of the lead, without damaging the body of lead itself. If traction also fails with a locking stylet, a dilator should be used. Several kind of dilators have been released onto the market, but – for the purpose of this chapter – we can divide them into two groups: mechanical and potentiated dilators (Figure 25.4). Mechanical sheaths use their cutting edge to disrupt fibrous adherences that tighten the lead to the vascular wall; potentiated sheaths use different energy sources to achieve this effect. The most common potentiated sheaths are laser, radiofrequency, and rotating threaded sheaths.

Removal is usually performed through the same venous access used at the time of implant, but if this approach fails, other approaches have been successful, mainly using the femoral or the internal jugular vein. If performed in an adequate hospital setting and by an experienced operator, the success rate (putting together

(a)

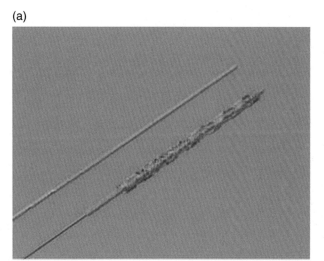

(b)

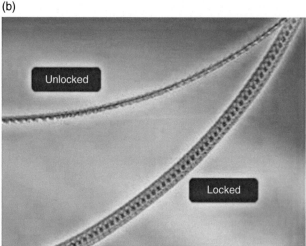

Figure 25.3 Locking stylets. (a) "Anchor tip" locking stylet: (b) "stenting" locking stylet.

(a)

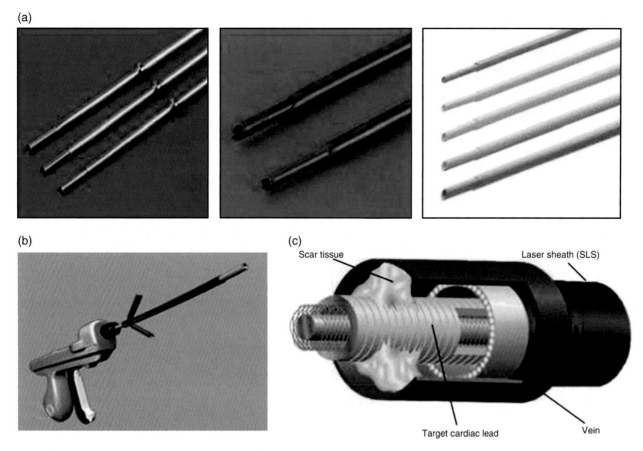

(b)

(c)

Scar tissue   Laser sheath (SLS)

Target cardiac lead   Vein

Figure 25.4 Dilators and sheaths for lead extraction. (a) Different types of mechanical dilators; (b) rotating threaded sheath; (c) laser sheath. Source: Reproduced with permission of The Spectranetics Corporation.

complete radiologic and clinical success) has been reported to be higher than 95% in many publications.

Major complication rate has been described to be as high as 1.6%, but it is strictly dependent on operator experience. Centers that perform more than 300 extraction procedures per year can reduce the major complication rate to less than 1%. Four major risk factors have been found to be related to higher complication rates: time from implant; female gender; ICD leads; and use of laser sheaths techniques, even if the last point is very much debated. Major complications include death, cardiac or vascular avulsion requiring immediate invasive intervention, pulmonary embolism, stroke and pacing system-related infection of a previously non-infected site. Other events are considered as minor complications: pericardial effusion, hematoma at the surgical site requiring drainage, arm swelling, migrated lead fragment without sequelae, and blood transfusion.

In patients who need temporary pacing, in addition to conventional temporary pacing catheter, a new technique has been demonstrated to be safe and effective.

A permanent active fixation lead is positioned into the right ventricle and connected to the removed device which is fixed over the patient's skin. This technique has the great advantage of allowing the patient's movement, avoiding confining the patient to bed, possibly for a long period of time.

Timing of Reimplantation

After having removed the pacing/ICD system, the indication to reimplant a new device should be carefully evaluated as not all patients still have an indication to pacing (less frequently, ICD) after removal. In some reports the proportion of patients not reimplanted with a new device is as high as 30–60%.

It should be remembered that after CIED removal for infection, it is mandatory to implant a new device contralaterally to the previous one. For this reason, it is important to reimplant a new device when the risk of infection has been lowered to the same risk the patient would have for a first procedure, with two aims: safety of the patient and avoidance of compromising the "last possible" pectoral site. In patients in whom both pectoral sites have already been used, the easiest and safest procedure probably remains the epicardial implant, even if new possibilities are offered by the new leadless devices (as the Nanostim) or the new subcutaneous ICDs. Use of the controlateral site and re-evaluation of the need for a new CIED are considered class I recommendations for the timing of reimplantation. Quite surprisingly, all the guidelines that refer to this issue have a level of evidence C, as no randomized clinical trials have been published. The class II (level of evidence C) recommendations are the following:

- A new CIED can be implanted in patients who have no vegetations on valve/leads, even if with positive pre-operative blood cultures of lead tip cultures, provided that there are no further clinical evidences of systemic infection and the blood cultures drawn within 24 hours of CIED system removal remain negative for at least 72 hours.
- Transvenous reimplant of a new CIED system in patients who presented with valvular or lead vegetations should be delayed for at least 14 days after CIED system removal, time that could be reduced in case of surgical debridement of vegetations, provided that there is no more instrumental evidence of vegetations and blood culture are negative.

As far as antibiotic therapy is concerned, its duration should be established on the basis of information in the relevant chapter.

References

1 Wazni O, Epstein LM, Carrillo RG, Love C, Adler SW, Riggio DW, *et al*. Lead extraction in the contemporary setting. The LExICon study: an observational retrospective study of consecutive lead extractions. J Am Coll Cardiol 2010;55(6):579–586.

2 Wilkoff BL, Love CJ, Byrd CL, Bongiorni MG, Carrillo RG, Crossley GH 3rd, *et al*. Transvenous lead extraction: Heart Rhythm Society expert consensus on facilities, training, indications, and patients management (endorsed by the American Heart Association, AHA). Heart Rhythm 2009;6(7):1085–1104.

3 Greenspon AJ, Patel JD, Lau E, Ochoa JA, Frisch DR, Ho RT, *et al*. 16-year trends in the infection burden for pacemakers and implantable cardioverter-defibrillators in the United States: 1993 to 2008. J Am Coll Cardiol 2011;58(10):1001–1006.

4 Sohail MR, Uslan DZ, Khan AH, Friedman PA, Hayes DL, Wilson WR, *et al*. Management and outcome of permanent pacemaker and implantable cardioverter-defibrillator infections. J Am Coll Cardiol 2007;49(18):1851–1859.

5 Le Dolley Y, Thuny F, Mancini J, Casalta JP, Riberi A, Gouriet F, *et al*. Diagnosis of cardiac device-related infective endocarditis after device removal. JACC Cardiovasc Imaging 2010;37(7):673–681.

6 Bongiorni MG, Di Cori A, Soldati E, Zucchelli G, Arena G, Segreti L, *et al*. Intracardiac echocardiography in patients with pacing and defibrillating leads: a feasibility study. Echocardiography 2008;25(6):632–638.

7 Dababneh AS, Sohail MR. Cardiovascular implantable electronic device infection: a stepwise approach to diagnosis and management. Cleve Clin J Med 2011;78(8):529–537.

26

How to Implement a Remote Follow-up Program for Patients with Cardiac Implantable Electronic Devices

George H. Crossley[1], April Bain[2], and Rachel Tidwell[2]

[1] *Vanderbilt Heart and Vascular Institute, Nashville, TN, USA*
[2] *Medtronic Inc., Nashville, TN, USA*

The Heart Rhythm Society/European Heart Rhythm Association (HRS/EHRA) Expert Consensus paper in 2008 codified remote follow-up of cardiac implantable electronic devices (CIEDs) as an excellent alternative to in-office follow-up when accompanied by intermittent office visits [1]. Since then, remote follow-up of patients with implanted pacemakers and defibrillators has become the standard of care. While each has different features and functionality, all manufacturers now offer such a program. The rationale for using remote follow-up is simple. First, it is significantly more convenient for the patients as well as their family members. The caregiver burden in pacemaker and defibrillator patient follow-up is significant because it is common for a patient to need a family member to take off from work to transport the patient to and from the device clinic. Secondly, it has been clearly demonstrated that remote follow-up is more effective than both trans-telephonic telemetry (TTM) and intermittent in-office follow-up [2–4]. TTM is effective in identifying the elective replacement indicator in most pacemakers but it is not very effective in managing other problems. Clinical problems are solved earlier with remote follow-up and the impact of those problems is lessened because of the rapid response. Certainly, remote follow-up allows for more effective problem-solving of patient issues such as shocks, atrial fibrillation, and the management of end of battery service. Finally, remote follow-up is significantly more convenient for the device clinic staff. It is unreasonable to expect device clinic staff to process more than three patients per hour in the office. However, a skilled follow-up nurse can process between six and nine patients per hour depending upon the "user friendliness" of the data recording system being used. In addition, this service can be performed at a time that is convenient for the staff or it can even be performed by a staff member who is working from home.

The data that are available by remote follow-up is the same information that is acquired in the office. There is a clinic splash screen that allows the staff to have an overview of the available data (Figure 26.1). Each patient will have an individual splash screen that gives the clinician an overview of the patient (Figure 26.2). Data are then available to allow for the detailed follow-up of the patient (Figure 26.3).

Staff

The opportunity to follow-up patients with devices remotely is widely available to clinics of all sizes. Access to remote monitoring services is currently provided free of charge by each major device manufacturer. The spectrum of devices that are eligible to be followed remotely vary by manufacturer. Some manufacturers limit remote follow-up technology to their newer device models, while other manufacturers have enabled nearly all of their devices to be followed remotely. Device manufacturers can provide a detailed list of their devices that are eligible for remote monitoring.

The staff required to launch a remote follow-up clinic varies depending on the clinic's device patient population and financial considerations. In smaller clinics, it is reasonable for an experienced device nurse to manage patients in the clinic and spend a portion of the work week managing the remote follow-up patient transmissions. For clinics whose device patient population exceeds 2000 patients, it may be more reasonable to employ a device

How-to Manual for Pacemaker and ICD Devices: Procedures and Programming, First Edition. Edited by Amin Al-Ahmad, Andrea Natale, Paul J. Wang, James P. Daubert, and Luigi Padeletti.
© 2018 John Wiley & Sons, Inc. Published 2018 by John Wiley & Sons, Inc.
Companion website: www.wiley.com/go/al-ahmad/pacemakers_and_icds

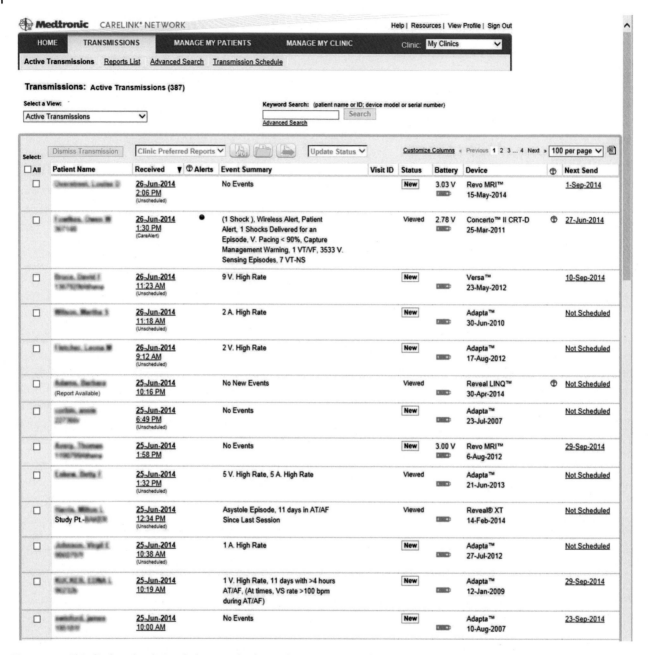

Figure 26.1 This displays the clinic splash screen for the Medtronic system. Red and yellow alerts are noted as are the transmissions that are new. Basic data are seen as well as the next scheduled transmission.

nurse whose sole responsibility is the remote follow-up of patients with CIEDs. This nurse may not necessarily be physically in the clinic each day, but can work from home or an alternate location. This may well be attractive in the current nursing employment environment. Some clinics may choose to explore more creative staffing models to manage their patients remotely. One model is to contract with one or more experienced nurses who may not work full time. This person could be paid on a salary basis or could be paid on a "piece-work" basis. This could be an experienced nurse who wants

more flexible working hours or a former device industry professional with the experience to process the transmissions in a fast and accurate manner.

Qualifications

Execution of a successful remote follow-up program certainly requires that the staff be experienced device specialists. In general, there is an experienced nurse or an extraordinarily experienced medical assistant or

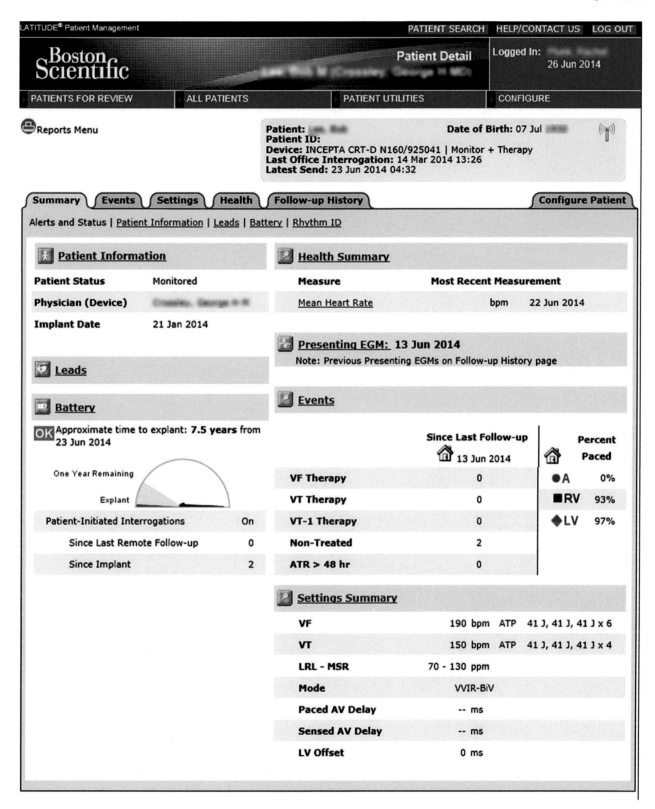

Figure 26.2 The patient splash screen for the Boston Scientific system is seen here. Basic settings are seen as well as recent arrhythmias, pacing history, and battery status.

(a)

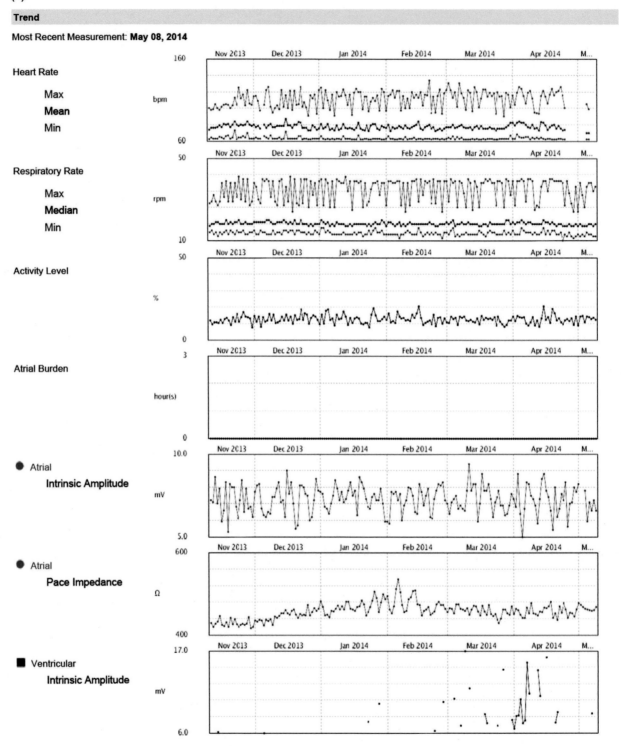

Figure 26.3 (a) A time-dependent trending view of numerical data is seen here in the Boston Scientific system. Heart rate, respiratory rate, and other data are graphed over time.

(b)

Device: Concerto™ II CRT-D D274TRK	Serial Number: ▓▓▓▓▓	Date of Interrogation: 26-Jun-2014 13:30:11
Patient: ▓▓▓▓▓	ID: 367148	Physician: Dr. ▓▓▓▓ 615-329-▓▓▓

LV Pace Polarity   **LVtip to RVcoil**
Lead Model   **4195**

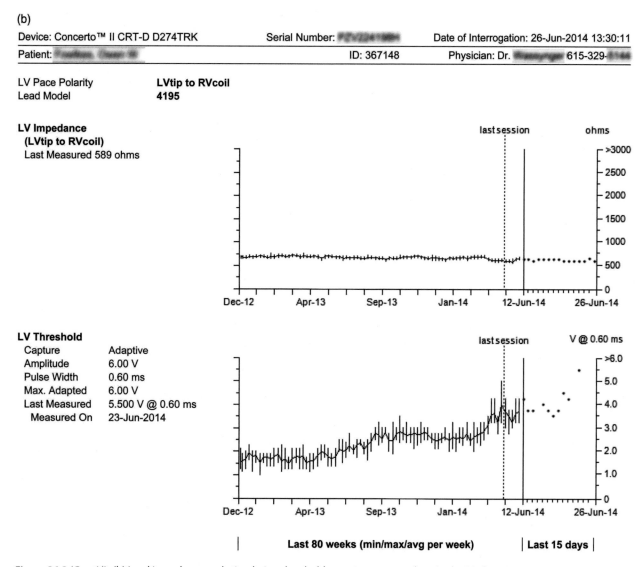

LV Impedance
  (LVtip to RVcoil)
  Last Measured 589 ohms

LV Threshold
  Capture   Adaptive
  Amplitude   6.00 V
  Pulse Width   0.60 ms
  Max. Adapted   6.00 V
  Last Measured   5.500 V @ 0.60 ms
    Measured On   23-Jun-2014

Last 80 weeks (min/max/avg per week) | Last 15 days |

Figure 26.3 (Cont'd) (b) Lead impedance and stimulation threshold over time are seen here in the Medtronic system.

technician who carries out an overview of the information. This person must be able to identify arrhythmias, determine nominal and unexpected device function, and be able to identify unexpected programmed parameters. A remote monitoring program will fail badly if this person is an inexperienced technician who only downloads and prints the reports. The best practice approach is for this person to create a "red light, green light" approach where one group of reports is sent through the process expecting an intense clinical and physician review and the other is reviewed by the physician but with the expectation that all is well. In the practice that we ran for 15 years, the initial review was carried out by a device nurse working from home. The green light reports go straight to the physician for review and signature. The red light reports go to the office nurse who couples that report with the appropriate clinical information and gives it to the physician.

Documentation and Data Management

For accurate documentation, it is necessary to utilize a standard report to summarize remote follow-up transmissions. This form should contain the patient's name, medical record number, date of remote transmission, and specific electrical and clinical data from the device interrogation. The form can be as simple as a paper document that is attached to the chart, or it can also be electronic. It is important to remember (in the USA) that for the purposes of coding a separate report is necessary

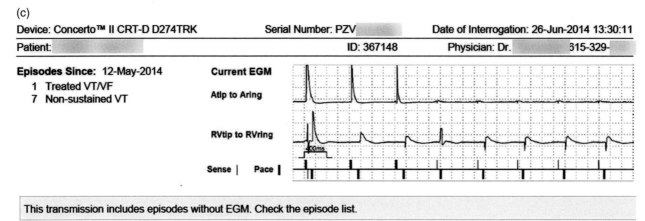

(c)

Figure 26.3 (Cont'd) (c) In this report of a patient with a Medtronic system it is seen that there was an episode of sustained VT where antitachycardia pacing failed and a high energy shock was efficacious.

for the reporting of physiologic information such as weight, blood pressure, or the measurement of fluid index. The definition of a separate report is that it must have a separate signature line. A separate piece of paper or screen in the electronic medical record (EMR) is not needed as long as the physician's signature is separate.

A central hub for device patient data can be valuable for remote follow-up documentation, scheduling, and billing. The Paceart™ system is compatible with all device manufacturers and acts as a central hub to store both in-office and remote follow-up patient data. This system can now be used to manage all device data and push the appropriate data to the patient's electronic health record (EHR). There are two methods for automatically pushing these data. It is certainly possible to create an interface between the Paceart™ system and the EHR such that discrete data is pushed over and all clinician–data interface is carried out on the EHR. While this is attractive, it creates a significant ongoing cost. That cost is created every time the device

data are changed (a new model with new data) and you will need to rebuild the HL-7 interface. This is quite costly. Another, more cost-effective approach, is to let the more esoteric data reside in the Paceart™ system and push over a 2-page summary the can be signed either in the Paceart™ system or in the EHR (Figure 26.4).

Transmission Devices

All major device manufacturers produce remote follow-up systems that transmit data to a secure server via landline. As technology continues to improve, many manufacturers have produced cellular adaptor accessories to enable remote transmissions via a cellular network. In fact, most manufacturers are now distributing remote follow-up boxes that will work with either a landline or a cellular network. In the future, devices may transmit data via different technologies (Figure 26.5).

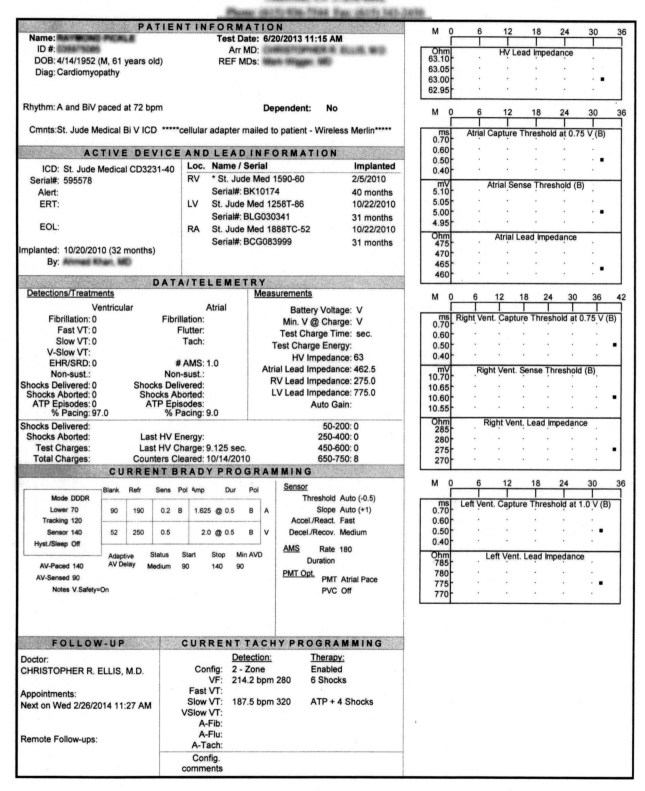

Figure 26.4 The two-page summary that is exported to the electronic medical record (EMR) is seen here.

| Patient Name: ███████ | Test Date: 6/20/2013 11:15 AM | Page 2 |

THERAPIES

DETECTION	DETAILS
VF Detect: 214.2 bpm 280 ms Duration: 12 Redetect: Committed: False	On: 15.0J Biphasic B > AX On: 36.0J Biphasic B > AX On: 40.0J Biphasic B > AX On: 40.0J Biphasic B > AX On: 40.0J Biphasic B > AX On: 40.0J Biphasic B > AX
Slow VT Detect: 187.5 bpm 320 ms Duration: 12 Redetect: 6 EHR/SRD: Onset: 100 Stability: 80 Morphology: On (60%, 5)	On: Burst, 5 sequences On: 10.0J Biphasic B > AX On: 36.0J Biphasic B > AX On: 40.0J Biphasic B > AX On: Biphasic B > AX

THRESHOLDS	SUMMARY
Atrial **Sensing** #1 5.0 mV (B) **Capture** #1 0.75 V @ 0.5 ms (B) **Ventricular (R)** **Sensing** #1 10.6 mV (B) **Capture** #1 0.75 V @ 0.5 ms (B) **Ventricular (L)** **Sensing** **Capture** #1 1 V @ 0.5 ms (B)	Underlying Rhythm: Sinus rhythm with BBB at 64 bpm AT/AF Burden: since 3-25-13 none VT/VF episodes: none Estimated battery longevity: 4.4 years Follow up: followed in ███████ here for transplant evaluation
Printed on: Thursday, September 11, 2014 Copyright © 2014 Medtronic, Inc.	Recorded by: ███████ RN MSN Reviewed/Signed By:

Figure 26.4 (Cont'd)

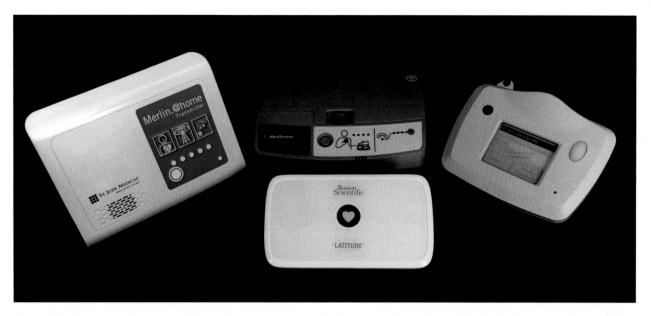

Figure 26.5 Examples of the remote follow-up home transmission devices are seen here. On the left is the St. Jude transmitter; middle upper is the Medtronic device; middle lower is the Boston Scientific pacemaker transmitter; and on the right is the Boston Scientific tachycardia ICD transmitter.

Conduct of the Remote Follow-up

Remote follow-up is not a substitute for good medical care. However, it is an excellent way to provide efficacious and efficient care of a patient's arrhythmias and to monitor the CIED function. The first part of any clinical encounter is taking a history. The history that is typically taken in a device follow-up clinic is brief and directed, but it must include questioning about arrhythmic symptoms and any new cardiac symptoms. We feel strongly that an integral part of providing good remote care of the patient is performing the same brief history by telephone. The importance of this two-way communication with each patient cannot be stressed enough. When patients are seen in the office they are interviewed before interrogation of their devices. In remote follow-up we typically reverse the order. We review the device interrogation and then interview the patient. The patient should never be left out of the puzzle. After all, he or she is the most important piece of this puzzle.

Scheduling and Managing the Patient's Expectations

When following hundreds or thousands of patients on remote monitoring, the likelihood of being able to analyze the device information and call every patient on the very day that a transmission is received is very low. The patients might envision that someone is sitting at the other end of their phone immediately processing their information and develop the expectation that an immediate response will occur. The expectations of the patient and family must be set by the clinicians. For routine transmissions with no alerts, we have our patients transmit one weekend and we tell them to expect to hear from us by the next weekend. They are clearly instructed that in the case of a perceived problem and a manual transmission, a different protocol is needed. Our practice for symptomatic transmissions sent by patients is to have them call the office after sending in the transmission to let the staff know the transmission was not routine and needs more immediate attention.

Managing Alerts

Alerts are typically divided into red alerts (urgent) and yellow alerts (important but not urgent). In our practice, red alerts are managed by having a staff member receive an immediate message by phone. Some of these alerts require immediate attention. An example of this is the Medtronic Lead Integrity Alert (LIA) that signals an impeding lead failure. The remote systems should be monitored at least several times daily and preferably continuously to observe for alerts. These alerts range from atrial arrhythmias for patients who are not anticoagulated to improperly programmed devices. The various companies have different methods of notifying the staff of an alert. The hours of notifications can be programmed. Clinicians can choose notifications of alerts for wireless devices in the following ways: online only, fax, email, phone, text, or a combination (Figure 26.6).

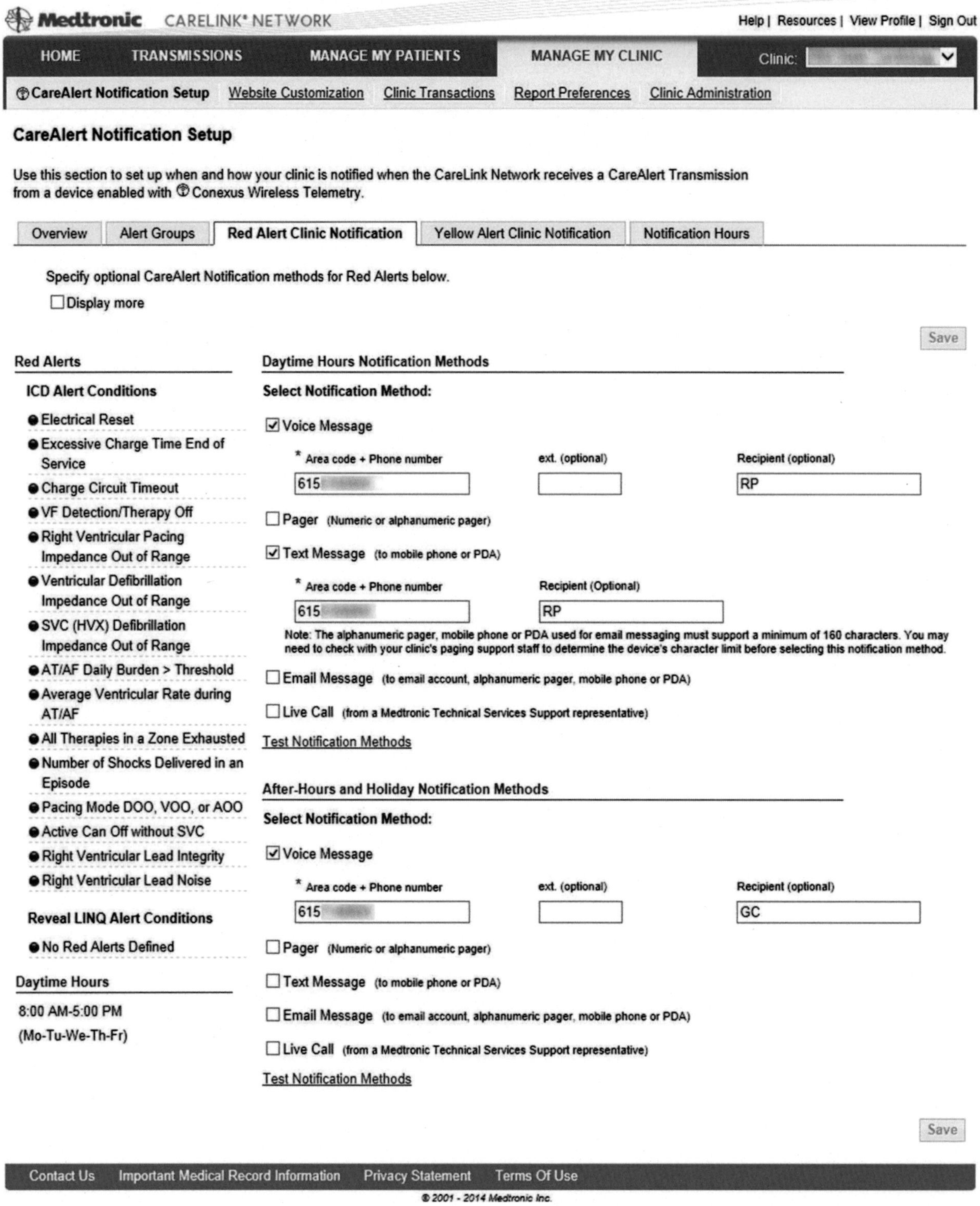

Medtronic CARELINK® NETWORK

Help | Resources | View Profile | Sign Out

HOME | TRANSMISSIONS | MANAGE MY PATIENTS | **MANAGE MY CLINIC** | Clinic:

⊕ **CareAlert Notification Setup** | Website Customization | Clinic Transactions | Report Preferences | Clinic Administration

CareAlert Notification Setup

Use this section to set up when and how your clinic is notified when the CareLink Network receives a CareAlert Transmission from a device enabled with ⊕ Conexus Wireless Telemetry.

| Overview | Alert Groups | **Red Alert Clinic Notification** | Yellow Alert Clinic Notification | Notification Hours |

Specify optional CareAlert Notification methods for Red Alerts below.

☐ Display more

Save

Red Alerts

ICD Alert Conditions

● Electrical Reset
● Excessive Charge Time End of Service
● Charge Circuit Timeout
● VF Detection/Therapy Off
● Right Ventricular Pacing Impedance Out of Range
● Ventricular Defibrillation Impedance Out of Range
● SVC (HVX) Defibrillation Impedance Out of Range
● AT/AF Daily Burden > Threshold
● Average Ventricular Rate during AT/AF
● All Therapies in a Zone Exhausted
● Number of Shocks Delivered in an Episode
● Pacing Mode DOO, VOO, or AOO
● Active Can Off without SVC
● Right Ventricular Lead Integrity
● Right Ventricular Lead Noise

Reveal LINQ Alert Conditions

● No Red Alerts Defined

Daytime Hours

8:00 AM-5:00 PM
(Mo-Tu-We-Th-Fr)

Daytime Hours Notification Methods

Select Notification Method:

☑ Voice Message

| * Area code + Phone number | ext. (optional) | Recipient (optional) |
| 615 | | RP |

☐ Pager (Numeric or alphanumeric pager)

☑ Text Message (to mobile phone or PDA)

| * Area code + Phone number | Recipient (Optional) |
| 615 | RP |

Note: The alphanumeric pager, mobile phone or PDA used for email messaging must support a minimum of 160 characters. You may need to check with your clinic's paging support staff to determine the device's character limit before selecting this notification method.

☐ Email Message (to email account, alphanumeric pager, mobile phone or PDA)

☐ Live Call (from a Medtronic Technical Services Support representative)

Test Notification Methods

After-Hours and Holiday Notification Methods

Select Notification Method:

☑ Voice Message

| * Area code + Phone number | ext. (optional) | Recipient (optional) |
| 615 | | GC |

☐ Pager (Numeric or alphanumeric pager)

☐ Text Message (to mobile phone or PDA)

☐ Email Message (to email account, alphanumeric pager, mobile phone or PDA)

☐ Live Call (from a Medtronic Technical Services Support representative)

Test Notification Methods

Save

Contact Us | Important Medical Record Information | Privacy Statement | Terms Of Use

® 2001 - 2014 Medtronic Inc.

Figure 26.6 This is the clinic notification programming screen where the method and timing of the notification is programmed.

Table 26.1 Alert notifications for the Medtronic system.

Alert	Red alert	Yellow alert	Patient notification
RV lead integrity	●		Beeping
RV lead noise	●		Beeping
Electrical reset	●		Beeping
Charge circuit time out	●		Beeping
Pacing mode set to DOO, VOO, or AOO	●		Beeping
Active can off without SVC	●		Beeping
Defibrillation impedance	●		
VF therapies off	●		
Excessive charge time	●		
Therapies exhausted	●		
AT/AF burden > threshold	●		
Fast ventricular rate during AT/AF	●		
Shocks delivered exceed threshold	●		
Lead impedance out of range (atrial, LV)		○	
Low battery voltage		○	

AF, atrial fibrillation; AT, tachycardia; LV, left ventricular; RV, right ventricular; SVC, superior vena cava; VF, ventricular fibrillation.

One of the important limitations of text messaging is a problem in the handling of failed text messaging. If a text message is issued and the receiving phone is unable to receive the message (e.g., in a shielded part of the hospital), the chance that the message will eventually be delivered is not 100%. In contrast, if a voice message fails, it will almost certainly eventually be received. Some manufacturers have technical staff who can receive the red alert information and phone the appropriate person. This can be helpful if the physicians covering the practice are not device experts.

Our approach is to have these alerts go to an office staff member during working hours and to a physician at night until 10 pm and on the weekend. We turn off the patient notification for all programmable alerts except those that require immediate attention, such as the LIA

alert. Our scheme of alert notifications for the Medtronic system can be seen in Table 26.1.

Missed Transmissions

Missed remote transmissions should be handled just as missed clinic visits. If patients are scheduled on the calendar in the remote system, the system will alert you when a transmission has been missed. Some clinics prefer to schedule in their EMR. Each method works as long as the clinicians are monitoring the remote schedules and ensuring no patient is being lost to follow-up. Clinics often have different processes for notifying patients of missed transmissions. Our protocol is to send a letter and ask the patient to send in a transmission. If the transmission is not received within 2 weeks, a phone call is then made to the patient. Documentation and follow through are imperative. Clinicians must document every effort that is made to obtain a remote transmission just as would be done to reschedule a missed office visit.

Coding and Reimbursement

This section applies only to the USA (Table 26.2). Remote follow-up reimbursement codes are time dependent. That is, each of the remote pacemaker and defibrillator codes specifies the reimbursement for a 90-day period that starts with the first remote follow-up. That reimbursement covers all remote follow-up activity for the next 90 days. It is perfectly allowable to perform more frequent transmissions in this period, but the reimbursement remains the same. Similarly, the follow-up codes for implanted cardiac monitoring and implanted loop monitoring are for a 30-day period. These timeframes do not limit the number of times a patient can transmit a remote transmission; they only limit the number of times a patient should be billed. For example, if a patient sends in a routine transmission on May 1 and then a symptomatic transmission on June 15, only one bill should be

Table 26.2 Remote follow-up reimbursement codes.

Device	Pacemaker	ICD	Loop recorder
Professional	93294	93295	93298
Technical	93296	93296	na
ICM	na	93297	na
TTM	93293	na	na

ICD, implantable cardioverter-defibrillator; ICM, implantable cardiovascular monitor; TTM, trans-telephonic telemetry.

submitted. Another example could be that a patient makes an error and sends in a transmission at 89 days after the previous transmission. Unfortunately, this transmission is still covered by the original billing because it is still within the 90-day timeframe. Therefore, wireless transmissions should be scheduled no more frequently than every 91 days. It is important that both clinicians and the billing departments are aware of the timeframes with the remote billing codes. CMS considers it fraud to bill more often than every 90 days, even if done in error.

Paceart™ provides an efficient method for billing remote transmissions. There is a Visit ID field that can be used to mark a transmission as billable or unbillable. The Medtronic Carelink remote system has a field for Visit ID as well. This field will automatically populate into Paceart when the remote transmissions are download into Paceart. Other company's remote systems typically do not have the Visit ID field and will have to be populated manually. A report for the billable transmissions can be run as often as needed. Depending on the clinics remote transmission volume, bi-weekly may be more manageable for the billing office.

Most CPT codes have a scheme where there is a global code such as the TTM code which is 93293. The professional component is specified by the use of the 26 modifier (93293-26) and the technical component is specified by the TC modifier (93293-TC). Currently, the average reimbursement for TTM in a pacemaker patient is about $15 for the professional fee and $39 for the technical fee. The scheme for remote follow-up is a bit different. Expecting that the standard practice would be for a practice to perform the professional work and that some commercial entity would provide the technical service, there are entirely separate codes for these services. The code 93296 is used for the technical support of remote follow-up regardless of whether the device is an ICD or a pacemaker. The average payment for this is about $30. This is a 90-day code. The professional analysis of a pacemaker remote follow-up is covered by code 93294 and averages about $33. It is also a 90-day code. The similar code for ICDs is 93295. It is a 90-day code and the average reimbursement for it is currently about $65. There is no difference in reimbursement for remote single, dual, or multiple lead systems.

The implantable loop recorder remote follow-up code is 93298. It is a 30-day code and there is no paired technical code. The average reimbursement for this code is currently about $25. There is also an add-on code for the use of reporting physiologic information. It is intended for the transmission of heart failure information such as Optivol™ and weights and blood pressures. That code is 93297. It is a 30-day code. It is quite important to know that this code is only appropriate in patients with a

diagnosis of heart failure. While most ICD patients have heart failure, all do not. It you were to implant a device capable of transmitting such data in a patient with the long QT syndrome and collect those data as a routine and then bill for it, it could well be considered to be fraudulent. Remember that to bill for this service there must be a separate report.

TTM

This 90-day timeframe also applies to the transtelephonic telemetry. As the pulse generator ages and the power source needs to be monitored more frequently, the timeframe still applies to the reimbursement. In a 10-year-old pacer, the power source should be checked monthly. However, the reimbursement code is a 90-day code. I suspect that this will create quite an issue for those of us who use an outside vendor for TTMs. The financial model for TTMs works well at quarterly and bimonthly transmission but seriously falls apart for the vendor when we need to do the transmission monthly. As we reach the point that almost all TTM transmissions involve devices that need monthly follow-up, I expect more of the vendors to cease offering this service.

Frequency

Practices differ somewhat in the frequency of pacemaker remote transmissions. Some practices follow pacemakers every 6 months, alternating between remote and in-office. Other practices follow pacemakers every 3 months with quarterly remote follow-ups and an annual office follow-up. Defibrillators should be followed quarterly as well, quarterly remotes with a yearly office follow-up. These frequencies are for devices with batteries at beginning of life. As the device ages and/or the battery voltage decreases, the frequency of monitoring should also increase. Fortunately, with current technology, devices give us an estimate on battery longevity. This can help determine when to increase remote transmission frequency. In devices with wireless technology it is not necessary to increase the frequency of follow-up evaluations because the clinic will be notified automatically when the device goes to its elective replacement indicator.

Conclusions

Remote follow-up is an effective method for following device patients. It provides timely transmission of appropriate data. It certainly improves the efficiency of the device clinic.

References

1 Wilkoff BL, Auricchio A, Brugada J, Cowie M, Ellenbogen KA, Gillis AM, *et al.* HRS/EHRA expert consensus on the monitoring of cardiovascular implantable electronic devices (CIEDs): description of techniques, indications, personnel, frequency and ethical considerations. Heart Rhythm 2008;5(6):907–925.

2 Crossley GH, Chen J, Choucair W, Cohen TJ, Gohn DC, Johnson WB, *et al.* Clinical benefits of remote versus transtelephonic monitoring of implanted pacemakers. J Am Coll Cardiol 2009;54(22):2012–2019.

3 Crossley GH, Boyle A, Vitense H, Chang Y, Mead RH; CONNECT Investigators. The CONNECT (Clinical Evaluation of Remote Notification to Reduce Time to Clinical Decision) Trial: the value of wireless remote monitoring with automatic clinician alerts. J Am Coll Cardiol 2011;j.

4 Varma N, Michalski J, Epstein AE, Schweikert R. Automatic remote monitoring of implantable cardioverter-defibrillator lead and generator performance: the Lumos-T Safely RedUceS RouTine Office Device Follow-Up (TRUST) trial. Circ Arrhythm Electrophysiol 2010;3(5):428–436.

27

How to Set Up an HF Monitoring Service

Edoardo Gronda[1], Emilio Vanoli[1,2], Margherita Padeletti[3], and Alessio Gargaro[4]

[1] *Cardiovascular Department, IRCCS MultiMedica, Sesto San Giovanni (Milan), Italy*
[2] *Department of Molecular Medicine, University of Pavia Margherita, Pavia, Italy*
[3] *Cardiology Unit, Borgo San Lorenzo Hospital, Florence, Italy*
[4] *Biotronik, Clinical Research Department, Vimodrone (MI), Italy*

Heart failure (HF) is a critical challenge in cardiology today. The primary economic and social-related burden is hospitalization rate which represents the highest costs within the entire healthcare management program in the western world and is currently extending into the eastern developing countries. HF is the most frequent cause of hospitalization in patients over the age of 65 years, whose numbers will almost double over the next 50 years [1], and poses an increasing problem for global healthcare systems. This burden is further worsened in those patients in whom the primary disease is complicated by comorbidities such as diabetes and renal failure.

Several models of remote care have been tried over the last decades in the attempt to improve patient outcomes while preventing hospitalizations. Models were essentially based on (Figure 27.1):

- Monitoring of physiologic data (e.g., blood pressure, weight, therapy compliance) by self-reporting via telephone calls;
- Invasive monitoring via implantable sensors;
- Automatic remote monitoring based on cardiac electronic implantable devices (CIEDs).

This chapter reviews the main results obtained with each model, and discusses future perspectives from recent evidence and ongoing trials.

Monitoring Based on Self-Reporting Via Telephone Contacts

Currently, a high level of real-time interaction between patients and the healthcare provider through phone conversations or online communications has been established and may represent a successful approach. The critical issue though, is whether the evidence documented is of real value in the remote management of chronic HF [2].

Telemonitoring has been accomplished, so far, by means of telephone-based interactive operator or voice response system-based interviews to periodically (even daily) record information about symptoms, weight, and other physiologic data, to be reviewed by the patients' clinicians.

A Cochrane review and meta-analysis reported that telemedicine (telephone assistance or remote monitoring) significantly reduced HF-related hospitalizations [3], but these results were not confirmed by two subsequent large randomized controlled trials [4,5]. A critical summary of the reviews and meta-analysis was recently published [6]. Out of 65 potentially relevant publications, the authors identified only 7 high quality reviews. Although the "meta-review" concluded that "remote monitoring reduced the relative risk of all-cause (0.52–0.96) and heart failure-related hospitalizations (0.72–0.79)", the authors also acknowledged the need for further research before considering an extensive distribution of such form of remote monitoring. In a recent study that enrolled 602 HF patients, changes in New York Heart Association (NYHA) class, left ventricular ejection fraction (LVEF), 6-minute walking distance (6MWD), and Minnesota Living with Heart Failure Questionnaire (MLHFQ) score were evaluated over 6 months follow-up with the support of home-based remote surveillance [7]. A significant reduction in clinical events occurred in association with a favorable response to the program (defined by an improvement in at least two of the outcomes). Of specific

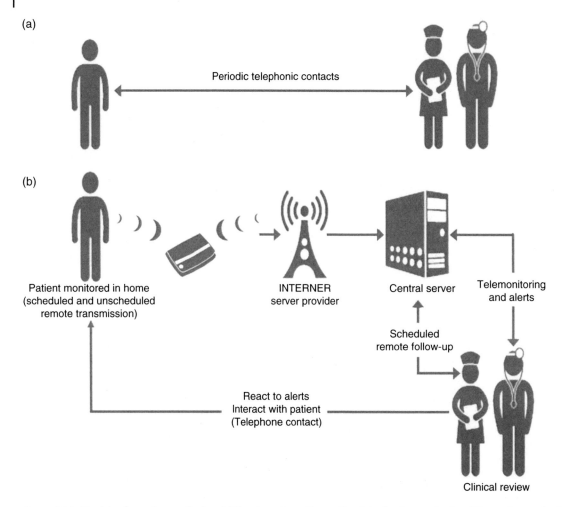

Figure 27.1 Models of remote monitoring. (a) Non-invasive self-reporting telephonic monitoring; (b) remote monitoring based on automatic transmissions from implantable/wareble devices. Source: Boriani [28], http://www.jmir.org/2013/8/e167/?trendmd-shared=1#Copyright used under CC BY S.A 2.0 https://creativecommons.org/licenses/by/2.0/

interest in this context is the HHH (Home or Hospital in Heart Failure) study [8], conducted between 2002 and 2004, where 461 patients with chronic HF with an average NYHA class 2.4 + 0.6 and a LVEF of 29 + 7% were enrolled at 11 centers in Italy, the UK, and Poland. The enrolled patients were randomized 1 : 2 to either standard outpatient care or home monitoring based on three randomized strategies involving the use of monthly telephone contact; associated or not with weekly transmission of vital signs; and monthly 24 h recording of cardiorespiratory activity. Over a 12-month follow-up, there were no significant reductions in hospitalization rate or duration for HF or cardiac death. Post hoc analysis revealed a trend towards a reduction of events in Italy, but not in the other participating countries.

A possible explanation for such contrasting results is related to patient compliance with remote monitoring. In monitoring approaches based on patients' self-reporting, patients generally have an active role, making

daily calls or collecting self-measurements. This may reduce compliance to the monitoring program, as in the Tele-HF study, where less than 80% of patients completed the study procedure in the short follow-up of 6 months [4].

Invasive Monitoring Via Implantable Sensors

The CardioMEMS Champion Heart Failure Monitoring System (CardioMEMS, Atlanta, GA, USA) is one of the first implantable devices for permanent pressure measurement designed to monitor pulmonary artery (PA) pressure and heart rate wirelessly in patients with HF. The system consists of an implantable sensor/monitor, which is a battery-free capacitive pressure sensor permanently implanted in the PA. The device is deployed in the distal PA by a transvenous delivery system and the Champion Electronics System (CardioMEMS) acquires and processes signals from the implantable sensor/ monitor and transfers them to a secure database accessed by the treating physician. This device is opening the way toward the extensive use of implantable monitoring to treat advanced HF patients, but had to overcome a number of issues before widespread use. The concept of right cardiac pressure measurements was already studied by the COMPASS HF study using the Chronicle device [9]. The results from this study suggested the potential contribution of continuous arterial pressure monitoring to optimal HF management, but the primary efficacy endpoint was not met as the Chronicle group had a non-significant 21% lower rate of all HF-related events compared with the control group (p = 0.33). The potential efficacy of right heart parameters in implementing HF management was there, but the sample size available was probably inadequate to prove it. Also, the Chronicle device required skill in implanting and was the size of a standard pacemaker. The CardioMEMS device offers a totally new prospective in view of its very small size and no need of a power supply. The monitoring system consists of a sensor, a delivery catheter, an interrogator, and a home-monitoring device. The HF sensor is implanted, via a transcutaneous procedure, into a distal branch of the PA. PA pressures can be monitored using the external device, which powers the HF sensor and transmits the hemodynamic data from the patient's home to a secure Internet database. The accuracy of the system has been extensively assessed by comparison with standard right heart catheterization. No safety issues have been raised about CardioMEMS but it took more than one study for the device to receive Food and Drug Administration (FDA) approval and to become available to HF patients as a standard of care.

The CHAMPION trial enrolled HF patients with NHYA class III, irrespective of LVEF, and with a previous hospital admission for HF in 64 centers in the USA [10]. Patients were randomly assigned to management with the wireless implantable hemodynamic monitoring (W-IHM) system (treatment group) or to a control group for at least 6 months. The conclusion was that "the addition of information about pulmonary artery pressure to clinical signs and symptoms allows for improved HF management." The study received several criticisms from the FDA [11]. Of note, as the CardioMEMS device detects PA pressure, but this might not mirror immediate changes in left ventricular filling pressure when pulmonary vascular resistances are elevated.

However, the pathophysiologic mechanisms underlying the concept of continuous pulmonary pressure monitoring are very straightforward: dilated hearts operate at the very end of the pressure–volume curve. In this setting, small increases in circulating volume are sufficient to produce significant pressure changes leading to acute decompensation and pulmonary edema. This is why

pulmonary pressure measurements can perceive risk for an upcoming acute HF much earlier than other traditional markers. One might say that CHAMPION merely duplicates what can be seen by measuring thorax impedance and even the most recent studies would support this hypothesis. However, chest impedance can be affected by many non-specific conditions such as pneumonia or a simple acute bronchitis and this lack of specificity constitutes a major limitation to its use. Furthermore, chest impedance can be effectively measured in device carrying patients only.

A second report of the CHAMPION trial provided details about the prospectively identified subgroup of HF patients characterized by LVEF ≥40% and further evaluated clinical outcomes in patients with LVEF ≥50% [12]. The primary efficacy endpoint of HF hospitalization rate at 6 months was 46% lower in the treatment group compared with the control group. After an average of 17.6 months of blinded follow-up, the hospitalization rate was 50% lower in the treatment arm. In response to pulmonary artery pressure information, more changes in diuretic and vasodilator therapies were made in the treatment group. Thus, the prognostic efficacy of CardioMEMS is related to the timely opportunity for appropriate therapeutic intervention.

Automatic Remote Monitoring Based on Cardiac Electronic Implantable Devices

The expanded capabilities of implantable cardioverter-defibrillators (ICD) and devices for cardiac resynchronization therapy (CRT) to monitor and store a number of parameters related to worsening HF can become an established tool to facilitate risk stratification and allow more efficient therapeutic interventions eventually leading to improved clinical outcomes and cost savings. Nonetheless, currently, the potential of remote monitoring has not been fully explored.

All the diagnostic variables containing information related to the compensation status of the patient are well-known predictors.

In the CIBIS II Trial, Lechat *et al.* [13] demonstrated that a 1 bpm reduction of the 2-month mean heart rate is associated with 1.8% risk reduction in HF hospitalization. Similarly, in the SHIFT study, Swedberg *et al.* [14] highlighted the important role of heart rate in the pathophysiology of HF by demonstrating the impact of heart-rate reduction by ivabradine in reducing mortality and hospitalizations in patients with EF <35%, HR >70 bpm, and optimized medical therapy. Last but not least, in the IN-CHF Registry, Opasich *et al.* [15] reported a 61% increase in the risk of short-term decompensation in patients with maximum heart rate (MHR) >100 bpm.

The close relationship between atrial fibrillation (AF) and HF has been extensively studied in recent years. AF correlates with unfavorable outcomes in HF patients and significantly increases the short-term risk of worsening HF. As early as in 1991, Middlekauff *et al.* [16] showed that AF is an independent predictor of both total mortality and sudden death in patients with advanced HF.

A long-term analysis of a cohort of 352 patients with HF showed that frequent premature ventricular contractions (PVC) at rest remained associated with a 5.5-fold increased risk of cardiovascular mortality, after adjusting for age, beta blocker use, rest ECG findings, resting and peak heart rate, ejection fraction, systolic pressure, and exercise capacity [17].

Reduced exercise capacity and short total daily activity time may be considered as potential indicators of worsening HF. Madsen *et al.* [18] showed that maximal exercise duration ≤4 minutes and inability to increase heart rate during exercise by >35 bpm were both independent risk factors of sudden death and pump failure.

A decrease in heart rate variability has been associated with an increased risk of cardiovascular events in patients with HF. In patients with sinus rhythm, the standard deviation of atrial interval (SDANN) is directly related to the sympathetic–vagal balance and it may be a promising prognostic indicator. In general, a reduced SDANN may be an indicator of negative short- and long-term prognosis. Fantoni *et al.* [19] observed that SDANN generally increases along with a reduction of the mean heart rate in CRT responders: failure to observe a SDANN increment after implant correlated with a significantly higher 2-year risk of all-cause mortality, hospitalization for cardiovascular causes, and need for heart transplantation. An analysis of the InSync Italian Registry cohort [20] also identified 65 and 76 ms as 1-week and 4-week lower thresholds, respectively, to stratify patients with a higher risk of cardiovascular events.

New devices can nowadays estimate thoracic impedance, a variable that is correlated with increased intrathoracic fluid [21]. The underlying hypothesis is that thoracic impedance may detect signs of precipitating HF episodes before hospitalization. However, it is worth noting that current implantable devices implementing intrathoracic impedance diagnostic features, do not really measure the overall chest impedance, but merely the electric impedance of tissues between the right ventricle lead and the pectoral device can. This limitation may result in misleading data about the true change of lung fluid concentration. Despite initial enthusiasm, thoracic impedance alone, not combined with other information, reaches fair but not excellent levels of

sensitivity and positive predictive value. In particular, specific threshold values and patient-tailored feature settings still need to be defined.

The mentioned studies demonstrate the importance of monitoring these parameters in HF patients and highlight the value of today's devices to do so. Nevertheless, we still need to define which parameters to monitor and what specific detection strategies should be used to prevent hospitalization. The value of monitoring several parameters in HF prediction has been demonstrated in the PARTNERS study [22] and in a more recent meta-analysis [23]. In these studies, two important insights were highlighted: (i) the use of a diagnostic algorithm based on multiple criteria increases the probability to predict HF hospitalization in comparison to individual measurements; (ii) the more frequent the monitoring, the higher the predictive capability of the algorithm. However, the 3.9% positive predictive value gained in the PARTNERS study still needs optimization, with only one correct alarm out of 27 and a resulting rate of 2.7 false alarms per patient per year. On the other hand, the predictor developed in the Home-CARE study could gain 65.4% sensitivity, despite a request of 99.5% specificity, by combining seven indexes daily sampled in a fixed time window of 25 days and ending 3 days before the event [24]. It is worth noting that 65% sensitivity is only slightly higher that 60% sensitivity reported in a recent large observational study on standard practice of Home Monitoring in which investigators acted on the basis of their individual experience without any predefined algorithms or protocols [25].

This suggests that despite an optimal algorithm not being developed yet, the potential of remote monitoring in improving HF management and patient care is there. An indirect indication has recently been obtained in the In-TIME trial [26], in which 664 ICD (with or without CRT) patients were randomly assigned to standard in-person visit follow-up or to multiparameter telemonitoring in addition to standard care with the primary outcome of a composite Packer's score combining all-cause death, overnight hospital admission for heart failure, change in NYHA class, and change in patient global self-assessment. After 1 year of follow-up, the combined Packer score worsened in 30% fewer patients in the telemonitoring group. Interestingly, the main drive was the reduction of all-cause and cardiovascular mortalities, which were significantly reduced by 61% and 60%, respectively.

Unfortunately, the study protocol did not enforce standardized treatment after telemonitoring observations nor did the authors thoroughly record clinical actions in response to remote observations. Therefore, the study cannot provide information on how to analyze remote monitoring data effectively and time trigger treatment changes to optimize clinical benefits. Authors could only speculate on three possible mechanisms that could explain the observed reduction in mortality associated with telemonitoring: (i) early detection of the onset or progression of ventricular and atrial tachyarrhythmias; (ii) early recognition of suboptimal device function (maximization of CRT, prevention of inappropriate shocks, etc.); (iii) increase in patient compliance induced "patient interviews raised patients' awareness of

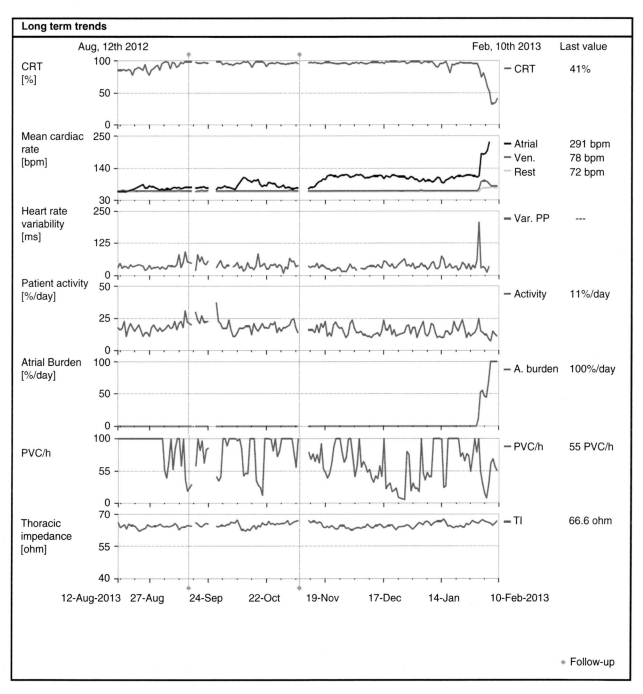

Figure 27.2 An example of 6-month trends of heart failure (HF)-related variables remotely collected with the remote monitoring system in a patient with a cardiac resynchronization therapy (CRT) device before a worsening HF episode. Note a smooth decrease in daily activity, starting about 3 months before the hospitalization date (right edge of the graph). A sudden onset 100% burden of atrial fibrillation occurred about 2 weeks before admission, resulting in sharp increases in atrial and ventricular rate and a reduction in CRT. The modest increase in atrial rate observed in November 2013 was caused by the onset of a retrograde conduction triggered by ventricular pacing.

relevant developments and encouraged them to take more responsibility for their own health, including adherence to prescribed treatments."

Currently, we still do not know how to reliably interpret remote transmitted trends of HF indexes.

Probably, the key is in the combination of more parameters (Figure 27.2) and in the daily sampling rate of HF indexes. This hypothesis is being explored by the ongoing Selene HF trial [27], whose results are expected by 2016.

References

1 Loh JC, Creaser J, Rourke DA, Livingston N, Harrison TK, Vandenbogaart E, *et al.* Temporal trends in treatment and outcomes for advanced heart failure with reduced ejection fraction from 1993–2010: findings from a university referral center. Circ Heart Fail 2013;6:411–419.

2 Wootton R. Twenty years of medicine in chronic disease management: an evidence synthesis. J Telemed Telecare 2012;18:211–220.

3 Inglis SC, Clark RA, McAlister FA, Stewart S, Cleland JG. Which components of heart failure programmes are effective? A systematic review and meta-analysis of the outcomes of structured telephone support or telemonitoring as the primary component of chronic heart failure management in 8323 patients: Abridged Cochrane Review. Eur J Heart Fail 2011;13:1028–1040.

4 Chaudhry SI, Mattera JA, Curtis JP, Spertus JA, Herrin J, Lin Z, *et al.* Telemonitoring in patients with heart failure. N Engl J Med 2010;363:2301–2309.

5 Koehler F, Winkler S, Schieber M, Sechtem U, Stangl K, Böhm M, *et al.* Telemedical Interventional Monitoring in Heart Failure Investigators. Impact of remote telemedical management on mortality and hospitalizations in ambulatory patients with chronic heart failure: the telemedical interventional monitoring in heart failure study. Circulation 2011;123:1873–1880.

6 Conway A, Inglis SC, Chang AM, Horton-Breshears M, Cleland JG, Clark RA. Not all systematic reviews are systematic: a meta-review of the quality of systematic reviews for non-invasive remote monitoring in heart failure. J Telemed Telecare 2013;19:326–337.

7 Giordano A, Scalvini S, Paganoni AM, Baraldo S, Frigerio M, Vittori C, *et al.* Home-based telesurveillance program in chronic heart failure: effects on clinical status and implications for 1-year prognosis. Telemed J E Health 2013;19:605–612.

8 Mortara A, Pinna GD, Johnson P, Maestri R, Capomolla S, La Rovere MT, *et al;* HHH Investigators. Home telemonitoring in heart failure patients: the HHH study (Home or Hospital in Heart Failure). Eur J Heart Fail 2009;11:312–318.

9 Bourge RC, Abraham WT, Adamson PB, Aaron MF, Aranda JM Jr, Magalski A, *et al;* COMPASS-HF Study Group. Randomized controlled trial of an implantable continuous hemodynamic monitor in patients with advanced heart failure: the COMPASS-HF study. J Am Coll Cardiol 2008;51:1073–1079.

10 Abraham WT, Adamson PB, Bourge RC, Aaron MF, Costanzo MR, Stevenson LW, *et al;* CHAMPION Trial Study Group. Wireless pulmonary artery haemodynamic monitoring in chronic heart failure: a randomised controlled trial. Lancet 2011;377:658–666.

11 Loh JP, Barbash IM, Waksman R. Overview of the 2011 Food and Drug Administration Circulatory System Devices Panel of the Medical Devices Advisory Committee Meeting on the CardioMEMS Champion Heart Failure Monitoring System. J Am Coll Cardiol 2013;61:1571–1576.

12 Adamson PB, Abraham WT, Bourge RC, Costanzo MR, Hasan A, Yadav C, *et al.* Wireless pulmonary artery pressure monitoring guides management to reduce decompensation in heart failure with preserved ejection fraction. Circ Heart Fail 2014;7:935–944.

13 Lechat P, Hulot J-S, Escolano S, Mallet A, Leizorovicz A, Werhlen-Grandjean M, *et al;* CIBIS II Investigators. Heart rate and cardiac rhythm relationship with bisoprolol benefit in chronic heart failure in CIBIS II Trial. Circulation 2001;103:1428–1433.

14 Swedberg K, Komajda M, Böhm M, Borer JS, Ford I, Dubost-Brama A, *et al;* SHIFT Investigators. Ivabradine and outcomes in chronic heart failure (SHIFT): a randomised placebo-controlled study. Lancet 2010;376(9744):875–885.

15 Opasich C, Rapezzi C, Lucci D, Pozzar F, Zanelli E, Tavazzi L, *et al;* Italian Network on Congestive Heart Failure (IN-CHF) Investigators. Precipitating factors and decision-making processes of short-term worsening heart failure despite "optimal" treatment (from the IN-CHF Registry). Am J Cardiol 2001;88(4):382–387.

16 Middlekauff HR, Stevenson WG, Stevenson LW. Prognostic significance of atrial fibrillation in advanced heart failure: a study of 390 patients. Circulation 1991;84:40–48.

17 Le VV, Mitiku T, Hadley D, Myers J, Froelicher VF. Rest premature ventricular contractions on routine ECG and prognosis in heart failure patients. Ann Noninvasive Electrocardiol 2010;15(1):56–62.

18 Madsen BK, Rasmussen V, Hansen JF. Predictors of sudden death and death from pump failure in congestive heart failure are different: analysis of 24 h Holter monitoring, clinical variables, blood chemistry, exercise test and radionuclide angiography. Int J Cardiol 1997;58(2):151–162.

19 Fantoni C, Raffa S, Regoli F, Giraldi F, La Rovere MT, Prentice J, *et al.* Cardiac resynchronization therapy improves heart rate profile and heart rate variability of patients with moderate to severe heart failure. J Am Coll Cardiol 2005;46(10):1875–1882.

20 Landolina M, Gasparini M, Lunati M, Santini M, Rordorf R, Vincenti A, *et al;* InSync/InSync ICD Italian Registry Investigators. Heart rate variability monitored by the implanted device predicts response to CRT and long-term clinical outcome in patients with advanced heart failure. Eur J Heart Fail 2008;10(11):1073–1079.

21 Yu CM, Wang L, Chau E, Chan RHW, Kong SL, Tang MO, *et al.* Intrathoracic impedance monitoring in patients with heart failure correlation with fluid status and feasibility of early warning preceding hospitalization. Circulation 2005;112:841–848.

22 Whellan DJ, Ousdigian KT, Al-Khatib SM, Pu W, Sarkar S, Porter CB, *et al;* PARTNERS Study Investigators. Combined heart failure device diagnostics identify patients at higher risk of subsequent heart failure hospitalizations: results from PARTNERS HF (Program to Access and Review Trending Information and Evaluate Correlation to Symptoms in Patients With Heart Failure) study. J Am Coll Cardiol 2010;55(17):1803–1810.

23 Cowie MR, Sarkar S, Koehler J, Whellan DJ, Crossley GH, Tang WH, *et al.* Development and validation of an integrated diagnostic algorithm derived from parameters monitored in implantable devices for identifying patients at risk for heart failure hospitalization in an ambulatory setting. Eur Heart J 2013;34(31):2472–2480.

24 Sack S, Wende CM, Nägele H, Katz A, Bauer WR, Barr CS, *et al.* Potential value of automated daily screening of cardiac resynchronization therapy defibrillator diagnostics for prediction of major cardiovascular events: results from Home-CARE (Home Monitoring in Cardiac Resynchronization Therapy) study. Eur J Heart Fail 2011;13(9):1019–1027.

25 Ricci RP, Morichelli L, D'Onofrio A, Calò L, Vaccari D, Zanotto G, *et al.* Effectiveness of remote monitoring of CIEDs in detection and treatment of clinical and device-related cardiovascular events in daily practice: the HomeGuide Registry. Europace 2013;15(7):970–977.

26 Hindricks G, Taborsky M, Glikson M, Heinrich U, Schumacher B, Katz A, *et al;* IN-TIME study group. Implant-based multiparameter telemonitoring of patients with heart failure (IN-TIME): a randomised controlled trial. Lancet 2014;384(9943):583–590.

27 Padeletti L, Botto GL, Curnis A, De Ruvo E, D'Onofrio A, Gronda E, *et al.* Selection of potential predictors of worsening heart failure: rational and design of the SELENE HF study. J Cardiovasc Med (Hagerstown) 2015;16(11):782–789.

28 Boriani G, Da Costa A, Ricci RP, Quesada A, Favale S, Iacopino S, *et al;* MORE-CARE Investigators. The MOnitoring Resynchronization dEvices and CARdiac patiEnts (MORE-CARE) randomized controlled trial: phase 1 results on dynamics of early intervention with remote monitoring. J Med Internet Res 2013;15(8):e167.

28

How to Deactivate Cardiac Implantable Electric Devices in Patients Nearing the End of Life and/or Requesting Withdrawal of Therapies

Rachel Lampert

Yale University School of Medicine, New Haven, CT, USA

As indications for the implantable cardioverter-defibrillator (ICD) have expanded, the population of patients living with these and other cardiac implantable electronic devices (CIEDs) has continued to grow, with over 12 000 implanted each month in the USA alone. While the efficacy of the ICD at preventing sudden cardiac death in patients at risk is well documented, all patients will eventually die, whether of their underlying heart disease, another fatal condition, or old age.

Why is ICD Deactivation Important?

Case reports in the palliative care literature describe, "Death and Dying, a Shocking Experience," and "And it can go on and on and on." The popular press has been even more sensational, "Devices wreak havoc at end of life" (*NY Times*). One family member described an ICD patient's last days, "His defibrillator kept going off...It went off 12 times in one night...He went in and they looked at it...they said they adjusted it and they sent him back home. The next day we had to take him back because it was happening again. It kept going off and going off and it wouldn't stop going off." ICD shocks are painful, described by patients as "a punch in the chest," "being kicked by a mule," and "putting a finger in a light socket," and have been shown to decrease quality of life. Thus, it is not surprising that receiving shocks at end of life is a distressing experience for the dying patient as well as his or her family.

* Relationships with industry: Dr. Lampert has received significant research funding from Boston Scientific, Medtronic, and St. Jude Medical.

Early reports of the frequency with which dying patients receive ICD shocks, relying on interviews with family members of deceased patients, suggested that 20% received shocks in the last weeks, days, or hours of their lives [1]. A recent prospective series of post-mortem ICD interrogations found that the true number is even higher – one-third of patients receive shocks in the last hours of life [2].

Legally and Ethically, Can CIEDs be Deactivated?

In order to define the legal and ethical underpinnings of CIED deactivation in the USA, as well as to define clinical management of deactivation, the Heart Rhythm Society (HRS) convened a multidisciplinary working group whose recommendations were published in 2010 [3]. The ethical and legal permission of discontinuation of life-sustaining therapies such such as hemodialysis, ventilators, feeding tubes, and cardiac rhythm devices is well described. The primary ethical principle supporting the withdrawal of life-sustaining therapies is respect for autonomy. In a series of cases addressing withdrawal of life-sustaining therapies, the US courts have ruled that the right to make decisions about medical treatments is both a common law right (derived from court decisions) based on bodily integrity and self-determination, and a constitutional right based on privacy and liberty. A patient has the right to refuse any treatment, even if the treatment prolongs life and death would follow a decision not to use it. Further, courts have ruled that there is no legal difference between withdrawing an ongoing treatment and not starting one in the first place. Granting requests

How-to Manual for Pacemaker and ICD Devices: Procedures and Programming, First Edition. Edited by Amin Al-Ahmad, Andrea Natale, Paul J. Wang, James P. Daubert, and Luigi Padeletti.
© 2018 John Wiley & Sons, Inc. Published 2018 by John Wiley & Sons, Inc.
Companion website: www.wiley.com/go/al-ahmad/pacemakers_and_icds

Table 28.1 Landmark legal cases confirming the right to withhold or withdraw life-sustaining therapies.

In re Quinlan	1976	Supreme Court of New Jersey	Withdrawal	Ventilator
Saikewicz	1977	Massachusetts Superior Judicial Court	Withholding	Chemotherapy
In the matter of Shirley Dinnerstein	1978	Massachusetts Court of Appeals	Withholding	Cardiopulmonary resuscitation
Spring	1980	Massachusetts Superior Judicial Court	Withdrawal	Hemodialysis
Barber	1983	California Court of Appeals	Withdrawal	Intravenous fluids
Bouvia	1985	California Court of Appeals	Both	Feeding tube
Cruzan vs Director, Missouri Department of Health	1990	US Supreme Court	Withdrawal	Feeding tube
Schiavo*	2005	Florida Court of Appeals*	Withdrawal	Feeding tube

* The Florida Supreme Court declined to consider case, the US Supreme Court declined to hear related case.
Source: Lampert (2011) [4]. Reproduced with permission of Elsevier.

to withdraw life-sustaining treatments from patients, who do not want them, is respecting a right to be left alone and to die naturally of the underlying disease, a legally protected right based on the right to privacy. This has been phrased, "a right to decide how to live the rest of one's life." The Supreme Court has not specifically addressed the question of pacemaker (PM) or ICD deactivation. However, the rulings described in Table 28.1 did not focus on the specific therapy under question, but rather, on "life-sustaining therapies." The law applies to the person, and informed consent is a right of the patient – it is not specific to any one medical intervention. Thus, because CIEDs deliver life-sustaining therapies, discontinuation of these therapies is clearly addressed by the Supreme Court precedents upholding the right to discontinue life-sustaining treatment: "Procedures don't have rights, patients do [3]." Finally, these rights extend to patients who lack decision-making capacity, through previously expressed statements (e.g., advance directives) and surrogate decision-makers.

While most physicians are comfortable with deactivation of an ICD, some are less comfortable with PM deactivation, especially in a dependent patient, and have questioned the difference between PM deactivation and assisted suicide or euthanasia. However, withdrawal of CIED therapies and assisted suicide differ in two key respects: first, the clinician's intent; and secondly, the cause of death. When a physician deactivates a device upon patient request, his or her intent is to remove a treatment which the patient finds an unwanted burden. While the effect of this may be that the patient dies of an underlying disease, hastening death is not the clinician's primary intent. In contrast, in assisted suicide, the patient intentionally terminates his own life using a lethal method provided or prescribed by a clinician. The second key difference between withdrawal of an unwanted therapy and assisted suicide lies in the cause of death. In assisted

suicide or euthanasia, death is caused by the intervention provided by the clinician. In contrast, when a patient dies after a treatment is refused or withdrawn, the cause of death is the underlying disease. These distinctions have been upheld by the US Supreme Court, which has ruled in the *Vacco vs Quill* case that while there is a constitutional right to refuse treatment based on the right to freedom from unwanted touching, there is not a constitutional right to hasten death by assisted suicide or euthanasia (i.e., the courts have not confirmed a legal "right to die," rather, there is a right to be left alone).

How to Communicate With Patients About CIED Deactivation

Only 15–27% of patients with ICDs have had their device deactivated, and even among patients who have chosen do not resuscitate (DNR) status, still only 50% have had the device deactivated, most in the last days of life. To what extent the failure to deactivate therapies stems from patient choice, versus failure of the physician to communicate this option, is unknown. Studies of patient preferences regarding ICD deactivation at end of life have shown mixed results. Several written surveys of patients with ICDs regarding preferences for ICD deactivation in hypothetical situations have found that patients may not wish deactivation, even in the setting of constant dyspnea or frequent shocks. In the only series of patients actually facing the decision in whom the option of deactivation was discussed – six patients with terminal malignancies, all with a history of treated ventricular arrhythmias – none chose to turn off shocking therapies. However, we found, in a recent interview study, again a survey of hypothetical situations, putting ICD deactivation in the context of health outcomes such as functional and cognitive disability known to influence

Table 28.2 Steps for communicating with patients and families about goals of care relating to cardiac implantable electronic devices (CIEDs).

	Sample phrases to use to begin conversation at each step
1) Determine what patients/families know about their illness	"What do you understand about your health and what is occurring in terms of your illness?"
2) Determine what patients/families know about the role the device plays in their health both now and in the future	"What do you understand the role of the [cardiac device] to be in your health now?"
3) Determine what additional information patients/families want to know about their illness	"What else would be helpful for you to know about your illness or the role the [cardiac device] plays within it?
4) Correcting or clarify any misunderstandings about the current illness and possible outcomes, including the role of the device	"I think you have a pretty good understanding of what is happening in terms of your health, but there are a few things I would like to clarify with you"
5) Determining the patient/family's overall goals of care and desired outcomes	"Given what we've discussed about your health and the potential likely outcomes of your illness, tell me what you want from your health care at this point." NB: Sometimes patients and families may need more guidance at this point, so some potential guiding language might be: "At this point some patients tell me they want to live as long as possible, regardless of the outcome, whereas other patients tell me that the goal is to be as comfortable as long as possible while also being able to interact with their family. Do you have a sense of what you want at this point?"
6) Using the stated goals as a guide, work to tailor treatments, and in this case management of the cardiac device, to those goals	Phrases to be used here depend on the goals as set by the patient and family For a patient who states that her desired goal is to live as comfortably as possible for whatever remaining time she has left: "Given what you've said about assuring that you are as comfortable as possible it might make sense to deactivate the shocking function of your ICD. What do you think about that?" *or* For a patient who states he wants all life-sustaining treatments to be continued, an appropriate response might be, "In that case, perhaps leaving the anti-arrhythmia function of the device active would best be in line with your goals. However, you should understand that this may cause you and your family discomfort at the end of life. We can make a decision at a future point in time about turning the device off. Tell me your thoughts about this"

Source: Lampert (2010) [1]. Reproduced with permission of Elsevier.

decision-making, that most would at least hypothetically choose deactivation in some situations [5]. Thus, it is more likely that the high number of patients who die with device therapies active do so not out of conscious choice, but because they did not know deactivation was an option. In the initial report by Goldstein *et al.* [1], only one-quarter of families of recently deceased patients with ICDs reported the patient or themselves having had a conversation with a healthcare provider about deactivation and, in most cases, it had been initiated by the family and not the healthcare provider team [1].

Timely and effective communication among patients, families, and healthcare providers is essential to prevent unwanted shocks at end of life. Most patients and families desire conversations about end-of-life care. Effective communication includes determining the patient's goals of care, helping the patient understand the role the device plays in his or her current medical care, and

weighing the benefits and burdens of device therapy as the clinical situation changes, clarifying the consequences of deactivation, and discussion of potential alternative treatments, as well as encouraging the patient to complete an advanced directive [3]. Clinicians must take a proactive role in discussions about the option of deactivation in the context of the patient's goals for care. Table 28.2 describes steps and suggested language to cover these points. These conversations should continue over the course of the patient's illness. As illness progresses, patient preferences for outcomes and the level of burden acceptable to the patient may change. Suggestions for ongoing conversations over the patient's life course are shown in Table 28.3.

Advanced care planning conversations improve outcomes for both patients and their families, as patients with ICDs who engage in advance care planning are less likely to experience shocks while dying because ICD deactivation has occurred. Completion of an advanced

Table 28.3 Adaptations of conversations over time.

Timing of conversation	Points to be covered	Helpful phrases to consider
Prior to implantation	● Clear discussion of the benefits and burdens of the device ● Brief discussion of potential future limitations or burdensome aspects of device therapy ● Encourage patients to have some form of advance directive ● Inform of option to deactivate in the future	"It seems clear at this point that this device is in your best interest, but you should know at some point if you become very ill from your heart disease or another process you develop in the future, the burden of this device may outweigh its benefit. While that point is hopefully a long way off, you should know that turning off your defibrillator is an option"
After an episode of increased or repeated firings from an ICD	● Discussion of possible alternatives, including adjusting medications, adjusting device settings, and cardiac procedures to reduce future shocks	"I know that your device caused you some recent discomfort and that you were quite distressed. I want to work with you to see if we can adjust the settings to assure that the device continues to work in the appropriate manner. If we can't get you to that point then we may want to consider turning it off altogether, but let's try some adjustments first"
Progression of cardiac disease, including repeated hospitalizations for heart failure and/or arrhythmias	● Re-evaluation of benefits and burdens of device ● Assessment of functional status, quality of life, and symptoms ● Referral to palliative and supportive care services	"It appears as though your heart disease is worsening. We should really talk about your thoughts and questions about your illness at this point and see if your goals have changed at all"
When patient/surrogate chooses a Do Not Resuscitate order*	● Re-evaluation of benefits and burdens of device ● Exploration of patient's understanding of device and how he/she conceptualizes it with regards to external defibrillation ● Referral to palliative care or supportive services	"Now that we've established that you would not want resuscitation in the event your heart were to go into an abnormal pattern of beating, we should reconsider the role of your device. In many ways it is also a form of resuscitation. Tell me your understanding of the device and let's talk about how it fits into the larger goals for your medical care at this point"
Patients at end of life	● Re-evaluation of benefits and burdens of device ● Discussion of option of deactivation addressed with all patients, though deactivation *not* required	"I think at this point we need to reconsider your [device]. Given how advanced your disease is we need to discuss whether it makes sense to keep it active. I know this may be upsetting to talk about, but can you tell me your thoughts at this point?"

* Patients may choose to forego intubation, CPR, and external defibrillation while at the same time decide to keep the defibrillation function of their ICD active. A patient's choice to be "DNR" may or may not be concomitant with a decision to withdraw CIED therapy, as resuscitation interventions and the ICD each carries its own benefits and burdens.
Source: Adapted from Lampert (2010) [1].

directive can often prevent ethical dilemmas at the end of life. In this process, which promotes patient autonomy, a patient identifies his or her values, preferences, and goals regarding future health care (e.g., at the end of life) and a surrogate decision-maker in the event he or she loses decision-making capacity. Studies have shown that advance directives are not common among patients with ICDs, and even those who have advance directives often do not mention their wishes regarding the ICD.

Effective discussion of device deactivation needs to occur in the context of overall goals of care. These conversations should include a discussion of quality of life, functional status, perceptions of dignity, and both current and potential future symptoms, as each of these elements can influence how patients set goals for their health care. It is critical to ensure that the patient understands the role the device has in their health, particularly in terms of care at the end of life. The role that each type of therapy – shocks, anti-tachycardia therapy, pacing, or cardiac resynchronization – has in the care of each specific patient, and the consequences of deactivation of each type of therapy, should be discussed in detail. For example, pacing and cardiac resynchronization therapy (CRT) are indicated for prevention of symptoms, and discontinuation can worsen underlying heart failure of lead to fatigue or syncope, worsening quality of life. ICDs alone do not improve symptoms, and shocks as the patient is nearing the end of life can increase emotional distress for both patients and families, and thus discontinuation of shocks can be said to improve quality of life.

These conversations should follow the model of "shared decision-making," in which clinicians work together with patients and families to ensure that patients understand in the context of their illness the benefits and burdens of a particular treatment and the potential outcomes that may occur as a result of its continued use or discontinuation. Once the patient understands the beneficial and negative effects of continuing or discontinuing device therapies, he or she can then assess how the benefits and burdens of continued therapy fit with his or her ongoing healthcare goals.

How to Deactivate a CIED

The HRS document lays out a series of steps for CIED deactivation, as shown in Table 28.4. First, the physician must confirm that the patient understands his or her medical condition and the consequences of deactivation and thus has capacity to make the decision. While legally, all adults are considered competent unless declared incompetent by courts, the AMA code of Medical Ethics [6] affirms that in most situations it is acceptable to act on the physician's determination of capacity without formal legal declaration of incompetence. If the physician does not feel able to determine decision-making capacity, either because of unclear cognitive or emotional state in the patient, a psychiatric colleague can be consulted, but psychiatric consultation is not required routinely.

Table 28.4 How to deactivate CIEDs.

Confirmation of decision-making capacity of patient

- Identification of surrogate if appropriate

Documentation

- Confirmation of patient/surrogate request
- Capacity
- Confirmation that alternative therapies have been discussed if relevant
- Confirmation that consequences of deactivation has been discussed
- Specific therapies to be discontinued

Preparation for palliative care and patient/family support if appropriate
Deactivation by electrophysiology personnel

- *or* by medical personnel with assistance from industry-employed allied professionals

If the patient lacks decision-making capacity, the next step is identification of the legal surrogate.

Next, documentation should include confirmation of the decision for deactivation, confirmation that alternative therapies have been discussed, if relevant, and that the consequences of deactivation have been discussed, and are understood by the patient. The specific therapies to be deactivated should be delineated – whether the patient wishes to deactivate just shocks, all tachyarrhythmia therapies, or bradycardia pacing in addition, following a conversation as described earlier.

Who Should Deactivate the ICD?

Deactivation should be performed, whenever possible, by individuals with electrophysiologic expertise such as physicians or device-clinic nurses or technicians. In cases in which this expertise is not available, deactivation should be performed by medical personnel (such as a hospice physician or nurse) with guidance from industry-employed allied professionals. Prior surveys have suggested that often, industry employees are asked to deactivate devices on their own, yet these are individuals who may have no clinical training. While there may be rare urgent situations in which it is necessary for an industry representative to perform deactivation alone, following transmission of specific orders from a medical physician, in most circumstances it can be arranged for medical personnel to take clinical responsibility for the deactivation by being present while the representative provides the technical assistance.

While carrying out requests to withdraw device therapies from patients who have (or their surrogate has) made this decision is ethical and legal, clinicians may have personal values and beliefs that lead them to prefer not to participate in device deactivation, particularly PM deactivation in dependent patients. As described in the AMA Code of Medical Ethics [6], clinicians and others, including industry employed allied professionals, should not be compelled to carry out any procedure they view as inconsistent with their personal values. Under these circumstances, the clinician should inform the patient of his or her preference not to perform device deactivation. However, as described in the AMA Code of Medical Ethics, the clinician should not impose his or her values on or abandon the patient, and should ensure that they do not cause the patient emotional distress [3]. If the primary clinician and patient can reach an acceptable plan, then the primary clinician should assist the patient in identifying another clinician who will deliver this legally permitted intervention.

Where Should Deactivation be Performed?

Device deactivation can be performed in multiple settings, but the logistics will vary depending on the location of the patient, his or her clinical situation, and what therapies are to be deactivated. For an inpatient hospitalized in a facility with electrophysiologic expertise, members of the electrophysiology team should be contacted. For outpatients who are ambulatory, deactivation of tachyarrhythmia therapies can be carried out in the electrophysiology clinic. If a decision is made to discontinue pacing in a dependent or very bradycardic patient, deactivation should be performed in a setting in which appropriate palliative care can be delivered, either as an inpatient or with the assistance of hospice services. For logistical reasons, this should not be performed in the outpatient setting where appropriate palliative care cannot be immediately put in place. For patients in facilities without electrophysiology expertise, such as long-term nursing facilities or hospices, deactivation should be carried out by medical personnel in conjunction with industry-employed personnel, after consultation with electrophysiologists who can assist in directing the plan. Deactivation for patients at home, such as those with home hospice, can be challenging, but can be managed with effective communication amongst members of the patient's healthcare team including hospice nurses, primary physicians, and electrophysiologists. Following direction from the electrophysiologist, the hospice team can perform deactivation in conjunction with industry representatives providing technical assistance in the home.

In summary, deactivation of ICDs and pacemakers is legal and ethic. Proactive communication by the healthcare team can help prevent painful shocks for patients nearing the end of life. Clinicians caring for patients with ICDs should have protocols in place for deactivation.

References

1 Goldstein NE, Lampert R, Bradley E, Lynn J, Krumholz HM. Management of implantable cardioverter defibrillators in end-of-life care. Ann Intern Med 2004;141:835–838.

2 Kinch Westerdahl A, Sjoblom J, Mattiasson AC, Rosenqvist M, Frykman V. Implantable cardioverter-defibrillator therapy before death: high risk for painful shocks at end of life. Circulation 2014;129:422–429.

3 Lampert R, Hayes DL, Annas GJ, Farley MA, Goldstein NE, Hamilton RM, *et al.* HRS Expert Consensus Statement on the Management of Cardiovascular Implantable Electronic Devices (CIEDs) in patients nearing end of life or requesting withdrawal of therapy. Heart Rhythm 2010;7:1008–1026.

4 Lampert R, Hayes D. Ethical issues. In Ellenbogen KA, Kay GN, Lau CP, Wilkoff BL (eds) Clinical Cardiac Pacing, Defibrillation, and Resynchronization Therapy, 4th edition. Elsevier: 2011.

5 Dodson JA, Fried TR, Van Ness PH, Goldstein N, Lampert R. Patient preferences for deactivation of implantable cardioverter defibrillators. JAMA Intern Med 2013;173(5):377–379.

6 AMA. Code of Medical Ethics: Current Opinions and Annotations. AMA Council on Ethical and Judicial Affairs. 2008–2009 edition. Chicago, IL: AMA Press, 2010.

Index

Page numbers in *italic* refer to figures.
Page numbers in **bold** refer to tables.

How-to Manual for Pacemaker and ICD Devices: Procedures and Programming, First Edition. Edited by Amin Al-Ahmad, Andrea Natale, Paul J. Wang, James P. Daubert, and Luigi Padeletti.
© 2018 John Wiley & Sons, Inc. Published 2018 by John Wiley & Sons, Inc.
Companion website: www.wiley.com/go/al-ahmad/pacemakers_and_icds